WORD BOOKS FROM SAUNDERS

Sloane: THE MEDICAL WORD BOOK, 2nd Edition

Sloane: MEDICAL ABBREVIATIONS AND EPONYMS

De Lorenzo: THE PHARMACEUTICAL WORD BOOK

Tessier: THE SURGICAL WORD BOOK

Sloane: A WORD BOOK IN PATHOLOGY AND
              LABORATORY MEDICINE

Medical Abbreviations and Eponyms

Sheila B. Sloane, C.M.T.

Formerly President, Medi-Phone, Inc.
Author, The Medical Word Book and
A Word Book in Pathology and Laboratory Medicine

1985

W. B. SAUNDERS COMPANY

PHILADELPHIA   RIO DE JANIERO
LONDON   SYDNEY
TORONTO   TOKYO
MEXICO CITY   HONG KONG

W. B. Saunders Company: West Washington Square
                           Philadelphia, PA 19105

Library of Congress Cataloging in Publication Data

Sloane, Sheila B.
  Medical abbreviations and eponyms.

  1. Medicine– Abbreviations–Dictionaries.
2. Eponyms–Dictionaries. I. Title. [DNLM:
1. Eponyms–dictionaries. 2. Medicine–abbreviations.
W 13 S634m]
R123.S569 1985   610'.148   85-2059
ISBN 0-7216-1522-8

Medical Abbreviations and Eponyms   ISBN   0–7216–1522–8

Last digit is the print number: 9   8   7   6   5   4   3   2   1

Dedicated
to
Ruth Huston
A loyal and devoted friend
who shared with me the
challenge and joys of
medical words

PREFACE

Since publication in 1973 of the first edition of The Medical Word Book, medical-record keeping has changed to a remarkable degree, becoming more sophisticated and expert than ever before. There are few more impressive success stories than that of the spectacular growth and professionalism achieved by the medical transcriptionist over these past years. A dramatic advancement in the practice of medicine, phenomenal progress in research, and the division of medicine into highly specialized fields have given birth to a vitally important new profession—that of the professional transcriptionist. It extends to all aspects of medicine, and two of its more difficult areas are in the use of medical abbreviations and eponyms.

It is, therefore, the purpose of this book to offer a comprehensive listing of medical abbreviations—in which are included chemical formulas, chemical symbols, many new biochemical terms, elements, acronyms, medical organizations, and some appropriate computer terms— and a complete listing of eponyms, which have long been a source of confusion to medical secretaries, transcriptionists, record librarians, physicians, nurses, and anyone involved directly or indirectly with medical terminology. Abbreviations are time-saving and space-saving as well as efficient, and therefore the attempt of the book is to be inclusive rather than selective. Often the same abbreviation has multiple meanings, and no attempt has been made to state which is the favored usage, all forms being listed. If there is any possibility of confusion in the significance of the abbreviation, its meaning should be spelled out in full.

Eponyms, too, are an ancient device for the storage and retrieval of information—a forerunner of the computer but considerably more handy. The very name Addison's disease brings to mind the whole complex field of diseases of the ductless glands and that Addison's great work on the subject was regarded in his day as merely a medical curiosity. The section on eponyms includes diseases, syndromes, positions, operations, instruments, stains, tests, signs, and any medical procedure or pathological condition named after the discoverer, the patient, or even mythological characters. In the case of diseases, syndromes and operations, a brief definition is given, whereas all other eponymic entries are simply listed alphabetically and characterized. No effort has been made to include under each eponymic entry all of its possible instruments; but rather, emphasis has been placed on completeness of the eponyms themselves for the purpose of correct spelling and identification. Occasionally the word "eponym" has been given a broad meaning to include difficult and obscure place names when they refer to diseases, viruses, and so on— for instance, O'nyong-nyong fever.

Every effort has been made to see that these listings are both accurate and current; thus many reference sources have been used to reach this goal. Nowhere was the question of proper usage more troublesome than in the use of upper and lower case letters and periods in listing the abbreviations. Since there are great differences in form from one reference to another, compilation of the book called for judgment and guidance. For their assistance I owe the Saunders editorial staff, particularly Wynette Kommer and Baxter Venable, my sincere thanks.

It is my hope that this book will provide a simple method of locating the sought-after abbreviation or eponym with ease and speed and eliminate the need to search through many reference books to achieve this end.

SHEILA B. SLOANE

CONTENTS

Medical Abbreviations

A

A — mass number
A or Å —
    Angström unit
    angstrom
$\tilde{A}$ — cumulated activity
A, α — alpha (first letter of the Greek alphabet)
AI — angiotensin I
AII — angiotensin II
AIII — angiotensin III
A_2 — aortic second sound
A. —
    absolute temperature
    absorbance
    acceptor
    accommodation
    acetum
    activity (radiation)
    adenine
    adenosine
    admittance
    adrenaline
    adult
    age
    alanine
    allergy
    alveolar gas
    ampere
    amphetamine

A. (*continued*)
    anaphylaxis
    anesthetic
    annum [L] year
    anode
    anterior
    aqueous
    area
    argon
    arteria
    artery
    atomic weight
    atropine
    start of anesthesia
    total acidity
A. —
    Actinomyces
    Anopheles
a — thermodynamic activity
a. —
    absorptivity
    acceleration
    acid
    acidity
    ampere
    annum
    anode
    anterior
    aqua [L] water

a. (*continued*)
   area
   arteria
   arterial blood
   artery
   asymmetric
   atto-
   axial
α — alpha (first letter of the Greek alphabet)
AA —
   acetic acid
   achievement age
   adenylic acid
   aggregated albumin
   alveolar-arterial
   aminoacetone
   amino acid
   anticipatory avoidance
   arachidonic acid
   ascending aorta
   atomic absorption
   Australia antigen
A & A — aid and attendance
$\overline{AA}$, $\overline{aa}$ — ana [Gr] of each
A.A. — Alcoholics Anonymous
aa — arteries
AAA —
   abdominal aortic aneurysm
   acute anxiety attack
   androgenic anabolic agent
A.A.A. —
   American Academy of Allergy
   American Association of Anatomists
aaa — amalgama, a variant of amalgam
AAAE — amino acid–activating enzymes
AA-AMP — amino acid adenylate
A.A.A.S. — American Association for the Advancement of Science

A.A.B. — American Association of Bioanalysts
A.A.B.B. — American Association of Blood Banks
AAC — antibiotic-associated pseudomembranous colitis
A.A.C.C. — American Association for Clinical Chemistry
A.A.C.I.A. — American Association for Clinical Immunology and Allergy
A.A.C.P. — American Academy of Cerebral Palsy
AAD — alloxazine adenine dinucleotide
A.A.D.R. — American Academy of Dental Radiology
A.A.D.S. — American Academy of Dental Schools
AAE —
   active assistive exercise
   acute allergic encephalitis
A.A.E.E. — American Association of Electromyography and Electrodiagnosis
AAF —
   acetic-alcohol-formalin
   acetylaminofluorene
   ascorbic acid factor
A.A.F.P. — American Academy of Family Physicians
A.A.G.P. — American Academy of General Practice
A.A.I. — American Association of Immunologists
A.A.I.N. — American Association of Industrial Nurses
AAL — anterior axillary line
A.A.M. — American Academy of Microbiology
A.A.M.A. — American Academy of Medical Assistants

A.A.M.C. —
American Association of
Medical Clinics
American Association of
Medical Colleges
AAME — acetylarginine methyl
ester
A.A.M.I. — Association for the
Advancement of Medical
Instrumentation
A.A.M.R.L. — American Academy
of Medical Record Librarians
A.A.M.T. — American Association
for Medical Transcription
AAN — alpha-amino nitrogen
A.A.N. — American Association
of Neuropathologists
AAO — amino acid oxidase
A.A.O. —
American Academy of Oste-
opathy
American Academy of Oto-
laryngology
A.A.O.O. — American Academy
of Ophthalmology and Oto-
laryngology
A.A.O.P. — American Academy of
Oral Pathology
AAP — air at atmospheric pressure
A.A.P. —
American Academy of Pedi-
atrics
American Academy of Pedo-
dontics
American Academy of Perio-
dontology
American Association of
Pathologists
A.A.P.A. — American Association
of Pathologist Assistants
A.A.P.B. — American Association
of Pathologists and Bacteriolo-
gists

$(A\text{-}a)P_{CO_2}$ — alveolar-arterial
carbon dioxide difference
A.A.P.H.P.— American Association
of Public Health Physicians
A.A.P.M.R. — American Academy
of Physical Medicine and Rehabilitation
A.A.P.S. —
American Association of
Physicians and Surgeons
American Association of
Plastic Surgeons
AAR — antigen-antiglobulin reaction
A.A.R.T. — American Association
for Respiratory Therapy
AAS —
anthrax antiserum
aortic arch syndrome
atomic absorption spectrophotometry
AAT — alpha-antitrypsin
AAV — adeno-associated virus
AB —
abnormal
abortion
Alcian blue
apex beat
asbestos body
asthmatic bronchitis
axiobuccal
A/B — acid-base ratio
A>B — air greater than bone
Ab — antibody
ab —
abortion
about
antibody
ABA —
abscissic acid
antibacterial activity
A.B.B. — American Board of Bio-
analysis

ABC —
    absolute basophil count
    aconite, belladonna, chloro-
        form
    antigen-binding capacity
    apnea, bradycardia, cyanosis
    aspiration biopsy cytology
    axiobuccocervical
A.B.C. — American Blood Com-
    mission
ABD, Abd or abd —
    abdomen
    abdominal
ABDOM, Abdom or abdom —
    abdomen
    abdominal
ABE — acute bacterial endo-
    carditis
ABG —
    arterial blood gases
    axiobuccogingival
ABL —
    abetalipoproteinemia
    axiobuccolingual
ABLB — alternate binaural loud-
    ness balance
A.B.M.S. — Advisory Board for
    Medical Specialties
ABN, Abn. or abn. — abnormal
ABO — blood groups (named for
    agglutinogens)
Abor. — abortion
ABP —
    androgen-binding protein
    arterial blood pressure
ABR — absolute bed rest
ABR test — abortus Bang ring test
ABr test — agglutination test for
    brucellosis
ABS —
    acrylonitrile-butadiene-styrene
    acute brain syndrome
    alkylbenzene sulfonate

abs. —
    absent
    absolute
abs. feb. — absente febre [L]
    while fever is absent
abst. or abstr. — abstract
ABVD — Adriamycin, bleomycin,
    vinblastine and dacarbazine
ABY — acid bismuth yeast (agar)
AC —
    acetylcholine
    acromioclavicular
    adrenal cortex
    air conduction
    alternating current
    anodal closure
    anterior chamber
    anticoagulant
    anticomplementary
    anti-inflammatory corticoid
    aortic closure
    atriocarotid
    auriculocarotid
    axiocervical
A/C — albumin-coagulin ratio
Ac —
    acetyl
    actinium
ac — acute
a.c. — ante cibum [L] before
    meals
ACA —
    adenocarcinoma
    Automatic Clinical Analyzer
A.C.A. —
    American College of Allergists
    American College of Anesthe-
        siologists
    American College of Angi-
        ology
    American College of Apothe-
        caries
AcAcOH — acetoacetic acid

acad. – academy

ACC –
adenoid cystic carcinoma
anodal closure contraction

A.C.C. – American College of Cardiology

acc. –
acceleration
accident
accommodation
according

AcCHS – acetylcholinesterase

ACCl – anodal closure clonus

AcCoA – acetylcoenzyme A

accom. – accommodation

accur. – accuratissime [L] most carefully, accurately

ACD –
absolute cardiac dullness
acid-citrate-dextrose
allergic contact dermatitis
anterior chest diameter

ACD solution – citric acid, tri-sodium citrate, dextrose solution

ACE –
actinium emanation
adrenocortical extract
alcohol, chloroform, ether

A.C.E.P. – American College of Emergency Physicians

acetyl-CoA – acetylcoenzyme A

ACF – accessory clinical findings

A.C.F.O. – American College of Foot Orthopedists

A.C.F.S. – American College of Foot Surgeons

ACG –
angiocardiography
apexcardiogram

A.C.G. – American College of Gastroenterology

AcG – accelerator globulin

A.C.G.P. – American College of General Practitioners

ACH –
adrenocortical hormone
arm, chest, height

ACh – acetylcholine

A.C.H.A. – American College of Hospital Administrators

AChE – acetylcholinesterase

AChRab – acetylcholine receptor antibody

ACI –
adrenal cortical insufficiency
anticlonus index

acid p'tase – acid phosphatase

A.C.I.P. – Advisory Committee on Immunization Practices

A.C.L.A. – American Clinical Laboratory Association

A.C.L.P.S. – Academy of Clinical Laboratory Physicians and Scientists

ACM – albumin-calcium-magnesium

A.C.N. – American College of Neuropsychiatrists

A.C.N.M. –
American College of Nuclear Medicine
American College of Nurse-Midwives

A.C.N.P. – American College of Nuclear Physicians

ACO – anodal-closing odor

A.C.O.G. – American College of Obstetricians and Gynecologists

A.C.O.H.A. – American College of Osteopathic Hospital Administrators

A.C.O.I. – American College of Osteopathic Internists

A.C.O.O.G. — American College of Osteopathic Obstetricians and Gynecologists

A.C.O.P. — American College of Osteopathic Pediatricians

A.C.O.S. — American College of Osteopathic Surgeons

ACP —
acid phosphatase
acyl-carrier protein
anodal-closing picture
aspirin, caffeine, phenacetin

A.C.P. —
Association of Clinical Pathologists
American College of Physicians
Association of Clinical Pathologists

A.C.P.M. — American College of Preventive Medicine

ACPP — adrenocorticopolypeptide

ACR — anticonstipation regimen

A.C.R. — American College of Radiology

ACS —
anodal-closing sound
antireticular cytotoxic serum
aperture current setting

A.C.S. —
American Cancer Society
American Chemical Society
American College of Surgeons
Association of Clinical Scientists

A.C.S.M. — American College of Sports Medicine

A.C.S.P. — Advisory Council on Scientific Policy

ACSV — aortocoronary saphenous vein

ACT —
activated coagulation time
anticoagulant therapy

act. — active

ACTe — anodal closure tetanus

ACTH — adrenocorticotropic hormone

ACTH-RF — adrenocorticotropic hormone–releasing factor

ACTN — adrenocorticotropin

ACTP — adrenocorticotropic polypeptide

ACVD — acute cardiovascular disease

AD —
adenoid degeneration
admitting diagnosis
alcohol dehydrogenase
Aleutian disease
anodal duration
antigenic determinant
average deviation
axiodistal
axis deviation

A.D. — auris dextra [L] right ear

A & D — ascending and descending

Ad. — adrenal

ad. — adde or addetur [L] let them be added

ADA —
adenosine deaminase
anterior descending artery

ADA# — American Diabetes Association diet number

A.D.A. —
American Dental Association
American Dermatological Association
American Diabetes Association
American Dietetic Association

A.D.A.M.H.A. — Alcohol, Drug Abuse and Mental Health Administration

ADC —
albumin, dextrose, catalase

ADC (*continued*)
   analog-to-digital converter
   anodal duration contraction
   average daily census
   axiodistocervical
A.D.C. — Aid to Dependent Children
AdC — adrenal cortex
ADCC — antibody-dependent cell-mediated cytotoxicity
add. —
   adde or addetur [L] let there be added
   addition
   adduction
add. c. trit. — adde cum tritu [L] add triturition
ad def. an. — ad defectionem animi [L] to the point of fainting
ad deliq. — ad deliquium [L] to the point of failure
ADE — acute disseminated encephalitis
ad effect. — ad effectum [L] until effectual
ADEM — acute disseminated encephalomyelitis
ad. feb. — adstante febre [L] fever being present
ADG —
   atrial diastolic gallop
   axiodistogingival
ad gr. acid. — ad gratum aciditatem [L] to an agreeable sourness
ad gr. gust. — ad gratum gustum [L] to an agreeable taste
ADH —
   alcohol dehydrogenase
   antidiuretic hormone
adhib. — adhibendus [L] to be administered

ADI —
   acceptable daily intake
   axiodistoincisal
ad int. — ad interim [L] meanwhile
adj. — adjoining
ADL — activities of daily living
ad lib. — ad libitum [L] as desired
ADM —
   administrative medicine
   administrator
AdM — adrenal medulla
adm. — admission
admov. — admove, admoveatur [L] let there be added
ad naus. — ad nauseam [L] to the extent of producing nausea
ad neut. — ad neutralizandum [L] to neutralization
ADO — axiodisto-occlusal
ADP —
   adenosine diphosphate
   automatic data processing
ad part. dolent. — ad partes dolentes [L] to the painful parts
ADPase — adenosinediphosphatase
ADPL — average daily patient load
ad pond. om. — ad pondus omnium [L] to the weight of the whole
Adr. — adrenaline
ADS —
   antibody deficiency syndrome
   antidiuretic substance
ad sat. — ad saturandum [L] to saturation
adst. feb. — adstante febre [L] fever being present
ADT —
   adenosine triphosphate
   agar-gel diffusion test
   alternate-day treatment

ADTe − tetanic contraction
ad us. − ad usum [L] according to custom
ad us. ext. − ad usum externum [L] for external use
A/DV − arterio/deep venous
adv. − adversum [L] against
ad 2 vic. −
    ad duas vices [L] at two times, for two doses
A5D5W − alcohol 5%, dextrose 5% in water
ADX − adrenalectomized
AE −
    above elbow
    apoenzyme
    energy of activation
A.E. − Antitoxineinheit [Ger] antitoxic unit
AEA − alcohol, ether, acetone
A.E.C. − Atomic Energy Commission
AEG − air encephalogram
aeg. − aeger, aegra [L] the patient
AEM − analytical electron microscope
AEP − average evoked potential
AEq − age equivalent
aeq. − aequales [L] equal
AER −
    aldosterone excretion rate
    auditory evoked response
    average evoked response
Aero. − *Aerobacter*
A.E.S. −
    American Encephalographic Society
    American Epidemiological Society
AET −
    absorption equivalent thickness

AET (*continued*)
    2-amino-ethyl-isothiouronium bromide
aet. − aetas [L] age
aetat. −
    aetatis [L] aged, of age
AF −
    acid-fast
    albumose-free
    aldehyde fuchsin
    amniotic fluid
    angiogenesis factor
    antibody-forming
    aortic flow
    atrial fibrillation
    atrial flutter
    auricular fibrillation
af. − audiofrequency
AFB − acid-fast bacilli
AFBG − aortofemoral bypass graft
AFC − antibody-forming cells
aff. −
    afferent
    affinis [L] having an affinity with but not identical with
AFI − amaurotic familial idiocy
AFIB − atrial fibrillation
A.F.I.P. − Armed Forces Institute of Pathology
AFL −
    anti-fatty liver
    atrial flutter
A.F.M.L. − Armed Forces Medical Library
AFP −
    alpha$_1$-fetoprotein
    anterior faucial pillar
AFR − ascorbic free radical
AFRD − acute febrile respiratory disease

AFRI — acute febrile respiratory illness

AFTC — apparent free testosterone concentration

AG —
   antiglobulin
   antigravity
   atrial gallop
   axiogingival

Ag —
   antigen
   argentum [L] silver

AGA —
   accelerated growth area
   appropriate for gestational age

A.G.A. —
   American Gastroenterological Association
   American Genetics Association
   American Geriatrics Association

AGCT — Army General Classification Test

AGD — agarose diffusion (method)

AGE —
   acrylamide gel electrophoresis
   agarose gel electrophoresis
   angle of greatest extension

AGF — angle of greatest flexion

ag. feb. — aggrediente febre [L] when the fever increases

AGG — agammaglobulinemia

agg. —
   agglutination
   aggravated
   aggregate

aggred. feb. — aggrediente febre [L] when the fever increases

AGGS — anti gas gangrene serum

AgI — silver iodide

agit. — agita [L] shake

agit. ante sum. — agita ante sumendum [L] shake before taking

agit. vas. — agitato vase [L] the vial being shaken

AGL —
   acute granulocytic leukemia
   aminoglutethimide

AGMK — African green monkey kidney

AGN — acute glomerulonephritis

agn. — agnosia

AgNO$_3$ — silver nitrate

Ag$_2$O — silver oxide

A/G ratio — albumin-globulin ratio

A/G ratio test — albumin/globulin ratio test

AGS — adrenogenital syndrome

A.G.S. — American Gynecological Society

Ag$_2$SO$_4$ — silver sulfate

AGT — antiglobulin test

AGTH — adrenoglomerulotropin hormone

AGTr — adrenoglomerulotropin

AGTT — abnormal glucose tolerance test

AGV — aniline gentian violet

AH —
   abdominal hysterectomy
   acetohexamide
   amenorrhea and hirsutism
   aminohippurate
   antihyaluronidase
   arterial hypertension

ah — hyperopic astigmatism

AHA —
   acquired hemolytic anemia
   aspartyl-hydroxamic acid
   autoimmune hemolytic anemia

A.H.A. —
   American Heart Association

A.H.A. (*continued*)
American Hospital Association
AHB — alpha-hydroxybutyric
dehydrogenase
AHD —
arteriosclerotic heart disease
atherosclerotic heart disease
autoimmune hemolytic disease
AHE — acute hemorrhagic encephalomyelitis
AHF —
American Hospital Formulary
antihemophilic factor
AHG —
antihemophilic globulin
antihuman globulin
AHGS — acute herpetic gingival
stomatitis
AHH —
alpha-hydrazine analogue of
histidine
arylhydrocarbon hydroxylase
AHLE — acute hemorrhagic leukoencephalitis
AHLS — antihuman lymphocyte
serum
AHP —
acute hemorrhagic pancreatitis
air at high pressure
Assistant House Physician
AHS — Assistant House Surgeon
A.H.S. — American Hearing Society
AHT —
antihyaluronidase titer
augmented histamine test
AHTG — antihuman thymocytic
globulin
AHTP — antihuman thymocytic
plasma
AI —
accidentally incurred
angiotensin I
aortic incompetence

AI (*continued*)
aortic insufficiency
apical impulse
artificial insemination
atherogenic index
axioincisal
AIA — allylisopropylacetamide
βAIB — β-aminoisobutyric acid
AIBA — aminoisobutyric acid
A.I.B.S. — American Institute of
Biological Sciences
AIC — amino-imidazole carboxamide
A.I.C. — Association des Infir-
mieres Canadiennes
AICAR — amino-imidazole
carboxamide ribonucleotide
AICF — autoimmune complement
fixation
AID —
acute infectious disease
artificial insemination donor
autoimmune disease
A.I.D. —
Agency for International
Development
America-India Dispensary
AIDS — acquired immune defi-
ciency syndrome
AIEP — amount of insulin extract-
able from the pancreas
AIH —
artificial insemination, homol-
ogous
homologous insemination
A.I.H. — American Institute of
Homeopathy
AIHA — autoimmune hemolytic
anemia
A.I.H.A. — American Industrial
Hygiene Association
AIL — angioimmunoblastic
lymphadenopathy

AIN — acute interstitial nephri-
tides
AIO — amyloid of immunoglobulin
origin
AIP —
acute intermittent porphyria
automated immunoprecipita-
tion
average intravascular pressure
AIR — amino-imidazole ribonucle-
otide
AIS — anti-insulin serum
AITT — arginine insulin tolerance
test
AIU — absolute iodine uptake
AIVR — accelerated idioventricu-
lar rhythm
AJ — ankle jerk
A.J.C.C.S. — American Joint
Committee on Cancer Staging
AK — above knee
AKA — above-knee amputation
AL —
adaptation level
albumin
alignment mark
axiolingual
A.L. — auris laeva [L] left ear
Al — aluminum
ALA —
δ-aminolevulinic acid
axiolabial
A.L.A. — American Laryngological
Association
Ala — alanine
ALAD —
abnormal left axis deviation
aminolevulinic acid dehydrase
ALAG — axiolabiogingival
ALAL — axiolabiolingual
ALAS — aminolevulinic acid syn-
thetase

alb. —
albumin
albus [L] white
ALC —
approximate lethal concentration
avian leukosis complex
axiolinguocervical
ALD —
alcoholic liver disease
aldolase
ALG —
antilymphocyte globulin
axiolinguogingival
ALGOL — *alg*orithmic *o*riented
*l*anguage
ALH —
anterior lobe hormone
anterior lobe of the hypophysis
alk. — alkaline
alk. phos. — alkaline phosphatase
ALL —
acute lymphoblastic leukemia
acute lymphocytic leukemia
all. — allergies
ALME — acetyl-lysine methyl
ester
ALMI — anterior lateral myocardial infarct
ALN — anterior lymph node
ALO — axiolinguo-occlusal
Al_2O_3 — aluminum oxide
$Al(OH)_3$ — aluminum hydroxide
ALP —
alkaline phosphatase
anterior lobe of pituitary
antilymphocyte plasma
A.L.R.O.S. — American Laryngological, Rhinological, and
Otological Society
ALS —
amyotrophic lateral sclerosis

ALS (*continued*)
  angiotensin-like substance
  antilymphatic serum
  antilymphocyte serum
ALT — alanine aminotransferase
alt. —
  alternate
  altitude
ALTB — acute laryngotracheobronchitis
alt. dieb. — alternis diebus [L]
  every other day
ALTEE — acetyl-L-tyrosine ethyl
  ester
alt. hor. — alternis horis [L] every
  other hour
alt. noc. — alternis nocta [L]
  every other night
ALU — arithmetic and logic unit
alv. — alveolar
alv. adst. — alvo adstricta [L] when
  the bowels are constipated
alv. deject. — alvi dejectiones [L]
  discharge from the bowels
ALW — arch-loop-whorl
AM —
  alveolar macrophage
  ammeter
  amperemeter
  amplitude modulation
  anovular menstruation
  arithmetic mean
  arousal mechanism
  aviation medicine
  axiomesial
  meter-angle
Am — americium
am —
  ametropia
  meter-angle
  myopic astigmatism
a.m. — ante meridiem [L] before
  noon

AMA — against medical advice
A.M.A. —
  American Medical Association
  Australian Medical Association
A.M.A.L. — Aero-Medical Acceler-
  ation Laboratory
amb. —
  ambulate
  ambulatory
AMC —
  arthrogryposis multiplex con-
   genita
  axiomesiocervical
AMD —
  alpha-methyldopa
  axiomesiodistal
A.M.D.S. — Association of Military
  Dental Surgeons
A.M.E.A. — American Medical
  Electroencephalographic
  Association
AMegL — acute megakaryoblastic
  leukemia
A.M.E.L. — Aero-Medical Equip-
  ment Laboratory
AMG —
  antimacrophage globulin
  axiomesiogingival
AMH — automated medical history
Amh — mixed astigmatism with
  myopia predominating
AMI —
  acute myocardial infarction
  amitriptyline
  axiomesioincisal
A.M.I. — Association of Medical
  Illustrators
AML —
  acute monocytic leukemia
  acute myeloblastic leukemia
  acute myelocytic leukemia
  acute myelogenous leukemia
  acute myeloid leukemia

AMLS – antimouse lymphocyte serum

AMM –
agnogenic myeloid metaplasia
ammonia

AMML – acute monomyelocytic leukemia

AMMOL – acute myelomono-blastic leukemia

AMO – axiomesio-occlusal

A-mode – amplitude modulation

AMOL –
acute monoblastic leukemia
acute monocytic leukemia

AMP –
acid mucopolysaccharide
adenosine monophosphate
amphetamine
ampicillin
amputation
average mean pressure

amp. –
ampere
amplification
ampule
amputation

ampl. – amplus [L] large

AMPS –
abnormal mucopolysac-chariduria
acid mucopolysaccharides

ampul. – ampulla [L] ampule

AMR – alternating motion reflexes

A.M.R.A. – American Medical Record Association

A.M.R.L. – Aerospace Medical Research Laboratories

AMS –
aggravated in military service
amylase
antimacrophage serum
auditory memory span

AMS (*continued*)
automated multiphasic screen-ing

A.M.S. –
American Microscopical Society
Army Medical Service
Association of Military Surgeons

ams. – *am*ount of a *s*ubstance

AMT –
alpha-methyltyrosine
amethopterin
amphetamine

A.M.T. – American Medical Tech-nologists

amt. – amount

amu – atomic mass unit

A.M.W.A. –
American Medical Women's Association
American Medical Writers Association

AMY – amylase

An – actinon

An. –
anisometropia
anodal
anode

A_n – normal atmosphere

ANA –
acetylneuraminic acid
antinuclear antibodies
aspartyl naphthylamide

A.N.A. –
American Neurological Asso-ciation
American Nurses Association

ana. – so much of each

anal. –
analgesic
analysis
analyst

ANAP — agglutination negative, absorption positive
anast. — anastomosis
anat. —
  anatomical
  anatomy
AnCC — anodal closure contraction
AnDTe — anodal duration tetanus
anes. —
  anesthesia
  anesthesiology
an. ex. — anode excitation
ANF —
  alpha-naphthoflavone
  antinuclear factor
ang. —
  angiogram
  angle
Ang GR — angiotensin generation rate
anh. — anhydrous
ANIT — alpha-naphthylisothiocyanate
ank. — ankle
ANLL — acute nonlymphocytic leukemia
AnOC — anodal opening contraction
ANOVA — analysis of variance
A.N.R.C. — American National Red Cross
ANRL — antihypertensive neutral renomedullary lipids
ANS —
  anterior nasal spine
  antineutrophilic serum
  arteriolonephrosclerosis
  autonomic nervous system
A.N.S.I. — American National Standards Institute
ANT — 2-amino-5-nitro-thiazol
ant. — anterior

ante — ante [L] before
anti-HAA — antibody hepatitis-associated antigen
ANTR — apparent net transfer rate
ANTU — alpha-naphthylthiourea
ANUG — acute necrotizing ulcerative gingivitis
AO —
  acridine orange
  anodal opening
  anterior oblique
  aorta
  aortic opening
  atomic orbital
  axio-occlusal
  opening of the atrioventricular valves
A.O.A. —
  American Optometric Association
  American Orthopedic Association
  American Orthopsychiatric Association
  American Osteopathic Association
AOAA — amino-oxyacetic acid
AOB — alcohol on breath
AOC — anodal opening contraction
A.O.C.A. — American Osteopathic College of Anesthesiologists
A.O.C.D. — American Osteopathic College of Dermatology
AOCl — anodal opening clonus
A.O.C.Pa. — American Osteopathic College of Pathologists
A.O.C.Pr. — American Osteopathic College of Proctology
A.O.C.R. — American Osteopathic College of Radiology
AOD — arterial occlusive disease
AODM — adult onset diabetes mellitus

AOL — acro-osteolysis
AOM — acute otitis media
AOO — anodal opening odor
AOP — anodal opening picture
AoP — left ventricle to aorta pressure gradient
A.O.P.A. — American Orthotics and Prosthetics Association
AOS — anodal opening sound
A.O.S. — American Otological Society
A.O.T. — Association of Occupational Therapists
A.O.T.A. — American Occupational Therapy Association
AOTe — anodal opening tetanus
AP —
  acid phosphatase
  action potential
  acute proliferative
  alkaline phosphatase
  alum-precipitated
  aminopeptidase
  angina pectoris
  antepartum
  anterior pituitary (gland)
  anteroposterior
  aortic pressure
  apical pulse
  appendix
  arterial pressure
  artificial pneumothorax
  association period
  axiopulpal
A/P — ascites-plasma ratio
A & P —
  anterior and posterior
  auscultation and palpation
  auscultation and percussion
3-AP — 3-acetylpyridine
$A_2 > P_2$ — aortic second sound greater than pulmonary second sound

$A_2 < P_2$ — aortic second sound less than pulmonary second sound
a.p. — ante pradium [L] before dinner
APA —
  aldosterone-producing adenoma
  aminopenicillanic acid
  antipernicious anemia factor
A.P.A. —
  American Pharmaceutical Association
  American Physiotherapy Association
  American Podiatric Association
  American Psychiatric Association
  American Psychoanalytic Association
  American Psychological Association
  American Psychopathological Association
APB —
  atrial premature beat
  auricular premature beat
APC —
  acetylsalicylic acid, phenacetin, caffeine
  adenoidal-pharyngeal-conjunctival
  antiphlogistic corticoid
  aspirin, phenacetin, caffeine
  atrial premature contraction
APC-C — aspirin, phenacetin, caffeine; with codeine
APC virus — adenoidal, pharyngeal, conjunctival virus
APD —
  action-potential duration
  atrial premature depolarization

A-PD — anteroposterior diameter
APE —
    acetone powder extract
    aminophylline, phenobarbital,
        ephedrine
    anterior pituitary extract
APF —
    anabolism-promoting factor
    animal protein factor
APGL — alkaline phosphatase
    activity of the granular
    leukocytes
APH —
    antepartum hemorrhage
    anterior pituitary hormone
A.P.H.A. —
    American Protestant Hospital
        Association
    American Public Health Asso-
        ciation
A.Ph.A. — American Pharmaceu-
    tical Association
APHP — anti-*Pseudomonas* human
    plasma
A.P.I.M. — Association Profession-
    nelle Internationale des
    Médecins
APL —
    accelerated painless labor
    acute promyelocytic leukemia
    anterior pituitary–like
AP & Lat. — anteroposterior and
    lateral
A.P.M. —
    Academy of Physical Medicine
    Academy of Psychosomatic
        Medicine
A.P.M.R. — Association for Physi-
    cal and Mental Rehabilitation
APN —
    acute pyelonephritis
    average peak noise

APP —
    alum-precipitated pyridine
    avian pancreatic polypeptide
app. — appendix
appl. —
    appliance
    applied
applan. — applantus [L] flattened
applicand. — applicandus [L] to
    be applied
approx. —
    approximately
    approximation
appt. — appointment
appy. — appendectomy
APR —
    amebic prevalence rate
    anterior pituitary resection
A.P.R.L. — American Prosthetic
    Research Laboratory
AProL — acute promyelocytic
    leukemia
APRT — adenine phosphoribosyl-
    transferase
APS — adenosine phosphosulfate
A.P.S. —
    American Pediatric Society
    American Physiological Soci-
        ety
    American Proctologic Society
    American Psychological Soci-
        ety
    American Psychosomatic Soci-
        ety
APT — alum-precipitated toxoid
A.P.T.A. — American Physical
    Therapy Association
aPTT — activated partial thrombo-
    plastin time
APUD — *a*mine *p*recursor *u*ptake
    (and) *d*ecarboxylation
AQ — achievement quotient

aq. −
    aqua [L] water
    aqueous
aq. astr. − aqua astricta [L]
    frozen water
aq. bull. − aqua bulliens [L] boil-
    ing water
aq. comm. − aqua communis [L]
    common water
aq. dest. − aqua destillata [L] dis-
    tilled water
aq. ferv. − aqua fervens [L] hot
    water
aq. fluv. − aqua fluvialis [L] river
    water
aq. font. − aqua fontana [L]
    spring water
aq. frig. − aqua frigida [L] cold
    water
aq. mar. − aqua marina [L] sea
    water
aq. niv. − aqua nivalis [L] snow
    water
aq. pluv. − aqua pluvialis [L] rain
    water
aq. pur. − aqua pura [L] pure
    water
AQS − additional qualifying
    symptoms
aq. tep. − aqua tepida [L] tepid
    water
AR −
    achievement ratio
    active resistance
    alarm reaction
    analytical reagent
    aortic regurgitation
    apical-radial (pulse)
    Argyll Robertson (pupil)
    arsphenamine
    articulare
    artificial respiration
    at risk

A/R − apical/radial
Ar − argon
A.R.A. − American Rheumatism
    Association
ara-A − adenine arabinoside
ara-C − cytosine arabinoside
ARBOR − arthropod-borne (virus)
ARC −
    anomalous retinal correspon-
        dence
    average response computer
A.R.C. − American Red Cross
A.R.C.S. − Associate of the Royal
    College of Science
ARD −
    absolute reaction of degenera-
        tion
    acute respiratory disease
    anorectal dressing
ARDS − adult respiratory distress
    syndrome
ARF −
    acute renal failure
    acute respiratory failure
    acute rheumatic fever
Arg − arginine
arg. − argentum [L] silver
AR grade − analytical reagent
    grade
A.R.I.C. − Associate of the Royal
    Institute of Chemistry
ARL − average remaining lifetime
ARM − artificial rupture of the
    membranes
A.R.M.H. − Academy of Religion
    and Mental Health
A.R.N.M.D. − Association for
    Research in Nervous and
    Mental Disease
A.R.O. − Association for Research
    in Ophthalmology
ARP −
    absolute refractory period

ARP (*continued*)
    at risk period
A.R.P. — American Registry of
    Pathologists
A.R.P.T. — American Registry of
    Physical Therapists
A.R.R.S. — American Roentgen
    Ray Society
A.R.R.T. —
    American Registered Respira-
    tory Therapist
    American Registry of Radio-
    logic Technologists
ARS — antirabies serum
A.R.S. —
    American Radium Society
    American Rhinologic Society
Ars. — arsphenamine
ART —
    absolute retention time
    automated reagin test
A.R.T. — Accredited Record
    Technicians
art. —
    artery
    articulation
AS —
    acetylstrophanthidin
    Adams-Stokes (disease) (syn-
    drome)
    alveolar sac
    androsterone sulfate
    ankylosing spondylitis
    antistreptolysin
    anxiety state
    aortic stenosis
    aqueous solution
    aqueous suspension
    arteriosclerosis
    atherosclerosis
A-S — ascendance-submission
A.S. — auris sinistra [L] left ear
As — arsenic

As. — astigmatism
ASA —
    acetylsalicylic acid
    Adams-Stokes attack
    argininosuccinic acid
    arylsulfatase-A
A.S.A. —
    American Society of Anesthe-
    siologists
    American Standards Associa-
    tion
    American Stomatological
    Association
    American Surgical Association
A.S.A.H.P. — American Society of
    Allied Health Professionals
ASAI — aortic stenosis and aortic
    insufficiency (murmurs)
A.S.A.I.O. — American Society
    for Artificial Internal Organs
ASAP — as soon as possible
A.S.B. — American Society of
    Bacteriologists
ASC — acetylsulfanilyl chloride
A.S.C. — American Society of
    Cytology
ASCAD — arteriosclerotic coro-
    nary artery disease
A.S.C.H. — American Society of
    Clinical Hypnosis
A.S.C.I. — American Society for
    Clinical Investigation
ASCII — American Standard Code
    for Information Interchange
Ascit. Fl. — ascitic fluid
A.S.C.L.T. — American Society of
    Clinical Laboratory Techni-
    cians
A.S.C.P. — American Society of
    Clinical Pathologists
A.S.C.P.C. — American Society of
    Clinical Pharmacology and
    Chemotherapy

ascr. – ascriptum [L] ascribed to
ASCVD –
    arteriosclerotic cardiovascular
      disease
    atherosclerotic cardiovascular
      disease
ASD –
    aldosterone secretion defect
    atrial septal defect
ASE – axilla, shoulder, elbow
    (bandage)
A.S.E.P. – American Society for
    Experimental Pathology
ASF – aniline, sulfur, formalde-
    hyde
A.S.G. – American Society for
    Genetics
A.S.G.E. – American Society of
    Gastrointestinal Endoscopy
ASH – asymmetrical septal hyper-
    trophy
A.S.H. – American Society for
    Hematology
As.H. – hypermetropic astigma-
    tism
A.S.H.A. –
    American School Health Asso-
      ciation
    American Speech and Hearing
      Association
ASHD – arteriosclerotic heart
    disease
A.S.H.I. – Association for the
    Study of Human Infertility
ASHN – acute sclerosing hyaline
    necrosis
A.S.H.P. – American Society of
    Hospital Pharmacists
A.S.I.I. – American Science In-
    formation Institute
A.S.I.M. – American Society of
    Internal Medicine
ASIS – anterior superior iliac spine

ASK – antistreptokinase
ASL – antistreptolysin
ASLO – antistreptolysin-O
A.S.M. – American Society for
    Microbiology
As.M. – myopic astigmatism
A.S.M.E. – Association for the
    Study of Medical Education
ASMI – anteroseptal myocardial
    infarct
A.S.M.T. – American Society for
    Medical Technology
ASN – alkali-soluble nitrogen
Asn – asparagine
ASO –
    antistreptolysin-O
    arteriosclerosis obliterans
A.S.O. – American Society of
    Orthodontics
As_2O_3 – arsenic trioxide
A.S.O.S. – American Society of
    Oral Surgeons
ASO titer – antistreptolysin-O
    titer
ASP – area systolic pressure
A.S.P. – American Society of
    Parasitologists
Asp – aspartic acid
ASR –
    aldosterone secretion rate
    aldosterone secretory rate
A.S.R.T. – American Society of
    Radiologic Technologists
ASS – anterior superior spine
Assn. – association
asst. – assistant
AST – aspartate aminotransferase
Ast. – astigmatism
A.S.T.C. – Association of Science
    Technology Centers
Asth. – asthenopia
A.S.T.H.O. – Association of State
    and Territorial Health Officials

ASTI — antispasticity index
A.S.T.M.H. — American Society of Tropical Medicine and Hygiene
ASTO — antistreptolysin-O
as tol. — as tolerated
ASV —
   anodic stripping voltammetry
   antisnake venom
   arterio-superficial venous difference
A/SV — arterio/superficial venous
asym. — asymmetrical
AT —
   achievement test
   adjunctive therapy
   air temperature
   aminotriazole
   antitrypsin
AT_7 — hexachlorophene
AT_{10} — dihydrotachysterol
AT-III — antithrombin III
A.T. — Alt Tuberculin [Ger] old tuberculin
At — astatine
ATA —
   alimentary toxic aleukia
   anti-*Toxoplasma* antibodies
   atmosphere absolute
   aurintricarboxylic acid
ATB — at the time of the bomb (A-bomb in Japan)
ATCC — American-Type Culture Collection
ATD — asphyxiating thoracic dystrophy
ATE — adipose tissue extract
ATEE — acetyltyrosine ethyl ester
at. fib. — atrial fibrillation
ATG —
   antithrombocyte globulin
   antithyroglobulin
ATH — acetyl-tyrosine hydrazide

ATHC — allotetrahydrocortisol
ATL —
   Achilles tendon lengthening
   antitension line
atm. — atmosphere
ATN — acute tubular necrosis
at. no. — atomic number
ATP — adenosine triphosphate
ATPase — adenosine triphosphatase
ATPD — ambient temperature and pressure, dry
ATPS — ambient temperature and pressure, saturated
ATR — Achilles tendon reflex
atr. — atrophy
atr. fib. — atrial fibrillation
ATS —
   antitetanic serum (tetanus antitoxin)
   antithymocyte serum
   anxiety tension state
   arteriosclerosis
   atherosclerosis
ATT — aspirin tolerance time
att. — attending
at. vol. — atomic volume
at. wt. — atomic weight
A.U. —
   Angström unit
   antitoxin unit
   arbitrary units
   aures unitas [L] both ears together
   auris uterque [L] each ear
   Australia (antigen)
   azauridine
Au —
   aurum [L] gold
   Australia antigen
^{198}Au — radioactive gold
A.U.A. — American Urological Association

Au Ag — Australia antigen
auct. — auctorum [L] of authors
aud. — auditory
AUHAA — Australia hepatitis
associated antigen
AUL — acute undifferentiated
leukemia
AUO — amyloid of unknown
origin
aur. fib. — auricular fibrillation
ausc. — auscultation
AuSH — Australia serum hepatitis
(antigen)
aux. — auxiliary
AV —
alveolar duct
anteversion
aortic valve
arteriovenous
atrioventricular
auriculoventricular
avoirdupois
A-V —
arteriovenous
atrioventricular
Av. —
average
avoirdupois
AVA — arteriovenous anastomosis
AV/AF — anteverted, anteflexed
AVC —
allantoin vaginal cream
atrioventricular canal
AVCS — atrioventricular conduction system
avdp. — avoirdupois
AVF — arteriovenous fistula
AVH — acute viral hepatitis
AVI — air velocity index
AVM — arteriovenous malformation

A.V.M.A. — American Veterinary
Medical Association
AVN — atrioventricular node
A-Vo$_2$ — arteriovenous oxygen
difference
AVP —
antiviral protein
arginine vasopressin
AVR — aortic valve replacement
AVRP — atrioventricular refractory period
AVS — arteriovenous shunt
A-V shunt — arteriovenous shunt
AVT —
Allen vision test
arginine vasotonin
AW —
above waist
anterior wall
atomic warfare
A & W — alive and well
A.W. — atomic weight
aw — airways
AWF — adrenal weight factor
AWI — anterior wall infarction
AWMI — anterior wall myocardial
infarction
awu — atomic weight unit
ax. —
axilla
axis
ax. grad. — axial gradient
AXM — acetoxycyclo-hexamide
Az. — azote [Fr] nitrogen
azg. — azaguanine
azo — indicates presence of the
group —N:N—
AZT — Aschheim-Zondek test
AZ test — Aschheim-Zondek test
AZUR — 6-azauridine

B

B −
bel
blood
boron
magnetic induction
B4 − before
B. −
bacillus
balneum [L] bath
barometric
base
Baumé scale
behavior
Benoist scale
benzoate
bicuspid
blue
boils at
brother
buccal
Bucky (film in cassette in
Potter-Bucky diaphragm)
symbol for gauss
tomogram with oscillating
Bucky
whole blood
B. − *Brucella*
b. −
barn
bis [L] twice
boils at
born
B, β − beta (second letter of the
Greek alphabet)
BA −
backache
bacterial agglutination
basion
betamethasone acetate
blocking antibody

BA (*continued*)
blood agar
bone age
boric acid
bovine albumin
brachial artery
bronchial asthma
buccoaxial
B > A − bone greater than air
B.A. −
Bachelor of Arts
balneum arenae [L] sand bath
Ba − barium
BAA − benzoyl arginine amide
Bab. − Babinski (reflex)
BAC −
bacterial antigen complex
blood alcohol concentration
buccoaxiocervical
BaCl$_2$ − barium chloride
Bact. − *Bacterium*
bact. −
bacteriology
bacterium
BaE − barium enema
BAEE −
benzoyl arginine ethyl ester
benzylarginine ethyl ester
BAEP − brain stem auditory
evoked potential
BAG − buccoaxiogingival
BAGG − buffered azide glucose
glycerol
BAIB − beta-aminoisobutyric
acid
BAL − British anti-lewisite
(dimercaprol)
bal. −
balance
balsam

bal. arenae — balneum arenae [L] sand bath

BALB — binaural alternate loudness balance (test)

bal. mar. — balneum maris [L] salt or sea-water bath

bals. — balsam

bal. vap. — balneum vapor [L] steam or vapor bath

BAm — mean brachial artery

BaM — barium meal

BAME — benzoyl arginine methyl ester

BAO — basal acid output

B.A.O. — Bachelor of the Art of Obstetrics

BAP —
blood agar plate
brachial artery pressure

bar. —
barometer
barometric

BAS — benzyl analogue of serotonin

BASH — body acceleration given synchronously with the heartbeat

Baso. or baso. — basophil

BaSO$_4$ — barium sulfate

BB —
bed bath
blanket bath
blood bank
blood buffer base
blue bloaters (emphysema)
both bones
breakthrough bleeding
breast biopsy
buffer base
isoenzyme of creatine kinase that contains two B subunits

BBA — born before arrival

BBB —
blood-brain barrier
bundle branch block

BBBB — bilateral bundle branch block

BBT — basal body temperature

BC —
bactericidal concentration
battle casualty
birth control
bone conduction
Bowman's capsule
buccocervical

B.C. — Bachelor of Surgery

BCB — brilliant cresyl blue

BC/BS — Blue Cross/Blue Shield

B.C.C. — Birth Control Clinic

BCD — binary coded decimal

BCE — basal cell epithelioma

BCF — basophil chemotactic factor

BCG —
bacille Calmette-Guérin (vaccine)
ballistocardiogram
bicolor guaiac (test)
bromocresol green

BCG test — bicolor guaiac test

BCH — basal cell hyperplasia

B.Ch. — Bachelor of Surgery

B.Ch.D. — Bachelor of Dental Surgery

B.C.I.C. — Birth Control Investigation Committee

BCM — birth control medication

BCME — bis chlormethyl ether

BCNU —
bischloroethylnitrosourea (carmustine)
bischloronitrosourea

BCP —
birth control pill
bromocresol purple

BCP-D — bromocresol purple desoxycholate (agar)
BCTF — Breast Cancer Task Force
BCW — biological and chemical warfare
BD —
   base deficit
   base (of prism) down
   bile duct
   borderline dull
   buccodistal
b.d. — bis die [L] twice a day
B.D.A. — British Dental Association
B.D.A.C. — Bureau of Drug Abuse Control
BDB — bis-diazotized-benzidine
BDC — burn-dressing change
BDE — bile duct exploration
BDG — buffered desoxycholate glucose (broth)
BDS — biological detection system
B.D.S. — Bachelor of Dental Surgery
BE —
   bacillary emulsion (tuberculin)
   bacterial endocarditis
   barium enema
   base excess
   below the elbow
   bile esculin
   bovine enteritis
   bronchoesophagology
Be — beryllium
BEAR — Biological Effects of Atomic Radiation
BEI — butanol-extractable iodine
ben. — bene [L] well, good
BES — balanced electrolyte solution
BeV — billion electron volts
BF —
   bentonite flocculation (test)

BF (continued)
   blastogenic factor
   blood flow
   bouillon filtre [Fr] bouillon filtrate (tuberculin)
   breakfast fed
   buffered
   butter fat
B/F — bound-free ratio
BFC — benign febrile convulsion
BFP —
   biologically false positivity
   biologic false-positive (reaction)
BFR —
   biologic false-positive reactor
   blood flow rate
   bone formation rate
BFT — bentonite flocculation test
BFU-E — burst-forming units — erythrocyte
BG —
   bicolor guaiac (test)
   blood glucose
   bone graft
   Bordet Gengou (test)
   buccogingival
BGD — blood group–degrading
BGE — butyl glycidyl ether
BGG — bovine gamma globulin
BGH — bovine growth hormone
BGLB — brilliant green lactose broth
BGlu — blood glucose
BGP — beta-glycerophosphatase
BGSA — blood granulocyte-specific activity
BGTT — borderline glucose tolerance test
BH —
   benzalkonium and heparin
   bill of health
   brain hormone

BH (*continued*)
    Bundle of His
BHA — butylated hydroxyanisole
BHBA — β-hydroxybutyric acid
BHC — benzene hexachloride
BHI — brain-heart infusion
BHIB — beef heart infusion broth
BHIS — beef heart infusion sup-
    plemented (broth)
BHL — biological half-life
BHN — bephenium hydroxynaph-
    thoate
BHS — beta-hemolytic strepto-
    coccus
BHT — butylated hydroxytoluene
BH/VH — body hematocrit–
    venous hematocrit ratio
BI —
    bacteriological index
    base (of prism) in
    bone injury
    burn index
Bi — bismuth
bib. — bibe [L] drink
BID — brought in dead
b.i.d. — bis in die [L] twice a day
BIDLB — block in the posteroin-
    ferior division of the left
    branch
BIH — benign intracranial hyper-
    tension
bihor. — bihorium [L] during two
    hours
Bi Isch. — between ischial tuber-
    osities
BIL — bilirubin
bil. or bilat. — bilateral
b.i.n. — bis in nocte [L] twice a
    night
$(BiO)_2CO_2$ — subcarbonate of
    bismuth
BIP —
    bacterial intravenous protein

BIP (*continued*)
    biparietal diameter
    bismuth iodoform paraffin
B.I.P.M. — Bureau International
    des Poids et Mesures (Inter-
    national Bureau of Weights
    and Measures)
BIPP — bismuth iodoform petro-
    latum paste
BIR — basic incidence rate
bis- — twice
BiSP — between ischial spines
Bisp. — bispinous or interspinous
    diameter
BiT — between great trochanters
BITU — benzyl-thiourea
BJ —
    Bence Jones
    biceps jerk
B&J — bone and joint
BJM — bones, joints and muscles
BJP — Bence Jones protein
BK — below knee
Bk — berkelium
BKA — below knee amputation
bkfst. — breakfast
BKTT — below knee to toe
BKWP — below knee walking
    plaster
BL —
    baseline
    Bessey-Lowry (unit)
    bleeding
    blood loss
    buccolingual
    Burkitt's lymphoma
B-L — bursa equivalent lympho-
    cyte
bl —
    bleeding
    blood
    blue

BLB — Boothby, Lovelace, Bulbulian (mask)
BLB unit —
Bessey-Lowry-Brock unit
Boothby, Lovelace, Bulbulian unit
bl. cult. — blood culture
BLG — beta-lactoglobulin
BLN — bronchial lymph nodes
bl. pr. — blood pressure
B.L.R.O.A. — British Laryngological, Rhinological, and Otological Association
BLT — blood-clot lysis time
BLU — Bessey-Lowry units
BM —
basal metabolism
basement membrane
body mass
bone marrow
bowel movement
buccomesial
B.M. — Bachelor of Medicine
b.m. — balneum maris [L] seawater bath
B.M.A. — British Medical Association
BME — basal medium, Eagle's
BMG — benign monoclonal gammopathy
bmk. — birthmark
BMMP — benign mucous membrane pemphigus
B-mode — brightness modulation
BMR — basal metabolic rate
B.M.S. — Bachelor of Medical Science
BN — brachial neuritis
BNA — Basle Nomina Anatomica
BNC — bladder neck contracture
B.N.D.D. — Bureau of Narcotics and Dangerous Drugs

BNG — bromo-naphthyl-beta-galactoside
BNGase — bromo-naphthyl-beta-galactosidase
BNO —
bladder neck obstruction
bowels not open
BNPA — binasal pharyngeal airway
BNS — benign nephrosclerosis
BO —
base (of prism) out
body odor
bowel obstruction
bowels open
bucco-occlusal
B & O — belladonna and opium
Bo — bohemium
BOA — born on arrival
B.O.A. — British Orthopaedic Association
BOBA — beta-oxybutyric acid
BOD — biochemical oxygen demand
Bod Units — Bodansky units
BOEA — ethyl biscoumacetate
bol. — bolus [L] pill
BOM — bilateral otitis media
BOP — Buffalo orphan prototype
BOR — bowels open regularly
BOW — bag of waters
BP —
back pressure
barometric pressure
bathroom privileges
bedpan
behavior pattern
benzopyrene
biotic potential
biparietal
birthplace
blood pressure
British Pharmacopoeia

BP (*continued*)
bronchopleural
buccopulpal
bypass
bp — base pair
b.p. — boiling point
B.P.A. — British Paediatric Association
BPB — bromophenol blue
BPC — British Pharmaceutical Codex
BPD —
biparietal diameter
blood pressure decreased
bronchopulmonary dysplasia
BPH —
benign prostatic hyperplasia
benign prostatic hypertrophy
B.Ph. — British Pharmacopoeia
BPI — blood pressure increased
BPL — β-propiolactone
BPO — benzylpenicilloyl
BPP — bovine pancreatic polypeptide
BPRS —
brief psychiatric rating scale
brief psychiatric reacting scale
BPV — bovine papilloma virus
Bq. — becquerel
BQC sol. — 2,6-dibromoquinone-chlorimide solution
BR —
bathroom
bedrest
bilirubin
Br —
bromine
bronchitis
brown
Br. — Brucella
br —
boiling range
branch

br (*continued*)
breath
brother
BRAT diet — bananas, rice, cereal, applesauce and toast
BRBC — bovine red blood cells
BrdU — 5-bromodeoxyuridine
B.R.H. — Bureau of Radiological Health
BRI — Bio-Research Index
brkf. — breakfast
BRM — biuret-reactive material
bron. — bronchial
BRP —
bathroom privileges
bilirubin production
B.R.S. — British Roentgen Society
brth. — breath
BS —
blood sugar
Blue Shield
bowel sounds
breaking strength
breath sounds
B.S. —
Bachelor of Science
Bachelor of Surgery
BSA —
benzenesulfonic acid
bismuth-sulfite agar
bis-trimethylsilylacetamide
body surface area
bovine serum albumin
BSAP —
brief short-action potential
brief, small, abundant potentials
BSB — body surface burned
B.Sc. — Bachelor of Science
BSDLB — block in the anterosuperior division of the left branch

BSE –
   bilateral, symmetrical and
      equal
   breast self-examination
BSF – back scatter factor
BSI – bound serum iron
BSL – blood sugar level
BSN – bowel sounds normal
BSO –
   bilateral sagittal osteotomy
   bilateral salpingo-oophorec-
      tomy
BSP – Bromsulphalein
BSp – bronchospasm
BSR –
   basal skin resistance
   blood sedimentation rate
BSS –
   balanced salt solution
   black silk suture
   buffered saline solution
BST –
   blood serological test
   brief stimulus therapy
BSTFA – bis-trimethylsilyl-
      trifluoroacetamide
BT –
   bedtime
   bitemporal
   bladder tremor
   bleeding time
   blue tetrazolium
   body temperature
   brain tumor
BTA – N-benzoyl-1-tyrosine
      amide
BTB –
   breakthrough bleeding
   bromothymol blue
BThU – British thermal unit
BTL – bilateral tubal ligation
BTPS – body temperature, ambi-
      ent pressure, saturated

BTR – Bezold-type reflex
BTSH –
   beef thyroid-stimulating hor-
      mone
   bovine thyroid-stimulating
      hormone
BTU – British thermal unit
BTX – benzene, toluene, xylene
BU –
   base (of prism) up
   Bodansky unit
   bromouracil
   burn unit
Bu – butyl
BUDR – bromodeoxyuracil
BUDU – bromodeoxyuridine
bull. – bulliat [L] let it boil
BUN – blood urea nitrogen
BUS – Bartholin's, urethral,
      Skene's (glands)
but. – butyrum [L] butter
BV –
   biological value
   blood vessel
   blood volume
   bronchovesicular
b.v. – balneum vaporis [L] vapor
      bath
BVH – biventricular hypertrophy
BVI – blood vessel invasion
BVM – bronchovascular markings
BVV – bovine vaginitis virus
BW –
   below waist
   biological warfare
   birth weight
   body water
   body weight
Bx – biopsy
BYE – Barile-Yaguchi-Eveland
      (agar)
BZ – benzoyl

C

C –
    calculus
    calorie (large)
    canine
    capacitance
    carbohydrate
    carbon
    carrier
    Caucasian
    central
    certified
    cervical
    chest
    clearance rate
    clonus
    cocaine
    coefficient
    complement
    compliance
    compound
    concentration
    constant
    contracture
    correct
    cortex
    coulomb
    cup
    curie
    cysteine
    cytidine
    cytochrome
    cytosine
    heat capacity
    hundred
    velocity of light
C′ – complement
C_I – first cranial nerve
C_{II} – second cranial nerve
C-1 – first cervical vertebra
C-2 – second cervical vertebra

C_3 – Collin's solution
C-6 – hexamethonium
C-10 – decamethonium
^{14}C – radioactive carbon
^{137}C – radioactive cesium
C. –
    cathodal
    cathode
    Celsius
    centigrade
    cervical
    clearance
    clonus
    closure
    color sense
    congius [L] gallon
    contraction
    cylinder
    speed of light
C. –
    Clostridium
    Cryptococcus
c. –
    calorie (small)
    candle
    capacity
    centi-
    centum [L] one hundred
    cibus [L] meal
    circa [L] about
    contact
    cubic
    cum [L] with
    cup
    curie
    cyclic
c̄. – cum [L] with
c′ – coefficient of partage
X, χ – chi (22nd letter of the Greek alphabet)

χ_e — electric susceptibility
χ_m — magnetic susceptibility
CA —
    cancer
    carbonic anhydrase
    carcinoma
    cardiac arrest
    catecholamine
    cathodal
    cathode
    cervicoaxial
    chronological age
    cold agglutinin
    common antigen
    coronary artery
    corpora amylacea
    cortisone acetate
    croup-associated (virus)
    cytosine arabinoside
Ca —
    calcium
    carcinoma
    cathode
^{45}Ca. — radioactive calcium
ca. —
    candle
    circa [L] about
CAAT — computer-assisted axial tomography
CAB — coronary artery bypass
CABG — coronary artery bypass graft
CaBP — calcium-binding protein
CAC — cardiac-accelerator center
CACC — cathodal closure contraction
$CaCl_2$ — calcium chloride
CaCl(OCl) — chlorinated lime
$CaCO_3$ — calcium carbonate
CaC_2O_4 — calcium oxalate
CACX — cancer of the cervix
CAD —
    computerized assisted design

CAD (*continued*)
    coronary artery disease
CADTe — cathodal duration tetanus
CAE —
    cellulose acetate electrophoresis
    contingent after-effects
CaEDTA —
    calcium disodium edetate
    edathamil calcium disodium
CaF_2 — calcium fluoride
CAG — chronic atrophic gastritis
CAH —
    chronic active hepatitis
    congenital adrenal hyperplasia
    cyanacetic acid hydrazine
CAHD — coronary atherosclerotic heart disease
C.A.H.E.A. — Committee on Allied Health Education and Accreditation
CaH_2O_2 — calcium hydroxide
CAI — computer-assisted instruction
CAL — computer-assisted learning
Cal. — large calorie
cal. — small calorie
C_{alb} — albumin clearance
calef. —
    calefac [L] make warm
    calefactus [L] warmed
CAM —
    chorioallantoic membrane
    contralateral axillary metastasis
C_{am} — amylase clearance
CAMP — computer-assisted menu planning
*c*AMP —
    adenosine $3',5'$-cyclic phosphate

cAMP (continued)
cyclic adenosine monophosphate
CAO — chronic airway obstruction
CaO — calcium oxide
CAOC — cathodal opening contraction
Ca(OH)$_2$ — calcium hydroxide
CAP —
cellulose acetate phthalate
chloramphenicol
cystine aminopeptidase
C.A.P. — College of American Pathologists
cap. —
capacity
capiat [L] let him take
capsula [L] capsule
cap. moll. — capsula mollis [L] soft capsule
Ca$_3$(PO$_4$)$_2$ — tribasic calcium phosphate
cap. quant. vult — capait quantum vult [L] let the patient take as much as he will
capsul. — capsule [L] capsule
C.A.R. — Canadian Association of Radiologists
card. or cardiol. — cardiology
C.A.R.F. — Commission on Accreditation of Rehabilitation Facilities
CAS —
Cancer Attitude Survey
cardiac surgery
cerebral arteriosclerosis
CASHD — coronary arteriosclerotic heart disease
CaSO$_4$ — calcium sulfate
CAT —
catecholamines
children's apperception test

CAT (continued)
chlormerodrin accumulation test
computed axial tomography
computerized axial tomography
computer of average transients
cath. —
catharticus [L] cathartic
catheter
catheterization
catheterize
Cauc. — Caucasian
CAV —
congenital absence of vagina
congenital adrenal virilism
CA virus — croup-associated virus
CB — chronic bronchitis
CB$_{11}$ — phenadoxone hydrochloride
C.B. — Chirurgiae Baccalaureus [L] Bachelor of Surgery
Cb — columbium
cb. — cardboard or plastic film holder without intensifying screens
CBA — chronic bronchitis with asthma
CB agar — chocolate blood agar
CBC — complete blood count
CBD —
closed bladder drainage
common bile duct
C.B.E. — Council of Biology Editors
CBF —
capillary blood flow
cerebral blood flow
coronary blood flow
CBG —
corticosteroid-binding globulin
cortisol-binding globulin

CBI — continuous bladder irrigation

C.B.N. — Commission on Biological Nomenclature

CBOC — completion bed occupancy care

CBR —
chemical, biological and radiological
complete bed rest
crude birth rate

CBS — chronic brain syndrome

CBV —
central blood volume
circulating blood volume
corrected blood volume

CBW —
chemical and biological warfare
critical band width

CBz — carbobenzoxychloride

CC —
cardiac cycle
chief complaint
circulatory collapse
classical conditioning
clinical course
coefficient of correlation
commission certified
compound cathartic
computer calculated
coracoclavicular
cord compression
corpus callosum
costochondral
creatinine clearance
critical condition
current complaints

Cc — concave

cc. — cubic centimeter

CCA —
cephalin cholesterol antigen

CCA (continued)
chick-cell agglutination
chimpanzee coryza agent
common carotid artery

CCAT — conglutinating complement absorption test

CCBV — central circulating blood volume

CCC —
calcium cyanamide
cathodal closing contraction
chronic calculous cholecystitis
consecutive case conference

C.C.C. — Commission on Clinical Chemistry

CCCl — cathodal closure clonus

CCCR — closed chest cardiac resuscitation

CCD — calibration curve data

CCE — cyanosis, clubbing or edema

CCF —
cephalin-cholesterol flocculation
compound comminuted fracture
congestive cardiac failure

CCHE — Central Council for Health Education

CCI — chronic coronary insufficiency

CCK — cholecystokinin

CCK-PZ — cholecystokinin-pancreozymin

CCl_4 — carbon tetrachloride

CCl_3CHO — chloral

$CCl_3CH(OH)_2$ — chloral hydrate

c. cm. — cubic centimeter

CCMSU — clean catch midstream urine

CCMT — catechol-O-methyl transferase

CCN — coronary care nursing

C.C.N.S.C. — Cancer Chemotherapy National Service Center

CCNU — code designation for lomustine

CCP — ciliocytophthoria

C_{cr} or c.cr. — creatinine clearance

CCS — casualty clearing station

CCT —
    composite cyclic therapy
    controlled cord traction

CCTe — cathodal closure tetanus

C.C.T.P. — Coronary Care Training Project

CCU —
    cardiac care unit
    Cherry-Crandall units
    community care unit
    coronary care unit

CCV — conductivity cell volume

CCW — counterclockwise

CD —
    cadaver donor
    canine distemper
    carbonate dehydratase
    cardiac disease
    cardiac dullness
    cardiovascular disease
    caudal
    cesarean-delivered
    circular dichroism
    colla dextra [L] with the right hand
    common duct
    communicable disease
    completely denatured
    conjugata diagonalis [L] the diagonal conjugate diameter of the pelvic inlet
    consanguineous donor
    contact dermatitis
    contagious disease
    convulsive disorder

CD (*continued*)
    curative dose
    cystic duct

C/D — cigarettes per day

C & D — cystoscopy and dilatation

CD_{50} — median curative dose

Cd —
    cadmium
    caudal
    coccygeal

^{115}Cd — radioactive cadmium

cd — candela

CDA —
    chenodeoxycholic acid
    congenital dyserythropoietic anemia

CDAA — chlorodiallylacetamide

C & DB — cough and deep breath

CDC —
    calculated date of confinement
    chenodeoxycholate

C.D.C. —
    Center(s) for Disease Control
    Communicable Disease Center

CDD — certificate of disability for discharge

CDE —
    canine distemper encephalitis
    chlordiazepoxide
    common duct exploration

CDH —
    ceramide dihexoside
    congenital dislocation of the hip

CDL — chlorodeoxylincomycin

cDNA — complementary DNA

CDP —
    continuous distending pressure
    coronary drug project
    cytidine diphosphate

CDPC — cytidine diphosphate choline

CDS — cul-de-sac

CDSS — clinical decision support system
CDT — carbon dioxide therapy
Cdyn. — dynamic compliance
CE —
  California encephalitis
  cardiac emergency
  cardiac enlargement
  chemical energy
  chick embryo
  cholesterol esters
  clinical emphysema
  constant error
  contractile element
  cytopathic effect
Ce — cerium
^{58}Ce — radioactive cerium
CEA —
  carcinoembryonic antigen
  crystalline egg albumin
CEEV — Central European encephalitis virus
CEF — chick embryo fibroblast
Cel. — Celsius
CELO — chicken-embryo-lethal-orphan (virus)
CEM — conventional-transmission electron microscope
C-E mixture — chloroform-ether mixture
Cent. — centigrade
cent. — centimeter
centi- — hundred
CEO — chick embryo origin
CEP — countercurrent electrophoresis
CEPA — chloroethane phosphoric acid
Ceph. floc. — cephalin flocculation (test)
CER — conditioned emotional response

cert. — certified
cerv. —
  cervical
  cervix
CES — central excitatory state
CF —
  cancer-free
  cardiac failure
  carrier-free
  chemotactic factor
  chest and left leg (ECG leads)
  Chiari-Frommel syndrome
  Christmas factor
  colicin factor
  complement fixation
  complement-fixing
  contractile force
  coronary flow
  cystic fibrosis
C.F. —
  carbolfuchsin
  citrovorum factor
Cf — californium
Cf. — carrier of iron (ferrum)
cf. — confer [L] compare
c.f. —
  count fingers
  counting finger
CFA —
  complement-fixing antibody
  complete Freund adjuvant
CFF — critical flicker fusion (test)
c.f.f. — critical fusion frequency
Cf-Fe — carrier-bound iron
CFI — complement-fixation inhibition (test)
CFM — chlorofluoromethane
cfm — cubic feet per minute
CFP —
  chronic false-positive
  cystic fibrosis of the pancreas
cfs — cubic feet per second

CFSE − crystal field stabilization energy

C.F.S.T.I. − Clearinghouse for Federal Scientific and Technical Information

CFT −
clinical full-time
complement-fixation test

CFU −
colony-forming units
color-forming units

CFU-C − colony-forming units - culture

CFU-E − colony-forming units - erythrocyte

CFU_{EOS} − colony-forming units − eosinophil

CFU_{MEG} − colony-forming units − megakaryocyte

CFU-mL − colony-forming units/ mL

CFU_{NM} − colony-forming units - neutrophil-monocyte

CFU-S − colony-forming units - spleen

CFWM − cancer-free white mouse

CG −
cardiogreen
choking gas (phosgene)
chorionic gonadotropin
chronic glomerulonephritis
colloidal gold

cg. − centigram

CGD − chronic granulomatous disease

CGH − chorionic gonadotropic hormone

CGI − clinical global impression

CGL − chronic granulocytic leukemia

c. gl. − correction with glasses

CGM − central gray matter

cgm. − centigram

cGMP − cyclic guanosine monophosphate

CGN − chronic glomerulonephritis

CG/OQ − cerebral glucose oxygen quotient

CGP −
N-carbobenzoyl-glycyl-L-phenylalanine
choline glycerophosphatide
chorionic growth hormone prolactin
circulating granulocyte pool

CGS − catgut suture

cgs system − centimeter-gram-second system

CGT −
N-carbobenzoyl-a-glutamyl-L-tyrosine
chorionic gonadotropin

CGTT − cortisone glucose tolerance test

CH −
cholesterol
crown-heel (length of fetus)
wheelchair

C & H − cocaine and heroin

CH_4 − methane

C_2H_2 − acetylene

C_2H_4 − ethylene

C_6H_6 − benzene

C.H. − Community Health

Ch^1 − Christchurch chromosome

cH − hydrogen ion concentration

ch. −
chest
chief
child
choline

CHA −
congenital hypoplastic anemia
cyclohexylamine

C.H.A. − Catholic Hospital Association

ChA − choline acetylase

C.H.A.M.P.U.S. − Civilian Health and Medical Program of the Uniformed Services

chart. − charta [L] paper

CHB − complete heart block

C_2H_5Br − ethyl bromide

Ch.B. − Chirurgiae Baccalaureus [L] Bachelor of Surgery

$CHCl_3$ − chloroform

$C_2H_4Cl_2$ − ethylene chloride

C_2H_5Cl − ethyl chloride

$C_2H_5CO_2NH_2$ − ethyl carbamate

$(CH_3 \cdot CO)_2O$ − acetic anhydride

$CH_3 \cdot COOH$ − acetic acid

$C_4H_9 \cdot COOH$ − valeric acid

CHD −
    Chediak-Higashi disease
    childhood disease
    congenital heart disease
    congestive heart disease
    coronary heart disease

Ch.D. − Chirurgiae Doctor [L] Doctor of Surgery

ChE − cholinesterase

Chem. − chemotherapy

CHF − congestive heart failure

CHH − cartilage-hair hypoplasia

CHI_3 − iodoform

C_2H_5I − ethyl iodide

χ_e − electric susceptibility

χ_m − magnetic susceptibility

Chir. Doct. − Chirurgiae Doctor [L] Doctor of Surgery

CHL − chloramphenicol

Chl. − chloroform

Ch.M. − Chirurgiae Magister [L] Master of Surgery

CHN −
    central hemorrhagic necrosis
    Child Neurology

$C_6H_5NH_2$ − aniline

$C_3H_5(NO_3)_3$ − glyceryl trinitrate (nitroglycerin)

$C_5H_4N_4O_3$ − uric acid

$C_5H_{11}NO_2$ − amyl nitrite

C_8H_9NO − acetanilid

$C_9H_9NO_3$ − hippuric acid

$C_6H_2(NO_2)_3OH$ − trinitrophenol (picric acid)

CHO − carbohydrate

CH_2O − formaldehyde

CH_2O_2 − formic acid

CH_4O − methyl alcohol

$C_2H_2O_4$ − oxalic acid

$C_2H_4O_2$ − acetic acid

C_2H_6O − ethyl alcohol

C_3H_6O − acetone

$C_3H_6O_3$ − lactic acid

$C_3H_8O_3$ − glycerin

$C_4H_6O_2$ − crotonic acid

$C_4H_6O_5$ − malic acid

$C_4H_6O_6$ − tartaric acid

$C_4H_8O_2$ − butyric acid; isobutyric acid

$C_4H_{10}O$ − ether (ethyl ether)

$C_5H_{10}O_2$ − valeric acid

$C_5H_{12}O$ − amyl alcohol

C_6H_6O − phenol

$C_6H_8O_7$ − citric acid

$C_6H_{12}O_6$ − dextrose (D-glucose)

$C_7H_4O_7$ − meconic acid

$C_7H_6O_2$ − benzoic acid

$C_7H_6O_3$ − salicylic acid

$C_7H_6O_5$ − gallic acid

$C_{12}H_{22}O_{11}$ − cane sugar

$C_{15}H_{10}O_4$ − chrysophanic acid

$C_{18}H_{34}O_2$ − oleic acid

$C_{18}H_{36}O_2$ − stearic acid

C_6H_5OH − phenol

chol. − cholesterol

chole. − cholecystectomy

Chol. est. − cholesterol esters

$(C_6H_{10}O_5)_n$ — starch, glycogen or other hexose polymers
CHOP — cyclophosphamide, hydroxydaunorubicin (Adriamycin), Oncovin and prednisone
CHP —
child psychiatry
comprehensive health planning
chpx. — chickenpox
CHR — cercarien hüllen reaction
Chr. — *Chromobacterium*
chr. — chronic
chron. — chronological
CHS —
Chediak-Higashi syndrome
cholinesterase
CI —
cardiac index
cardiac insufficiency
cerebral infarction
chemotherapeutic index
clinical investigation
clonus index
coefficient of intelligence
colloidal iron
color index
contamination index
coronary insufficiency
crystalline insulin
Ci — curie
cib. — cibus [L] food
CIBHA — congenital inclusion body hemolytic anemia
CICU —
cardiac intensive care unit
coronary intensive care unit
CID —
chick infective dose
cytomegalic inclusion disease
CIDS — cellular immunity deficiency syndrome
CIE — counterimmunoelectrophoresis

C.I.E.B.M. — Committee on the Interplay of Engineering with Biology and Medicine
CIEP — counterimmunoelectrophoresis
CIF — cloning inhibitory factor
C.I.F.C. — Council for the Investigation of Fertility Control
CIH — carbohydrate-induced hyperglyceridemia
C.I.H. — Certificate in Industrial Health
Ci-hr. — curie-hour
CIM — cortically-induced movement
CIN —
cervical intraepithelial neoplasia
chronic interstitial nephritis
C_{in} — insulin clearance
C.I.O.M.S. — Council for International Organizations of Medical Sciences
circ. —
circulation
circumcision
CIS —
carcinoma in situ
central inhibitory state
cit. — citrate
cito disp. — cito dispensetur [L] dispense quickly
CIXU — constant infusion excretory urogram
CJD — Creutzfeldt-Jakob disease
CK — creatine kinase
CK_1, CK_2, CK_3 — isoenzymes of creatine kinase
ck. — check
CL —
chest and left arm
cholesterol-lecithin (test)
corpus luteum

CL (*continued*)
  critical list
Cl –
  chloride
  chlorine
  clavicle
  clinic
  closure
Cl. – Clostridium
cl. – centiliter
CLA – cervicolinguoaxial
C.L.A. – Certified Laboratory
  Assistant
CLAS – congenital localized absence of skin
CLBBB – complete left bundle
  branch block
$Cl_3C \cdot CHO$ – chloral
CL/CP – cleft lip and cleft palate
CLD –
  chronic liver disease
  chronic lung disease
cldy. – cloudy
CLE – centrilobular emphysema
CLH – chronic lobular hepatitis
clin. –
  clinic
  clinical
CLIP – corticotropin-like intermediate lobe peptide
CLL –
  cholesterol-lowering lipid
  chronic lymphatic leukemia
  chronic lymphocytic leukemia
C.L.M.A. – Clinical Laboratory
  Management Association
CLML – Current List of Medical
  Literature
CLO – cod liver oil
C.L.S. – Clinical Laboratory
  Scientist
CLSL – chronic lymphosarcoma
  (cell) leukemia

CLT – clot-lysis time
CM –
  capreomycin
  carboxymethyl cellulose
  cardiac monitor
  Chick-Martin (coefficient)
  chloroquine-mepacrine
  chondromalacia
  cochlear microphonic
  complications
  congenital malformation
  costal margin
  cow's milk
C & M – cocaine and morphine
  mixed
C.M. – Chirurgiae Magister [L]
  Master in Surgery
Cm – curium
C_m – maximum clearance with
  reference to urea clearance
cm. – centimeter
$cm.^2$ – square centimeter
$cm.^3$ – cubic centimeter
c.m. –
  costal margin
  cras mane [L] tomorrow
    morning
C.M.A. –
  Canadian Medical Association
  Certified Medical Assistant
CMB –
  carbolic methylene blue
  chloromercuribenzoate
CMC –
  carboxymethylcellulose
  carpometacarpal
cmc. – critical micelle concentration
CM-cellulose – carboxymethylcellulose
CMD – count median diameter
CME – continuing medical education

CMF –
    chondromyxoid fibroma
    cyclophosphamide, metho-
        trexate and fluorouracil
    Cytoxan, methotrexate, 5-
        fluorouracil
CMFVP – cyclophosphamide,
    methotrexate, fluorouracil,
    vincristine and prednisone
CMG –
    chopped meat glucose (agar)
    cystometrogram
CMGN – chronic membranous
    glomerulonephritis
CMH – congenital malformation
    of heart
CMI –
    carbohydrate metabolism
        index
    cell-mediated immunity
CMID – cytomegalic inclusion
    disease
c/min. – cycles per minute
CML –
    chronic myelocytic leukemia
    chronic myelogenous leukemia
CMM – cutaneous malignant
    melanoma
c.mm. – cubic millimeter
CMN – cystic medial necrosis
CMN-AA – cystic medial necrosis
    of the ascending aorta
CMO – cardiac minute output
C.M.O. – Chief Medical Officer
cMo. – centimorgan
CMoL – chronic monocytic
    (monoblastic) leukemia
C-MOPP – cyclophosphamide,
    nitrogen mustard, vincristine
    (Oncovin), procarbazine and
    prednisone
CMOS – complementary metal
    oxide semiconductor logic

CMP –
    cardiomyopathy
    cytidine monophosphate
    cytidine-5'-phosphate
cmp'd. – compound
CMR –
    cerebral metabolic rate
    crude mortality ratio
C.M.R. – Certified Medical Repre-
    sentative
CMRG – cerebral metabolic rate
    of glucose
CMRO – cerebral metabolic rate
    of oxygen
CMRR – common mode rejection
    ratio
CMS – Clyde Mood Scale
c.m.s. – cras mane sumendus [L]
    to be taken tomorrow morning
CMT –
    California mastitis test
    catechol-O-methyl transferase
    current medical terminology
C.M.T. – Certified Medical Tran-
    scriptionist
CMU – chlorophenyldimethylurea
CMV – cytomegalovirus
CN –
    clinical nursing
    cranial nerve(s)
    cyanide anion
    cyanogen
c.n. – cras nocte [L] tomorrow
    night
C.N.A. – Canadian Nurses' Asso-
    ciation
C.N.C. – Clinical Nursing Confer-
    ence
CNE – chronic nervous exhaus-
    tion
CNH – community nursing home
CNHD – congenital nonsphero-
    cytic hemolytic disease

C.N.H.I. – Committee for National Health Insurance
CNL – cardiolipin natural lecithin
C.N.M. – Certified Nurse-Midwife
C.N.M.T. – Certified Nuclear Medicine Technologist
CNOH – cyanic acid
CNP – continuous negative pressure
CNS –
    central nervous system
    sulfocyanate
c.n.s. – cras nocte sumendus [L] to be taken tomorrow night
CNV –
    conative negative variation
    contingent negative variation
CO –
    carbon monoxide
    cardiac output
    castor oil
    centric occlusion
    cervicoaxial
    coenzyme
    compound
    corneal opacity
    crossover
C/O –
    check out
    complains of
CO_2 – carbon dioxide
Co – cobalt
Co I – coenzyme I (nicotinamide adenine dinucleotide)
Co II – coenzyme II (nicotinamide adenine dinucleotide phosphate)
^{60}Co – radioactive cobalt
co. – compositus [L] a compound
C.O.A. – Canadian Orthopaedic Association
CoA – coenzyme A

COAD – chronic obstructive airway disease
coag. – coagulation
COBOL – common business oriented language
COBS – cesarean-obtained barrier-sustained
COBT – chronic obstruction of biliary tract
COC –
    cathodal opening clonus
    cathodal opening contraction
    coccygeal
    combination-type oral contraceptive
cochl. – cochleare [L] spoonful
cochl. amp. – cochleare amplum [L] heaping spoonful
cochl. mag. – cochleare magnum [L] tablespoonful
cochl. med. – cochleare medium [L] dessertspoonful
cochl. parv. – cochleare parvum [L] teaspoonful
COCL – cathodal opening clonus
coct. – coctio [L] boiling
COD –
    cause of death
    chemical oxygen demand
cod. – codeine
C of A – coarctation of aorta
COGTT – cortisone-primed oral glucose tolerance test
COH – carbohydrate
COHb – carboxyhemoglobin
$C_4O_6H_4NaK$ – potassium sodium tartrate
col. –
    cola [L] strain
    colony
    colored
    column

colat. – colatus [L] strained
COLD – chronic obstructive lung disease
colet. – coletur [L] let it be strained
coll. – collyrium [L] eyewash
collun. – collunarium [L] nose wash
collut. – collutorium [L] mouthwash
collyr. – collyrium [L] eyewash
color. –
  coloretur [L] let it be colored
  colorimetry, including spectrophotometry and photometry
C.O.M. – College of Osteopathic Medicine
comp. –
  compare
  compensated
  complaint
  composition
  compositus [L] compound
COMT – catechol-*O*-methyl transferase
CON – certificate of need
con. – contra [L] against
ConA – concanavalin A
conc. –
  concentrated
  concentration
concis. – concisus [L] cut
cond. –
  condensed
  condition
  conditional
  conductivity
conf. –
  confectio [L] a confection
  conference
cong. – congius [L] gallon
CO(NH$_2$)$_2$ – urea

cons. – conserva [L] keep
cont. –
  containing
  continue
  continuously
  contra [L] against
  contusus [L] bruised
contin. – continuetur [L] let it be continued
contra. – contraindicated
contralat. – contralateral
cont. rem. – continuetur remedium [L] let the medicine be continued
contus. – contusus [L] bruised
conv. –
  convalescent
  conventional (rat)
COP –
  colloid osmotic pressure
  Cytoxan, Oncovin, prednisone
COP-BLAM – Cytoxan, Oncovin, prednisone and procarbazine, bleomycin, Adriamycin
COPD – chronic obstructive pulmonary disease
COPE – chronic obstructive pulmonary emphysema
C.O.P.E. – Committee on Political Education
coq. – coque [L] boil
coq. in s.a. – coque in sufficiente aqua [L] boil in sufficient water
coq. s.a. – coque secundum artem [L] boil properly
CORA – conditioned orientation reflex audiometry
Cort. – cortex (bark)
C.O.S. –
  Canadian Ophthalmological Society
  Clinical Orthopaedic Society

cos. — cosine
COT — critical off-time
COTe — cathodal opening tetanus
C.O.T.H. — Council of Teaching
    Hospitals
COV — cross-over value
CP —
    capillary pressure
    cerebral palsy
    chemically pure
    chest pains
    chloropurine
    chloroquine and primaquine
    chronic pyelonephritis
    cleft palate
    closing pressure
    clottable protein
    cochlear potential
    combination product
    combining power
    constant pressure
    coproporphyrin
    cor pulmonale
    creatine phosphate
C/P — cholesterol-phospholipid
    ratio
C & P —
    compensation and pension
    cystoscopy and pyelogram
C_p — phosphate clearance
cP. — centipoise
c.p. — candle power
CPA —
    cerebellar pontine angle
    chlorophenylalanine
    cyclophosphamide
Cpah — p-aminohippuric acid
    clearance
C_{pah} — para-aminohippurate clear-
    ance
CPAP — continuous positive air-
    way pressure

CPB —
    cardiopulmonary bypass
    cetyl pyridinium bromide
    competitive protein-binding
CPC —
    cetylpyridinium chloride
    chronic passive congestion
    clinicopathological conference
CPD —
    cephalopelvic disproportion
    citrate-phosphate-dextrose
    contagious pustular dermatitis
    cyclopentadiene
cpd. — compound
CPDA-1 — citrate-phosphate-dex-
    trose-adenine
CPE —
    chronic pulmonary emphy-
      sema
    compensation, pension and
      education
    corona penetrating enzyme
    cytopathic effect
C. Ped. — Certified Pedorthist
C.P.E.H.S. — Consumer Protection
    and Environmental Health
    Service
CPF — clot-promoting factor
CPH — chronic persistent hepatitis
C.P.H. — Certificate in Public
    Health
C.P.H.A. — Committee on Profes-
    sional and Hospital Activities
CPI —
    constitutional psychopathic
      inferiority
    coronary prognostic index
CPIB — chlorophenoxyisobutyrate
CPK — creatine phosphokinase
CPLM — cysteine-peptone-liver in-
    fusion media

cpm. —
    counts per minute
    cycles per minute
CPN — chronic pyelonephritis
CPP —
    cerebral perfusion pressure
    cyclopentenophenanthrene
CPPB — continuous positive-pressure breathing
CPPD — calcium pyrophosphate dihydrate
CPPV — continuous positive pressure ventilation
CPR —
    cardiopulmonary resuscitation
    cerebral cortex perfusion rate
    chlorophenyl red
    cortisol production rate
CPS —
    chloroquine, pyrimethamine, sulfisoxazole
    clinical performance score
    constitutional psychopathic state
    cumulative probability of success
cps. —
    counts per second
    cycles per second
CPT —
    chest physiotherapy
    combining power test
CPU — central processing unit
CPZ — chlorpromazine
CQ —
    chloroquine-quinine
    circadian quotient
    conceptual quotient
CQM — chloroquine mustard
C.Q.U.C.C. — Commission on Quantities and Units in Clinical Chemistry

CR —
    calculus removal
    cardiorespiratory
    centric relation
    chest and right arm
    clinical research
    clot retraction
    colon resection
    complete remission
    conditioned reflex
    creatinine
    cresyl red
    critical ratio
    crown rump (length of fetus)
CR_1 — first cranial nerve
CR_2 — second cranial nerve
Cr —
    chromium
    cranial
    creatinine
    crown
^{51}Cr — radioactive sodium chromate
cr. — cras [L] tomorrow
CRA — central retinal artery
cran. — cranial
crast. — crastinus [L] for tomorrow
CRBBB — complete right bundle branch block
CRD —
    chronic renal disease
    chronic respiratory disease
    complete reaction of degeneration
CRE — cumulative radiation effect
creat. — creatinine
crep. — crepitus [L] crepitation
CRF —
    chronic renal failure
    coagulase-reacting factor
    corticotropin-releasing factor

CRH – corticotropin-releasing hormone
CRI – concentrated rust inhibitor
crit. – hematocrit
CRM – cross-reacting material
C.R.M. – Certified Reference Materials
C.R.N.A. – Certified Registered Nurse Anesthetist
cRNA – chromosomal RNA
cr. ns. – cranial nerves
CRO –
    cathode ray oscillograph
    centric relation occlusion
CROS – contralateral routing of signal
CRP – C-reactive protein
Cr. P. –
    creatine phosphate
    phosphocreatine
CRPA – C-reactive protein antiserum
CRS –
    Chinese restaurant syndrome
    colon-rectal surgery
CRST – calcinosis cutis, Raynaud's phenomenon, sclerodactyly and telangiectasia
CRT –
    cardiac resuscitation team
    cathode-ray tube
    complex reaction timer
    corrected retention time
CRU – Clinical Research Unit
CRV – central retinal vein
crys. – crystal
CS –
    cerebrospinal
    cesarean section
    chondroitin sulfate
    chorionic somatomammotropin

CS (continued)
    colla sinistra [L] with the left hand
    conditioned stimulus
    congenital syphilis
    conscious
    coronary sclerosis
    coronary sinus
    corpus striatum
    corticosteroid
    current strength
    cycloserine
C & S –
    conjunctiva and sclera
    culture and sensitivity
CS_2 – carbon disulfide
C.S. –
    Central Service
    Central Supply
Cs – cesium
cS – centistoke
CSA –
    canavaninosuccinic acid
    chondroitin sulfate A
    colony-stimulating activity
    compressed spectral assay
C.S.A.A. – Child Study Association of America
C.S.C. – coup sur coup [Fr] in small doses at short intervals
CSF –
    cerebrospinal fluid
    colony-stimulating factor
C.S.G.B.I. – Cardiac Society of Great Britain and Ireland
CSH –
    chronic subdural hematoma
    cortical stromal hyperplasia
CSL – cardiolipin synthetic lecithin
CSM –
    cerebrospinal meningitis
    corn-soy milk

CSN − carotid sinus nerve
CSOM − chronic suppurative otitis media
C/spine − cervical spine
CSR −
Central Supply Room
Cheyne-Stokes respiration
corrected sedimentation rate
cortisol secretion rate
CSS −
carotid sinus stimulation
Central Sterile Supply
chewing, sucking, swallowing
subclinical scurvy syndrome
CST −
cardiac stress test
convulsive shock therapy
Cst. − static compliance
cSt. − centistoke
CSU − catheter specimen of urine
C.S.W. − Certified Social Worker
CT −
cardiothoracic (ratio)
carotid tracing
carpal tunnel
cerebral thrombosis
chlorothiazide
circulation time
classic technique
clotting time
coagulation time
collecting tubule
computed tomography
computerized tomography
connective tissue
contraction time
Coombs' test
corneal transplant
coronary thrombosis
corrected transposition
corrective therapy
crest time
cystine-tellurite (medium)

CT (*continued*)
cytotechnologist
C_{T-1824} − clearance of Evans blue
CTA −
chromotropic acid
cyproterone acetate
cytotoxic assay
C.T.A. −
Canadian Tuberculosis Association
Committee on Thrombolytic Agents (units)
CTAB − cetyltrimethylammonium bromide
C.T.A.C. − Cancer Treatment Advisory Committee
CTAT − computerized transaxial tomography
CTBA − cetrimonium bromide
CTC − chlortetracycline
$ctCO_2$ − concentration of total carbon dioxide
CTD −
carpal tunnel decompression
congenital thymic dysplasia
C.T.D. − Corrective Therapy Department
C-terminal − carboxyl terminal
CTFE − chlorotrifluoroethylene
CTH − ceramide trihexoside
CTL − cytologic T lymphocyte
CTP − cytidine triphosphate
$CTP-^3H$ − cytidine triphosphate tritium-labeled
CTR − cardiothoracic ratio
CTS −
carpal tunnel syndrome
computerized topographic scanner
CT scan − computed tomography scan
CTT −
compressed tablet titurate

CTT (*continued*)
    computed transaxial tomography
CTU — centigrade thermal unit
CTX — Cytoxan (cyclophosphamide)
CTZ — chlorothiazide
CU —
    color unit
    convalescent unit
Cu — cuprum [L] copper
^{61}Cu, ^{64}Cu — radioactive copper
C_u — urea clearance
CUC — chronic ulcerative colitis
cu. cm. — cubic centimeter
cu. ft. — cubic foot
CUG — cystourethrogram
cu. in. — cubic inch
cuj. — cujus [L] of which
cuj. lib. — cujus libet [L] of any
    you desire
cu. m. — cubic meter
cu. mm. — cubic millimeter
CuO — cupric oxide
Cu_2O — cuprous oxide
curat. — curatio [L] a dressing
CUSA — Cavitron ultrasonic
    aspirator
CV —
    cardiovascular
    cell volume
    central venous
    cerebrovascular
    coefficient of variation
    color vision
    concentrated volume
    conjugata vera [L] conjugate
      diameter of pelvic inlet
    conversational voice
    corpuscular volume
    cresyl violet
c.v. — cras vespere [L] tomorrow
    evening

CVA —
    cardiovascular accident
    cerebrovascular accident
    costovertebral angle
CVAT — costovertebral angle
    tenderness
CVD —
    cardiovascular disease
    color vision deviant
    color vision deviate
cvd. — curved
CVH —
    combined ventricular hypertrophy
    common variable hypogamma-
      globulinemia
C virus — Coxsackie virus
CVO — conjugata vera obstetrica
    [L] obstetric conjugate diameter of pelvic inlet
CVOD — cerebrovascular obstructive disease
CVP —
    cell volume profile
    central venous pressure
    cyclophosphamide, vincristine,
      prednisone
    Cytoxan, vincristine, prednisone
CVP lab. — cardiovascular pulmonary laboratory
CVR —
    cardiovascular-renal
    cardiovascular-respiratory
    cerebrovascular resistance
CVRD — cardiovascular renal
    disease
CVS —
    cardiovascular surgery
    cardiovascular system
    clean-voided specimen
CW —
    cardiac work

CW (*continued*)
 casework
 chemical warfare
 chest wall
 children's ward
 continuous wave
cw. – clockwise
CWDF – cell wall-deficient
 bacterial forms
CWI – cardiac work index
CWP –
 childbirth without pain
 coal workers' pneumoconi-
  osis
CWS – cold-water soluble
cwt. – hundredweight
Cx. –
 cervix
 chest x-ray
 convex
CXR – chest x-ray

Cy –
 cyanogen
 cyclonium
cy. – copy
cyath. – cyathus [L] a glassful
cyclic AMP – cyclic adenosine
 monophosphate
cyclic GMP – cyclic guanosine
 monophosphate
Cyclo. –
 cyclophosphamide
 cyclopropane
cyl. –
 cylinder
 cylindrical lens
Cys or Cys. – cystine
cys. – cysteine
cysto. –
 cystoscopic examination
 cystoscopy
CZI – crystalline zinc insulin

D

$\underline{D}$ – deuterium
$\overline{D}$ – mean dose
D_1 – first dorsal vertebra
D_2 – second dorsal vertebra
3-D – delayed double diffusion
 (test)
D. –
 aspartic acid
 daughter
 day
 dead air space
 debye
 deciduous
 decimal reduction time
 degree
 density
 dermatology
 deuteron

D. (*continued*)
 dextro
 dextrose
 diagnosis
 didymium
 died
 diffusing capacity
 diopter
 diplomate
 disease
 distal
 divorced
 donor
 dorsal
 duration
 electric displacement
 mean dose
 vitamin D potency

D — chemical prefix

d —

    atomic orbital with angular momentum quantum number 2

    deci-

    density

    deoxyribose

    dextro rotary

    diameter

    diurnal

    dyne

    relative to rotation of a beam of polarized light

d. —

    dare [L] to give

    detur [L] let it be given

    dexter [L] right

    dies [L] day

    dosis [L] dose

Δ, δ — delta (fourth letter of the Greek alphabet)

DA —

    degenerative arthritis

    delayed action

    dental assistant

    developmental age

    diphenylchlorarsine

    direct agglutination

    disaggregated

    dopamine

    ductus arteriosus

D/A — discharge and advise

da — deca-

DAB — dimethylaminoazobenzene

DAC — digital-to-analog converter

DACA — Drug Abuse Control Amendments

DAD — dispense as directed

DADDS — diacetyl diaminodiphenylsulfone

DAGT — direct antiglobulin test

DAH — disordered action of the heart

DALA — delta-aminolevulinic acid

DAM —

    degraded amyloid

    diacetyl monoxime

dAMP —

    deoxyadenosine monophosphate

    deoxyadenosine-5'-phosphate

D and C —

    dilatation and curettage

    dilation and curettage

DANS — 1-dimethylaminonaphthalene-5-sulfonyl chloride

DAO — diamine oxidase

DAP —

    dihydroxyacetone phosphate

    direct agglutination pregnancy (test)

DAPT — direct agglutination pregnancy test

Dapt — Daptazole

DAS — dextroamphetamine sulfate

DAT —

    differential agglutination titer

    differential aptitude test

    diphtheria antitoxin

    direct agglutination test

DB —

    date of birth

    dextran blue

    disability

    distobuccal

db. — decibel

DBA — dibenzanthracene

DBC — dye-binding capacity

DBCL — dilute blood clot lysis (method)

DBI — development-at-birth index

DBM —

    diabetic management

    dibromomannitol

DBO − distobucco-occlusal
DBP −
   diastolic blood pressure
   dibutylphthalate
   distobuccopulpal
DBS − despeciated bovine serum
D.B.S. − Division of Biological
   Standards
DBT − dry blood temperature
DC −
   daily census
   deoxycholate
   diagnostic code
   diphenylarsine cyanide
   direct current
   discontinue
   distocervical
D/C −
   discharge
   discontinue
D & C −
   dilatation and curettage
   dilation and curettage
D.C. − Doctor of Chiropractic
d.c. − direct current
DCA −
   deoxycholate-citrate agar
   desoxycorticosterone acetate
D.Cc. − double concave
DCF − direct centrifugal flotation
DCG −
   deoxycorticosterone glucoside
   disodium cromoglycate
D.C.H. − Diploma in Child Health
D.Ch. − Doctor Chirurgiae [L]
   Doctor of Surgery
DCHFB − dichlorohexafluorobu-
   tane
DCHN − dicyclohexylamine ni-
   trite
DCI − dichloroisoproterenol
DCLS − deoxycholate citrate lac-
   tose saccharose (agar)

dCMP −
   deoxycytidine monophosphate
   deoxycytidine-5′-phosphate
DCN − delayed conditional necrosis
D_{CO} − diffusing capacity for carbon monoxide
D.C.O.G. − Diploma of the College of Obstetricians and
   Gynaecologists (British)
DCP − dicalcium phosphate
DCR − direct cortical response
DCT −
   direct Coombs' test
   distal convoluted tubule
DCTMA − desoxycorticosterone
   trimethylacetate
DCTPA − desoxycorticosterone
   triphenylacetate
DCU − dichloral urea
D.Cx. − double convex
DD −
   dependent drainage
   developmental disability
   died of the disease
   differential diagnosis
   disk diameter
   double diffusion (test)
   dry dressing
d.d. − detur ad [L] let it be given
   to
DDAVP − 1-deamino-(8-D-argi-
   nine)-vasopressin
DDC −
   diethyldithiocarbamic acid
   dihydrocollidine
   direct display console
DDD −
   degenerative disk disease
   dense deposit disease
   dichlorodiphenyldichloroeth-
   ane

DDD (*continued*)
 dihydroxydinaphthyl disulfide
DDE — dichlorodiphenyldichloro-
 ethylene
D.D.H. — Division of Dental
 Health
DDI — dressing, dry and intact
dd. in d. — de die in diem [L]
 from day to day
DDS —
 diaminodiphenylsulfone
 dystrophy-dystocia syndrome
D.D.S. — Doctor of Dental Surgery
D.D.Sc. — Doctor of Dental Science
DDSO — diamino diphenylsulfox-
 ide
DDT —
 chlorophenothane
 dichlorodiphenyltrichloro-
 ethane
DDVP — dichlorvos
DE —
 digestive energy
 dream elements
 duration of ejection
D & E — dilation and evacuation
DEA —
 dehydroepiandrosterone
 diethanolamine
DEAE —
 diethylaminoethanol
 diethylaminoethyl
 diethylaminoethylcellulose
DEAE-D — diethylaminoethyl
 dextran
dearg. pil. — deargentur pilulae
 [L] let the pills be silverized
deaur. pil. — deaurentur pilulae
 [L] let the pills be gilded
DEB — diethylbutanediol
DEBA — diethylbarbituric acid

deb. spis. — debita spissitudine
 [L] of the proper consistency
dec. —
 decanta [L] pour off
 deceased
 deciduous
 decompose
 decrease
deca- — ten
deci- — a tenth
decoct. — decoctum [L] a decoction
decr. — decrease(d)
decub. — decubitus [L] lying
 down
DED — delayed erythema dose
de d. in d. — de die in diem [L]
 from day to day
DEEG —
 depth electroencephalogram
 depth electroencephalography
 depth electrography
def. —
 defecation
 deficiency
defib. — defibrillate
deg. —
 degeneration
 degree
deglut. — deglutiatur [L] let it be
 swallowed
D.E.H.S. — Division of Emergency
 Health Service
deka- — ten
del. — delivery
Dem — Demerol (meperidine)
Dent. —
 dental
 dentistry
 dentition
dent. — dentur [L] let it be given
DEP — diethylpropanediol

dep. —
  dependents
  depuratus [L] purified
DeR — reaction of degeneration
der — derivative chromosome
derm. — dermatology
DES — diethylstilbestrol
D.E.S. — Doctors' Emergency
  Service
dest. —
  destilla [L] distil
  destillatus [L] distilled
DET — diethyltryptamine
det. — detur [L] let it be given
det. in dup., det. in 2 plo. — detur
  in duplo [L] let twice as
  much be given
d. et s. — detur et signetur [L] let
  it be given and labeled
DEV — duck embryo vaccine
DF —
  decapacitation factor
  deficiency factor
  desferrioxamine
  diabetic father
  discriminant function
  disseminated foci
  dorsiflexion
df. — degrees of freedom
DFA — direct fluorescent antibody (test)
DFDD — difluoro-diphenyl-
  dichloroethane
DFDT — difluoro-diphenyl-tri-
  chloroethane
DFOM — deferoxamine
$DF^{32}P$ — diisopropyl phospho-
  fluoridate
DFU —
  dead fetus in utero
  dideoxyfluorouridine
DG —
  deoxyglucose

DG (*continued*)
  diagnosis
  diastolic gallop
  diglyceride
  distogingival
2DG — 2-deoxy-D-glucose
dg. — decigram
dGMP —
  deoxyguanosine monophos-
    phate
  deoxyguanosine-5'-phosphate
dGTP — 2-deoxyguanosine-5'-tri-
  phosphate
DGVB — dextrose, gelatin, Veronal buffer
DH —
  dehydrocholic acid
  dehydrogenase
  delayed hypersensitivity
DHA —
  dehydroepiandrosterone
  dihydroxyacetone
DHAP — dihydroxyacetone
  phosphate
DHAS — dehydroepiandrosterone
  sulfate
DHE-45 — dihydroergotamine
DHEA — dehydroepiandrosterone
DHEAS — dehydroepiandrosterone sulfate
D.H.E.W. — Department of Health,
  Education and Welfare
DHFR — dihydrofolate reductase
D.Hg. — Doctor of Hygiene
DHIA — dehydrosoandrosterone
DHIC — dihydroisocodeine
DHL — diffuse histiocytic lym-
  phoma
DHMA — 3,4-dihydroxymandelic
  acid
D.H.N. — Department of Hospital
  Nursing
DHO — deuterium hydrogen oxide

DHO 180 — dihydroergocornine
DHPG — dehydroxyphenylglycol
DHR — delayed hypersensitivity
    reaction
DHSM — dihydrostreptomycin
DHT —
    dihydrotachysterol
    dihydrotestosterone
    dihydrothymine
D.Hy. — Doctor of Hygiene
DI —
    deterioration index
    diabetes insipidus
    diagnostic imaging
    distoincisal
D_I — inulin dialysance
Di — didymium
diab. — diabetic
DIAC — diiodothyroacetic acid
diag. — diagnosis
diam. — diameter
diaph. —
    diaphragm
    diaphragmatic
dias. — diastolic
DIC —
    diffuse intravascular coagula-
        tion
    disseminated intravascular co-
        agulation
dic. — dicentric
DID — dead of intercurrent disease
DIE — died in Emergency Room
dieb. alt. — diebus alternis [L] on
    alternate days
dieb. tert. — diebus tertiis [L]
    every third day
diff. — differential count
DIFP — diisopropyl fluorophos-
    phonate
dig. —
    digeratur [L] let it be digested
    digoxin

dil. — dilue [L] dilute or dissolve
DILD — diffuse infiltrative lung
    disease
diluc. — diluculo [L] at daybreak
dilut. — dilutus [L] diluted
DIM — divalent ion metabolism
dim. —
    dimidius [L] one half
    diminutus [L] diminished
D.I.M.E. — Division of Interna-
    tional Medical Education
DIMOAD syndrome — diabetes in-
    sipidus, diabetes mellitus,
    optic atrophy and deafness
d. in p. aeq. — dividatur in partes
    aequales [L] divide into equal
    parts
DIP —
    desquamative interstitial
        pneumonia
    desquamative interstitial
        pneumonitis
    diisopropyl phosphate
    distal interphalangeal
    dual-in-line package
diph. — diphtheria
DIPJ — distal interphalangeal joint
dir. — directione [L] directions
dir. prop. — directione propria
    [L] with a proper direction
dis. —
    disabled
    disease
    distance
disc. — discontinue
disch. — discharge
disp. —
    dispensare [L] to dispense
    dispensatory
dist. —
    distance
    distilla [L] distil
DIT — diiodotyrosine

div. –
 divido [L] to divide
 division
div. in par. aeq. – dividatur in
 partes aequales [L] divide
 into equal parts
DJD – degenerative joint disease
DK –
 decay
 diseased kidney
 dog kidney
DKA – diabetic ketoacidosis
dkg. – decagram
dkm. – decameter
DL –
 danger list
 difference limen
 diffusing capacity of the lung
 distolingual
 Donath-Landsteiner (test)
D_L – diffusing capacity of the
 lungs
dl. – deciliter
DLA – distolabial
D-L Ab – Donath-Landsteiner
 antibody
DLAI – distolabioincisal
DLAP – distolabiopulpal
DL_{CO} – diffusing capacity of the
 lungs for carbon monoxide
$DL_{CO}SB$ – single breath diffusing
 capacity of the lungs
$DL_{CO}SS$ – steady state diffusing
 capacity of the lungs
DLE –
 discoid lupus erythematosus
 disseminated lupus erythematosus
DLI – distolinguoincisal
DLL – dihomo-gammalinoleic
 acid
DLLI – dulcitol lysine lactose
 iron (agar)

DLO – distolinguo-occlusal
DL_{O_2} – diffusing capacity of the
 lungs for oxygen
DLP – distolinguopulpal
DM –
 diabetes mellitus
 diabetic mother
 diastolic murmur
 diphenylamine-arsine
 chloride
 diphenylaminechlorarsine
 dopamine
D_M – membrane component of
 diffusion
D.M. – Doctor Medicinae [L]
 Doctor of Medicine
dm. – decimeter
DMA –
 dimethyladenosine
 direct memory access
DMAB – dimethylaminobenzalde-
 hyde
DMAC – *N,N*-dimethylacetamide
DMBA – 7,12-dimethylbenz[a] -
 anthracene
DMC – di(*p*-chlorophenyl)
 methylcarbinol
DMCT – demethylchlortetracy-
 cline
DMD – Duchenne's muscular dystrophy
D.M.D. – Doctor of Dental Medicine
DME – dimethyl ether (of
 D-tubocurarine)
D.M.E. – Director of Medical
 Education
DMF –
 decayed, missing or filled
 (teeth)
 N,N-dimethylformamide
D.M.H. – Department of Mental
 Health

DMI — diaphragmatic myocardial
infarct
DMM — dimethylmyleran
DMN — dimethylnitrosamine
DMO — 5,5-dimethyl-2,4-oxazoli-
dinedione
DMP — dimethylphthalate
DMPA — depomedroxyprogester-
one acetate
DMPE — 3,4-dimethoxyphenyl-
ethylamine
DMPP — dimethylphenylpipera-
zinium
D.M.R. — Diploma in Medical
Radiology
D.M.R.D. — Diploma in Medical
Radio-Diagnosis (British)
D.M.R.T. — Diploma in Medical
Radio-Therapy (British)
DMS —
dermatomyositis
dimethyl sulfoxide
D.M.S. — Department of Medicine
and Surgery
DMSO — dimethyl sulfoxide
DMT — N,N-dimethyltryptamine
DN —
dextrose-nitrogen (ratio)
dibucaine number
dicrotic notch
D/N — dextrose-nitrogen (ratio)
Dn. — dekanem
dn. — decinem
DNA — deoxyribonucleic acid
DNA-P — deoxyribonucleic acid-
phosphorus
DNase — deoxyribonuclease
DNB — dinitrobenzene
D.N.B. — Diplomate of the
National Board (of Medical
Examiners)
DNC — dinitrocarbanilide
DNCB — dinitrochlorobenzene

DND — died a natural death
DNFB — dinitrofluorobenzene
DNOC — dinitro-orthocresol
DNP —
deoxyribonucleoprotein
dinitrophenol
DNPH — dinitrophenylhydrazine
DNPM — dinitrophenylmorphine
D5/NS — 5 per cent dextrose in
normal saline
DNT — did not test
DNTP — diethylnitrophenyl thio-
phosphate
DO —
diamine oxidase
dissolved oxygen
disto-occlusal
doctor's orders
D_2O — heavy water
D.O. — Doctor of Osteopathy
DOA —
dead on arrival
driver of automobile
DOB — date of birth
DOC —
deoxycholate
11-desoxycorticosterone
died of other causes
DOCA — deoxycorticosterone
acetate
DOCs — deoxycorticoids
DOC-SR — desoxycorticosterone
secretion rate
DOD —
date of death
dead of disease
DOE —
desoxyephedrine hydrochloride
dyspnea on exercise
dyspnea on exertion
DOET — 2,5-dimethoxy-4-ethyl
amphetamine

DOM –
  deaminated-*O*-methyl metab-
    olite
  dimethoxymethylampheta-
    mine
  2,5-dimethoxy-4-methylam-
    phetamine
DOMA – dihydroxymandelic acid
DON – diazo-oxonorleucine
don. – donec [L] until
donec alv. sol. fuerit – donec
  alvus soluta fuerit [L] until
  the bowels are opened
DOPA – dihydroxyphenylalanine
DOPAC – dihydroxyphenylacetic
  acid
DOPS – diffuse obstructive pulmonary syndrome
D.O.S. – Division of Operational
  Safety
dos. –
  dosage
  dosis [L] dose
DOSC – Dubois oleic serum complex
DP –
  deep pulse
  dementia praecox
  diastolic pressure
  diffusion pressure
  digestible protein
  diphosgene
  diphosphate
  dipropionate
  directional preponderance
  disability pension
  displaced person
  distopulpal
  donor's plasma
  dorsalis pedis
D.P. –
  Doctor of Pharmacy
  Doctor of Podiatry

d.p. – directione propria [L] with
  proper direction
DPA –
  diphenylamine
  dipropylacetate
DPC – delayed primary closure
DPD –
  desoxypyridoxine hydrochlo-
    ride
  diffuse pulmonary disease
DPDL – diffuse, poorly differen-
  tiated lymphoma
dpdt switch – double-pole double-
  throw switch
DPG – displacement placento-
  gram
DPG or 2,3-DPG – 2,3-diphos-
  phoglycerate
2,3-DPGM – 2,3-diphosphoglycer-
  ate mutase
DPGP – diphosphoglycerate phos-
  phatase
DPH – diphenylhydantoin
D.P.H. – Diploma in Public Health
D.Ph. – Doctor of Philosophy
D.P.H.N. – Department of Public
  Health Nursing
DPI – disposable personal income
DPL –
  dipalmityl lecithin
  distopulpolingual
D.P.M. –
  Diploma in Psychological
    Medicine
  Doctor of Podiatric Medicine
dpm. – disintegration per minute
DPN – diphosphopyridine nucleo-
  tide
DPNH – diphosphopyridine nu-
  cleotide (reduced form)
DPP – dimethoxyphenyl penicillin
DPS – dimethylpolysiloxane
dps. – disintegration per second

dpst switch — double-pole single-throw switch

DPT —
 diphosphothiamine
 diphtheria, pertussis and tetanus
 dipropyltryptamine

DPTA — diethylenetriamine penta-acetic acid

DQ —
 deterioration quotient
 developmental quotient

DR —
 delivery room
 diabetic retinopathy
 diagnostic radiology
 dorsal root
 reaction of degeneration

Dr. — doctor

dr. —
 drachm
 dram
 dressing

DREZ — dorsal root entry zone

DRF —
 daily replacement factor
 dose-reduction factor

D.R.F. — Deafness Research Foundation

DRG — Diagnosis-Related Groups

D.R.I. — Discharge Readiness Inventory

Dr.P.H. — Doctor of Public Health

DS —
 defined substrate
 dehydroepiandrosterone sulfate
 density standard
 dextrose-saline
 dilute strength
 dioptric strength
 donor's serum
 Down's syndrome

DS (continued)
 dry swallow
 duration of systole

D/S — dextrose in saline

D & S — dermatology and syphilology

DSA — digital subtraction angiography

DSAP — disseminated superficial actinic porokeratosis

DSC or DSCG — disodium cromoglycate

D.S.C. — Doctor of Surgical Chiropody

DSD — dry sterile dressing

dsDNA — double-stranded deoxyribonucleic acid

dsg. — dressing(s)

DSM — dextrose solution mixture

D/spine — dorsal spine

DSS — dioctyl sodium sulfosuccinate

DST —
 desensitization test
 dexamethasone suppression test
 donor-specific transfusion

DSVP — downstream venous pressure

DT —
 delirium tremens
 distance test
 duration tetany
 dye test

DTBC — D-tubocurarine

DTBN — di-t-butyl nitroxide

DTC — D-tubocurarine

d.t.d. — datur talis dosis [L] let such a dose be given

dTDP — thymidine diphosphate

DTF — detector transfer function

DTH — delayed-type hypersensitivity reaction

DTIC – dacarbazine
D time – dream time
DTM – dermatophyte test medium
DTMP – deoxythymidine monophosphate
dTMP – thymidine-5'-phosphate
DTN – diphtheria toxin normal
DTNB – dithiobisnitrobenzoic
acid
DTP –
diphtheria, tetanus and pertussis
distal tingling on percussion
DTPA – diethylenetriaminepenta-
acetic acid
DTR – deep tendon reflex
DTT –
diphtheria-tetanus toxoid
dithiothreitol
dTTP – thymidine triphosphate
DTV – due to void
D.T.V.M. – Diploma in Tropical
Veterinary Medicine
DTZ – diatrizoate
DU –
density unknown
diagnosis undetermined
dog unit
duodenal ulcer
D_U – urea dialysance
dU – deoxyuridine
d.u. – dial unit
DUB – dysfunctional uterine
bleeding
dUMP –
deoxyuridine monophosphate
deoxyuridine-5'-phosphate
duod. – duodenum
dur. – durus [L] hard
dur. dolor. – durante dolore [L]
while the pain lasts
DV –
dependent variable

DV (continued)
dilute volume
D & V – diarrhea and vomiting
d.v. – double vibrations
DVA –
distance visual acuity
duration of voluntary apnea
D value – decimal reduction
time
DVD – dissociated vertical diverg-
ence
DVIU – direct vision internal
urethrotomy
DVM – digital voltmeter
D.V.M. – Doctor of Veterinary
Medicine
D.V.M.S. – Doctor of Veterinary
Medicine and Surgery
DVPL-ASP – daunorubicin, vin-
cristine, prednisone, L-aspar-
aginase
D.V.S. –
Division of Vital Statistics
Doctor of Veterinary Science
Doctor of Veterinary Surgery
DVT – deep venous thrombosis
DW –
distilled water
dry weight
D/W – dextrose in water
D5W, D5 & W or D_5W – 5 per
cent dextrose in water
dwt. – pennyweight
DX – dextran
Dx. – diagnosis
Dxd. – discontinued
DXM – dexamethasone
DXT – deep x-ray therapy
Dy – dysprosium
dyn – dyne
DZ –
dizygotic
dizygous

E −
  air dose
  cortisone (compound E)
  elastance
  electric field vector
  electrode potential
  electromotive force
  emmetropia
  energy
  enzyme
  epinephrine
  erythrocyte
  ester
  exa-
  experimenter
  expired gas
  extraction fraction
  eye
  glutamic acid
  internal energy
  mathematical expectation
  redox potential
E° − standard potential
E⁺ − positron (positive electron)
E⁻ − negative electron
E_1 − estrone
E_2 − 17 β-estradiol
E_3 − estriol
E_4 − estetrol
4E − four plus edema
E. −
  Entamoeba
  Escherichia
e −
  base of natural logarithms
  electric charge
  electron
  elementary charge
  ex [L] from

E, ε − epsilon (fifth letter of the
    Greek alphabet)
H, η − eta (seventh letter of the
    Greek alphabet)
EA −
  early antigen
  educational age
  erythrocyte antibody
  estivoautumnal
  ethacrynic acid
ea. − each
EAA − essential amino acid
EAC −
  Ehrlich ascites carcinoma
  erythrocyte antibody comple-
    ment
  external auditory canal
EACA − epsilon-aminocaproic
    acid
EACD − eczematous allergic con-
    tact dermatitis
ead. − eadem [L] the same
EAE − experimental allergic en-
    cephalomyelitis
EAHF − *e*czema, *a*sthma, *h*ay
    *f*ever
EAHLG − equine antihuman
    lymphoblast globulin
EAHLS − equine antihuman
    lymphoblast serum
EAM − external auditory meatus
EAN − experimental allergic
    neuritis
EAP − epiallopregnanolone
Ea. R. − Entartungs-Reaktion
    [Ger] reaction of degenera-
    tion
EB −
  elementary body

EB (*continued*)
    epidermolysis bullosa
    Epstein-Barr (virus)
    estradiol benzoate
E.B.A.A. — Eye Bank Association of America
EBCDIC — *e*xtended *b*inary *c*oded *d*ecimal *i*nterchange *c*ode
EBF — erythroblastosis fetalis
EBI — emetine bismuth iodide
EBL — estimated blood loss
EBM — expressed breast milk
EBNA — Epstein-Barr (virus) nuclear antigen
EBS — electric brain stimulator
EBV — Epstein-Barr virus
EC —
    electron capture
    enteric-coated
    entrance complaint
    Escherichia coli
    excitation-contraction
    experimental control
    extracellular
    eyes closed
E/C —
    endo/cystoscopy
    estrogen to creatinine (ratio)
E.C. — Enzyme Commission
ECA — ethacrynic acid
ECBO virus — enteric cytopathogenic bovine orphan virus
ECBV — effective circulating blood volume
ECC — extracorporeal circulation
E.C.C.L.S. — European Committee for Clinical Laboratory Standards
ECD — electron capture detector
ECDO virus — enteric cytopathogenic dog orphan virus
ECF —
    effective capillary flow

ECF (*continued*)
    extended care facility
    extracellular fluid
ECF-A — eosinophil chemotactic factor of anaphylaxis
ECFV — extracellular fluid volume
ECG — electrocardiogram
Echo —
    echocardiogram
    echoencephalogram
ECHO virus — enteric cytopathogenic human orphan virus
ECI —
    electrocerebral inactivity
    extracorporeal irradiation
ECIB — extracorporeal irradiation of blood
ECIL — extracorporeal irradiation of lymph
ECL — emitter-coupled logic
eclec. — eclectic
ECLT — euglobulin clot lysis time
ECM —
    erythema chronicum migrans
    extracellular material
E-C mixture — ether-chloroform mixture
ECMO virus — enteric cytopathogenic monkey orphan virus
ECoG —
    electrocorticogram
    electrocorticography
E. coli — *Escherichia coli*
ECP —
    erythrocyte coproporphyrin
    estradiol cyclopentaneopropionate
ECPOG — electrochemical potential gradient
ECPO virus — enteric cytopathogenic porcine orphan virus
ECS — electroconvulsive shock

ECSO virus — enteric cytopathogenic swine orphan virus
ECT —
electroconvulsive therapy
enteric-coated tablet
euglobulin clot test
ECV —
extracellular volume
extracorporeal volume
ECVE — extracellular volume
expansion
ECW — extracellular water
ED —
effective dose
Ehlers-Danlos syndrome
epidural
epileptiform discharge
erythema dose
ED_{50} — median effective dose
E_d — depth dose
EDB — early dry breakfast
EDC —
estimated date of confinement
expected date of confinement
EDD —
effective drug duration
enzyme-digested delta
expected date of delivery
EDN — electrodesiccation
EDP —
electronic data processing
end-diastolic pressure
EDR —
effective direct radiation
electrodermal response
EDS — Ehlers-Danlos syndrome
EDTA —
edathamil
edetic acid
ethylenediaminetetra-acetic
acid
EDV — end-diastolic volume
EDX — electrodiagnosis

EE —
embryo extract
end-to-end
equine encephalitis
eye and ear
E-E — erythematous-edematous
(reaction)
EEA — electroencephalic audiometry
EEC — enteropathogenic *Escherichia coli*
EEC syndrome — ectrodactyly-
ectodermal dysplasia–clefting
syndrome
EEEP — end-expiratory esophageal
pressure
EEE virus — eastern equine encephalomyelitis virus
EEG — electroencephalogram
EEME — ethinylestradiol methyl
ether
EENT — eyes, ears, nose and
throat
EER — electroencephalic response
EES — ethyl ethanesulfate
EF —
ectopic focus
edema factor
ejection fraction
encephalitogenic factor
equivalent focus
extrinsic factor
EFA —
essential fatty acids
extrafamily adoptees
EFC — endogenous fecal calcium
EFE — endocardial fibroelastosis
EFP — effective filtration pressure
EFR — effective filtration rate
EFV — extracellular fluid volume
EFVC — expiratory flow-volume
curve
EG — esophagogastrectomy

e.g. — exempli gratia [L] for example

EGD — esophagogastroduodenoscopy

EGF — epidermal growth factor

EGG — electrogastrogram

EGL — eosinophilic granuloma of the lung

EGM — electrogram

EGOT — erythrocyte glutamic oxaloacetic transaminase

EGS — ethylene glycol succinate

EGTA — ethylene glycol tetraacetic acid

EH —
enlarged heart
essential hypertension

E & H — environment and heredity

E_h — redox potential

eH — oxidation-reduction potential

EHBF —
estimated hepatic blood flow
exercise hyperemia blood flow

EHC —
enterohepatic circulation
essential hypercholesterolemia

EHDP — ethane hydroxydiphosphate

EHF — exophthalmos-hyperthyroid factor

EHL —
effective half-life
endogenous hyperlipidemia

EHO — extrahepatic obstruction

EHP —
di-(2-ethylhexyl) hydrogen phosphate
excessive heat production
extra high potency

EHPH — extrahepatic portal hypertension

EI —
enzyme inhibitor
eosinophilic index

E/I — expiration-inspiration ratio

EIA — enzyme immunoassay

E.I.A. — Electronics Industries Association

EID —
egg-infective dose
electroimmunodiffusion

EIP — extensor indicis proprius

EIT — erythroid iron turnover

EJ — elbow jerk

EJP — excitatory junction potential

ejusd. — ejusdem [L] of the same

EK — erythrokinase

EKC — epidemic keratoconjunctivitis

EKG — electrocardiogram

EKY — electrokymogram

EL — erythroleukemia

el. — elixir

ELB — early light breakfast

elb. — elbow

ELISA — enzyme-linked immunosorbent assay

elix. — elixir [L] elixir

ELT — euglobulin lysis time

EM —
ejection murmur
electron microscopy
erythrocyte mass

E-M — Embden-Meyerhof (pathway)

Em. — emmetropia

e/m — ratio of charge to mass

EMB —
embryology
eosin-methylene blue (agar)
ethambutol
Myambutol (ethambutol)

EMC –
    electron microscopy
    encephalomyocarditis
EMC virus – encephalomyocarditis
    virus
emer. – emergency
EMF –
    electromagnetic flowmeter
    electromotive force
    endomyocardial fibrosis
    erythrocyte maturation factor
EMG –
    electromyelography
    electromyogram
    electromyography
    exophthalmos, macroglossia,
      gigantism
EMI – Electric and Musical Indus-
    tries
EMIC – emergency maternity and
    infant care
EMIT – enzyme-multiplied im-
    munoassay technique
emp. –
    emplastrum [L] a plaster
    ex modo prescripto [L] as
      directed
emp. vesic. – emplastrum vesica-
    torium [L] a blistering plaster
EMS –
    early morning specimen
    ethyl methane sulfonate
EMT – emergency medical tech-
    nician
emu – electromagnetic unit
emul. – emulsio [L] an emulsion
EN –
    enema
    erythema nodosum
en. – enema
ENA – extractable nuclear antigen
end – endoreduplication
enem. – enema

ENG –
    electronystagmogram
    electronystagmograph
    electronystagmography
ENL – erythema nodosum lepro-
    ticum
enl. – enlargement
ENP – ethyl-p-nitrophenylthio-
    benzene phosphate
ENR – extrathyroidal neck radio-
    activity
ENT – ear, nose and throat
enz. – enzymatic
EO –
    eosinophils
    ethylene oxide
    eyes open
E_o –
    electric affinity
    skin dose (of radiation)
EOD – entry on duty
e.o.d. – every other day
EOG –
    electro-oculogram
    electro-olfactogram
EOM – extraocular movement
EOR – exclusive OR
eos. – eosinophil
EOT – effective oxygen transport
EP –
    ectopic pregnancy
    electrophoresis
    endogenous pyrogen
    end point
    erythrocyte protoporphyrin
    extreme pressure
EPA – eicosapentaenoic acid
EPC – epilepsia partialis
    continua
EPE – erythropoietin-producing
    enzyme
EPEC – enteropathogenic *Esche-
richia coli*

EPF – exophthalmos-producing factor

EPG – eggs per gram

epi. – epinephrine

epith. –
epithelial
epithelium

EPP –
end-plate potential
equal pressure point
erythropoietic protoporphyria

EPR –
electron paramagnetic resonance
electrophrenic respiration
estradiol production rate

EPROM – erasable programmable read-only memory

EPS – exophthalmos-producing substance

EPSP – excitatory postsynaptic potential

EPTE – existed prior to enlistment

EPTS – existed prior to service

Eq. – equivalent

ER –
ejection rate
emergency room
endoplasmic reticulum
environmental resistance
equivalent roentgen
estrogen receptor
evoked response
extended release
external resistance

Er – erbium

ERA – evoked response audiometry

E.R.A. – Electroshock Research Association

ERBF – effective renal blood flow

ERC – erythropoietin-responsive cell

ERCP – endoscopic retrograde cholangiopancreatography

ERD – evoked response detector

E.R.F. – Education and Research Foundation

ERG – electroretinogram

ERIA – electroradioimmunoassay

ERP –
effective refractory period
equine rhinopneumonitis

ERPF – effective renal plasma flow

ERV – expiratory reserve volume

ES –
emission spectrometry
end-to-side
enzyme substrate
Expectation Score

Es – einsteinium

ESB – electrical stimulation to brain

ESC – electromechanical slope computer

Esch. – Escherichia

ESCN – electrolyte- and steroid-produced cardiopathy characterized by necrosis

ESD – electronic summation device

ESE – electrostatische Einheit [Ger] electrostatic unit

ESF – erythropoietic-stimulating factor

ESL – end-systolic length

ESM – ejection systolic murmur

eso. –
esophagoscopy
esophagus

esoph. – esophagus

ESP –
end-systolic pressure

ESP (*continued*)
 eosinophil stimulation pro-
  moter
 extrasensory perception
ESR — erythrocyte sedimentation
  rate
esr — electron spin resonance
ESS — erythrocyte-sensitizing
  substance
ess. — essential
ess. neg. — essentially negative
EST — electroshock therapy
est. — estimated
e.s.u. — electrostatic unit
E-substance — excitor substance
ESV — end-systolic volume
ET —
 effective temperature
 ejection time
 endotracheal tube
 etiology
 eustachian tube
Et — ethyl
et — and
ETA — ethionamide
eta (η) — viscosity
et al. —
 et alibi [L] and elsewhere
 et alii [L] and others
etc. — et cetera [L] and so forth
ETEC — enterotoxic *Escherichia
  coli*
ETF —
 electron-transferring flavopro-
  tein
 eustachian tube function
ETH — elixir of terpin hydrate
ETH/C — elixir of terpin hydrate
  with codeine
ETIO — etiocholanolone
etiol. — etiology
ETKM — every test known to
  mankind

ETM — erythromycin
ETOH — ethyl alcohol
ETOX — ethylene oxide
ETP —
 electron transport particle
 entire treatment period
 eustachian tube pressure
ETT —
 exercise tolerance test
 extrathyroidal thyroxine
ETU —
 Emergency and Trauma Unit
 Emergency Treatment Unit
ETV — educational television
EU —
 Ehrlich unit
 enzyme unit
Eu — europium
EUA — examination under anesthesia
EUV — extreme ultraviolet laser
EV —
 evoked response
 extravascular
ev. or eV. — electron volt
EVA —
 ethylene vinyl acetate
 ethyl violet azide
evac. — evacuated
eval. — evaluation
evap. — evaporated
evisc. — evisceration
EVM — electronic voltmeter
EW — Emergency Ward
ew. — elsewhere
EWB — estrogen withdrawal
  bleeding
EWL —
 egg-white lysozyme
 evaporative water loss
ex — [L] from
ex. —
 excision

ex. (*continued*)
   exophthalmos
exam. – examination
EXBF – exercise hyperemia
   blood flow
exc. – excision
exer. – exercise
exhib. – exhibeatur [L] let it be
   given
exp. –
   expired
   exploration
   exponential function
   exposure
expir. –
   expiration

expir. (*continued*)
   expiratory
   expired
exp. lap. – exploratory laparotomy
EXREM – external radiation dose
ext. –
   extende [L] spread
   extensor
   exterior
   external
   extractum [L] extract
   extremities
ext. rot. – external rotation
Ez. – eczema

F

F –
   facies
   family
   farad
   Faraday constant
   fat
   father
   feces
   Fellow
   female
   fertility
   fetal
   finger
   fluorine
   focal length
   foramen
   force
   formula
   fractional
   fragment of an antibody
   frontal

F (*continued*)
   gilbert (unit of magnetomotive
      force)
   hydrocortisone (compound F)
   inbreeding coefficient
   phenylalanine
   variance ratio
F_1 – first filial generation
F_2 – second filial generation
F. –
   Fahrenheit
   field of vision
   French (catheter size)
F. –
   Filaria
   Fusiformis
   Fusobacterium
f –
   atomic orbital with angular
      momentum quantum num-
      ber 3

f (*continued*)
  breathing frequency
  femto-
  fluid
  frequency
  frequently
f-12 — freon
f. —
  fiat, fiant [L] let there be made
  forma [L] form
FA —
  far advanced
  fatty acid
  febrile antigens
  femoral artery
  field ambulance
  filterable agent
  first aid
  fluorescent antibody (technique)
  folic acid
  forearm
  fortified aqueous
  free acid
  Freund's adjuvant
  functional activities
FAA sol. — formalin, acetic, alcohol solution
FAB —
  formalin ammonium bromide
  functional arm brace
Fab — *f*ragment, *a*ntigen-*b*inding
F.A.C.A. — Fellow of the American College of Anesthesiologists
F.A.C.C. — Fellow of the American College of Cardiologists
F.A.C.C.P. — Fellow of the American College of Chest Physicians
F.A.C.D. — Fellow of the American College of Dentists

F.A.C.F.S. — Fellow of the American College of Foot Surgeons
F.A.C.H.A. — Fellow of the American College of Hospital Administrators
F.A.C.O.G. — Fellow of the American College of Obstetricians and Gynecologists
F.A.C.P. — Fellow of the American College of Physicians
F.A.C.R. — Fellow of the American College of Radiologists
F.A.C.S. — Fellow of the American College of Surgeons
F.A.C.S.M. — Fellow of the American College of Sports Medicine
FAD — flavin adenine dinucleotide
FADF — fluorescent antibody darkfield
$FADH_2$ — flavin adenine dinucleotide (reduced form)
FADN — flavin adenine dinucleotide
Fahr. — Fahrenheit
F.A.M.A. — Fellow of the American Medical Association
fam. doc. — family doctor
Fam. per. par. — familial periodic paralysis
fam. phys. — family physician
FAN — fuchsin, amido black and naphthol yellow
FANA — fluorescent antinuclear antibody
F.A.N.S. — Fellow of the American Neurological Society
F.A.P.A. —
  Fellow of the American Psychiatric Association
  Fellow of the American Psychoanalytical Association

F.A.P.H.A. — Fellow of the American Public Health Association

far. — faradic

F.A.S. — Federation of American Scientists

fasc. — fasciculus [L] bundle

F.A.S.E.B. — Federation of American Societies for Experimental Biology

FAT — fluorescent antibody test

FAV — feline ataxia virus

FB —
finger breadth
foreign body

FBD — functional bowel disorder

FBE — full blood examination

FBF — forearm blood flow

F.B.N. — Federal Bureau of Narcotics

FBP —
femoral blood pressure
fibrinogen breakdown products

FBS —
fasting blood sugar
feedback system
fetal bovine serum

FC —
finger clubbing
finger counting

5-FC — 5-fluorocytosine

Fc. — crystallizable fragment

fc. — foot candle

FCA — ferritin-conjugated antibodies

F.C.A.P. — Fellow of the College of American Pathologists

FCC — follicular center cells

FCG — French catheter gauge

F.C.G.P. — Fellow of the College of General Practitioners

FCP — final common pathway

F.C.P.S. — Fellow of the College of Physicians and Surgeons

FCS — fetal calf serum

FCT — food composition table

FD —
fatal dose
focal distance
foot drape
forceps delivery
freeze-dried

FD$_{50}$ — median fatal dose

F.D.A. —
Food and Drug Administration
fronto-dextra anterior [L] right frontoanterior; a presentation of the fetus

FDDC — ferric dimethyl dithiocarbonate

FDE — final drug evaluation

FDF — fast death factor

FDIU — fetal death in utero

FDNB — 1-fluoro-2,4-dinitrobenzene

FDP —
fibrin degradation products
flexor digitorum profundus
fructose 1,6-diphosphate

F.D.P. — fronto-dextra posterior [L] right frontoposterior; a presentation of the fetus

FDS — flexor digitorum superficialis

F.D.S. — Fellow in Dental Surgery

F.D.T. — fronto-dextra transversa [L] right frontotransverse; a presentation of the fetus

FE — fetal erythroblastosis

Fe — ferrum [L] iron

Fe$_2$ — ferrous

Fe$_3$ — ferric

^{59}Fe − radioactive iron
feb. dur. − febre durante [L] while the fever lasts
F.E.B.S. − Federation of European Biochemical Societies
FEC − free erythrocyte coproporphyrin
FECG − fetal electrocardiogram
FeCO$_3$ − ferrous carbonate
FECP − free erythrocyte coproporphyria
FECT − fibro-elastic connective tissue
FECV − functional extracellular fluid volume
FEF − forced expiratory flow
FEKG − fetal electrocardiogram
FEL − familial erythrophagocytic lymphohistiocytosis
fem. −
  female
  feminine
  femoral
  femoris [L] thigh
  femur
fem. intern. − femoribus internus [L] at the inner side of the thighs
FE$_{NA}$ test − excreted fraction of filtered sodium test
Fe$_2$O$_3$ − ferric oxide
Fe(OH)$_3$ − ferric hydroxide
FEP or FEPP − free erythrocyte protoporphyrin
ferv. − fervens [L] boiling
FES −
  flame emission spectroscopy
  forced expiratory spirogram
FET −
  field effect transistor
  forced expiratory time
FETS − forced expiratory time, in seconds

FEV − forced expiratory volume
FEV$_1$ − forced expiratory volume in one second
FEV$_1$/VC − forced expiratory volume (in one second) vital capacity
FF −
  fat free
  father factor
  fecal frequency
  filtration fraction
  finger-to-finger
  fixing fluid
  flat feet
  flip-flop
  force fluids
  forearm flow
  foster father
  fresh frozen
FFA − free fatty acids
F factor − fertility factor
FFC − free from chlorine
FFD − focus film distance
FFDW − fat-free dry weight
FFI − free from infection
FFM − fat-free mass
FFP − fresh frozen plasma
FFS − fat-free supper
FFT − flicker fusion threshold
FFWW − fat-free wet weight
FG − fibrinogen
FGAR − formylglycinamide ribonucleotide
FGD − fatal granulomatous disease
FGF − father's grandfather
FGM − father's grandmother
FH −
  family history
  fetal head
  fetal heart
  Frankfort horizontal

f.h. – fiat haustus [L] let a
draught be made
FHNH – fetal heart not heard
FHR – fetal heart rate
FHS – fetal heart sound
FHT –
fetal heart
fetal heart tone
FHVP – free hepatic vein pressure
FI –
fever caused by infection
fibrinogen
fixed internal
forced inspiration
FIA – fluorescent immunoassay
fib. –
fibrillation
fibrinogen
F.I.C.D. – Fellow of the Inter-
national College of Dentists
F.I.C.S. – Fellow of the Inter-
national College of Surgeons
FID – flame ionization detector
FIF – forced inspiratory flow
FIFR – fasting intestinal flow
rate
fig. – figure
FIGLU – formiminoglutamic acid
F.I.G.O –
International Federation of
Gynecology and Obstetrics
International Federation of
Gynecology and Obstetrics
Staging Classification
FIH – fat-induced hyperglycemia
filt. – filtra [L] filter
F.I.M.L.T. – Fellow of the Insti-
tute of Medical Laboratory
Technology
FIN – fine intestinal needle
F-insulin – fibrous insulin
FIO$_2$ –
fractional inspired oxygen

FIO$_2$ (*continued*)
inspired flow of oxygen
fist. – fistula
FIT – fusion inferred threshold
(test)
FITC – fluorescein isothiocyanate
F-J – Fisher-John (melting point
method)
FJN – familial juvenile nephro-
phthisis
FJRM – full joint range of movement
FL –
filtered load
focal length
fl. –
femtoliter
flexion
fluidus [L] fluid
F.L.A. – fronto-laeva anterior
[L] left frontoanterior; a
presentation of the fetus
f.l.a. – fiat lege artis [L] let it be
done according to rule
flac. – flaccid
flav. – flavus [L] yellow
fld. – fluid
fl. dr. – fluid dram
fldxt. – fluidextractum [L]
fluidextract
flex. – flexion
FLK – funny looking kid
flor. – flores [L] flowers
fl. oz. – fluid ounce
F.L.P. – fronto-laeva posterior
[L] left frontoposterior; a
presentation of the fetus
FLS – fibrous long-spacing (collagen)
FLSA – follicular lymphosarcoma
F.L.T. – fronto-laeva transversa
[L] left frontotransverse; a
presentation of the fetus

flu − influenza
fluor. − fluorometry
fluoro. − fluoroscopy
fl.-up −
    flare-up
    follow-up
FM −
    flavin mononucleotide
    flowmeter
    formerly married
    foster mother
    frequency modulation
    Fusobacterium micro-orga-
      nisms
Fm − fermium
fm − femtometer
fm. − fiat mistura [L] make a
    mixture
FMD − foot-and-mouth disease
FME − full-mouth extraction
FMF −
    familial Mediterranean fever
    fetal movement felt
FMG − foreign medical graduate
f-MLP − formyl-methionyleucyl-
    phenylalanine
FMN − flavin mononucleotide
fmol − femtomole
FMP − first menstrual period
FMS −
    fat-mobilizing substance
    full-mouth series
FN −
    false-negative
    finger-to-nose
    fluoride number
FNa − filtered sodium
FO −
    foramen ovale
    fronto-occipital
FOAVF − failure of all vital forces
FOB −
    fecal occult blood

FOB (*continued*)
    feet out of bed
FOCAL − *fo*rmula *cal*culation
FOD − free of disease
fol. − folia [L] leaves
FOR − forensic
fort. − fortis [L] strong
FORTRAN − *fo*rmula *tran*slation
FP −
    false-positive
    family practice
    family practitioner
    flat plate
    flavin phosphate
    flavoprotein
    freezing point
    frontoparietal
    frozen plasma
    fundal pressure
F-P − femoral-popliteal
Fp − filtered phosphate
fp. −
    fiat potio [L] let a potion be
      made
    forearm pronated
    freezing point
f.p. − foot pound
FPA − fluorophenylalanine
F.P.A. − Family Planning Associa-
    tion
FPC − fish protein concentrate
FPG − fasting plasma glucose
FPH_2 − flavin phosphate, reduced
f. pil. − fiat pilulae [L] let pills
    be made
f. pil. xi − fac pilulae xi [L] make
    11 pills
FPM − filter paper microscopic
    (test)
fpm. − feet per minute
FPM test − filter paper micro-
    scopic test
fps. − frames per second

FR –
  Fisher-Race (notation)
  fixed ratio
  flocculation reaction
  flow rate
F & R – force and rhythm (of
  pulse)
Fr –
  francium
  franklin
Fr. – French (catheter gauge)
fract. – fracture
fract. dos. – fracta dosi [L] in
  divided doses
frag. – fragility
Fr BB – fracture of both bones
FRC –
  frozen red cells
  functional reserve capacity
  functional residual capacity
F.R.C.P. – Fellow of the Royal
  College of Physicians
F.R.C.S. – Fellow of the Royal
  College of Surgeons
frem. – fremitus vocalis [L] vocal
  fremitus
freq. – frequent
FRF – follicle-stimulating hormone–releasing factor
FRH – follicle-stimulating hormone–releasing hormone
frict. – friction
frig. – frigidus [L] cold
FRJM – full range joint movement
FROM – full range of motion
FRP – functional refractory
  period
FRS –
  ferredoxin-reducing substance
  furosemide
FRT – full recovery time
fru. – fructose

frust. – frustillatim [L] in small
  pieces
FS –
  frozen section
  full scale (IQ)
  function study
f.s.a. – fiat secundum artem [L]
  let it be made skillfully
FSD – focal skin distance
FSF – fibrin-stabilizing factor
FSH – follicle-stimulating hormone
FSH/LH-RH – follicle-stimulating
  hormone and luteinizing hormone–releasing hormone
FSH-RF – follicle-stimulating
  hormone–releasing factor
FSH-RH – follicle-stimulating
  hormone–releasing hormone
F.S.M.B. – Federation of State
  Medical Boards
FSP –
  fibrinogen split products
  fibrinolytic split products
FSR – fusiform skin revision
FSR-3 – isoniazid
FSU – Family Service Unit
FSW – Field Service Worker
FT –
  false transmitter
  family therapy
  fibrous tissue
  follow through
  formol toxoid
  free thyroxine
  full-term
FT_4 – free (unbound) thyroxine
ft. –
  feet
  ıt or fiant [L] let there be
  made
  foot

FTA — fluorescent treponemal antibody

FTA-ABS — fluorescent treponemal antibody absorption (test)

FTBD — full-term born dead

ft.-c. — foot-candle

ft. collyr. — fiat collyrium [L] let an eyewash be made

FTG — full-thickness graft

ft. garg. — fiat gargarisma [L] let a gargle be made

FTI — free thyroxine index

FT_3 index — free triiodothyronine index

FT_4 index — free thyroxine index

FTLB — full-term living birth

ft.-lb. — foot-pound

ft. mas. div. in pil. — fiat massa dividenda in pilulae [L] let a mass be made and divided into pills

FTND — full-term normal delivery

ft. pulv. — fiat pulvis [L] let a powder be made

ft. solut. — fiat solutio [L] let a solution be made

FTT — failure to thrive

FU —
fecal urobilinogen
fluorouracil
follow-up
fractional urinalysis

F/U — follow-up

5-FU — 5-fluorouracil

FUB — functional uterine bleeding

FUDR —
floxuridine
fluorodeoxyuridine

FUM — fumarate

FUO —
fever of undetermined origin
fever of unknown origin

FUR — fluorouracil riboside

FV — fluid volume

FVC — forced vital capacity

FVL — femoral vein ligation

FVR — forearm vascular resistance

f.vs. — fiat venaesectio [L] let the patient be bled

FW —
Felix-Weil (reaction)
Folin and Wu's (method)
forced whisper
fragment wound

FWHM — full width half-maximum

FWR — Felix-Weil reaction

fx. —
fractional
fracture
frozen section

FY — fiscal year

FYI — for your information

FZ — focal zone

G

G —
an immunoglobulin
conductance
force (pull of gravity)
gap
gas

G (*continued*)
gastrin
gauge
gauss
Gibbs free energy
giga-

G (*continued*)
  gingival
  globular
  globulin
  glucose
  glycine
  gonidial (in colony cultures)
  good
  gravida
  gravitational constant
  Greek
  green
  guanine
  guanosine
G_4 — dichlorophen (dihydroxy-dichlorodiphenyl urethane)
G_{11} — hexachlorophene
g —
  gender
  gravity
  group
g. — gram(s)
Γ, γ — gamma (third letter of the Greek alphabet)
γ —
  immunoglobulin
  microgram
GA —
  gastric analysis
  general anesthesia
  gestational age
  gingivoaxial
  glucuronic acid
  gut-associated
Ga — gallium
ga. — gauge
GABA — gamma-aminobutyric acid
GABHS — group A beta-hemolytic streptococcus
GAD — glutamic acid decarboxylase

gal. —
  galactose
  gallon
gal-1-P — galactose-1-phosphate
GALT — gut-associated lymphoid tissue
GaLV — gibbon ape lymphosarcoma virus
galv. — galvanic
gang. — ganglion
GAPD or GAPDH — glyceraldehyde-phosphate dehydrogenase
garg. — gargarismus [L] gargle
GAS —
  general adaptation syndrome
  generalized arteriosclerosis
GAW — airway conductance
GB —
  gallbladder
  Guillain-Barré syndrome
GBA —
  ganglionic-blocking agent
  gingivobuccoaxial
GBH —
  gamma benzene hydrochloride
  graphite-benzalkonium-heparin
GBIA — Guthrie bacterial inhibition assay
GBM — glomerular basement membrane
GBS —
  gallbladder series
  glycerine buffered saline
GC —
  ganglion cells
  gas chromatography
  glucocorticoid
  gonococcal
  gonococcus
  gonorrhea

GC (*continued*)
    granular cysts
    guanine cytosine
g-cal. — gram-calorie
G.C.F. — greatest common factor
GCFT — gonorrhea complement-fixation test
g-cm. — gram-centimeter
GC-MS — gas chromatography—mass spectrometry
GCS — general clinical service
Gc/s — gigacycles per second
GC type — guanine, cytosine type
G.C.W.M. — General Conference on Weights and Measures
Gd — gadolinium
GDA — germine diacetate
GDH —
    glutamic acid dehydrogenase
    glycerophosphate dehydrogenase
GDP — guanosine diphosphate
GDS — gradual dosage schedule
GE —
    gastroemotional
    gastroenterology
    gastroenterostomy
G/E — granulocyte-erythroid ratio
Ge — germanium
GEE — glycine ethyl ester
GEF — gonadotropin-enhancing factor
gel. — gelatin
gel. quav. — gelatina quavis [L] in any kind of jelly
GEMS — good emergency mother substitute
gen. —
    general
    genus [L] genus
gen. et sp. nov. — genus et species nova [L] new genus and species

gen. nov. — genus novum [L] new genus
GEP — gastroenteropancreatic
ger. — geriatrics
GET — gastric emptying time
GET½ — gastric emptying half-time
GeV — giga electron volt
GF —
    gastric fluid
    germ-free
    glass factor
    glomerular filtrate
    gluten-free
    grandfather
    growth fraction
GFD — gluten-free diet
GFR — glomerular filtration rate
GG —
    gamma globulin
    glycylglycine
GGA — general gonadotropic activity
GGE — general gland enlargement
GGG — gummi guttae gambiae [L] gamboge
GG or S — glands, goiter or stiffness
GGT —
    gamma glutamyltransferase
GGTP — gamma-glutamyl transpeptidase
GH — growth hormone
G.H.A.A. — Group Health Association of America
GHD — growth hormone deficiency
GH-RF — growth hormone–releasing factor
GH-RH — growth hormone–releasing hormone
GH-RIH — growth hormone-release-inhibiting hormone

GHz – gigahertz
GI –
    gastrointestinal
    globulin insulin
    growth-inhibiting
GIF – growth hormone–inhibiting factor
GIGO – garbage in, garbage out
GIH – growth-inhibiting hormone
GIK – glucose, insulin and potassium
GIM – gonadotropin-inhibitory material
ging. – gingiva [L] gum
GIP –
    gastric inhibitory polypeptide
    giant cell interstitial pneumonia
GIS –
    gas in stomach
    gastrointestinal system
GI series – gastrointestinal series
GIT –
    gastrointestinal tract
    glutathione-insulin transhydrogenase
GITT – glucose-insulin tolerance test
GK – glycerol kinase
GL – greatest length
GL 54 – athomin
Gl – glucinium (beryllium)
g/l – grams per liter
gl. –
    gill
    gland(s) (glandula and glandulae)
GLA – gingivolinguoaxial
gland. –
    glandula [L] a gland
    glandular
GLC – gas-liquid chromatography

GLI – glucagon-like immunoreactivity
Gln – glutamine
glob. – globulin
GLP – group-living program
Glu –
    glutamic acid
    glutamine
glu. or gluc. – glucose
Gly – glycine
glyc. –
    glycerin
    glyceritum [L] glycerite
GM –
    gastric mucosa
    Geiger-Müller counter
    general medical
    geometric mean
    grandmother
    grand multiparity
Gm – gamma
g-m – gram-meter
g/m – gallons per minute
gm. – gram(s)
GMA – glyceryl methacrylate
G.M.C. – General Medical Council (British)
GMK – green monkey kidney (cells)
gm/l – grams per liter
gm-m. – gram-meter
g-mol. – gram-molecule
GMP –
    guanosine monophosphate
    guanosine-5-phosphate
GM & S – general medical and surgical
G.M.S. – General Medical Services
GMT –
    geometric mean titer
    Greenwich Mean Time
GMW – gram-molecular weight

GN —
    glomerulonephritis
    gram-negative
G/N — glucose nitrogen (ratio)
Gn. — gonadotropin
G.N.C. — General Nursing Council
GNID — gram-negative intracellular diplococci
Gn-RH — gonadotropin-releasing hormone
G&O — gas and oxygen
GΩ — gigohm
GOE — gas, oxygen and ether
GOK — God only knows
GOT — glutamic-oxaloacetic transaminase
GP —
    general paralysis
    general paresis
    general practice
    general practitioner
    geometric progression
    glutathione peroxidase
    glycoprotein
    gram-positive
    guinea pig
    gutta-percha
G-1-P — glucose-1-phosphate
G-6-P — glucose-6-phosphate
gp. — group (muscle)
GPA — grade-point averages
GPAIS — guinea pig anti-insulin serum
GPB — glossopharyngeal breathing
GPC —
    gastric parietal cell
    glycerylphosphorylcholine
GPD or GPDH — glucose-6-phosphate dehydrogenase
G-6-PD or G-6-PDH — glucose-6-phosphate dehydrogenase

G-6-PDHA — glucose-6-phosphate dehydrogenase enzyme variant A
GPE — glycerylphosphorylethanolamine
GPI —
    general paralysis of the insane
    glucosephosphate isomerase
GPIMH — guinea pig intestinal mucosal homogenate
GPIPID — ginea pig intraperitoneal infectious dose
GPK — guinea pig kidney (antigen)
GPKA — guinea pig kidney absorption (test)
GPM — general preventive medicine
GPS — guinea pig serum
GPT — glutamate pyruvate transaminase
GPU — guinea pig unit
GPUT — galactose phosphate uridyl transferase
GR —
    gamma ray
    gastric resection
    general research
    glutathione reductase
gr. —
    gamma roentgen
    grain(s)
    gravity
GRA — gonadotropin-releasing agent
grad. —
    gradatim [L] by degrees
    gradient
    graduate
GRAE — generally regarded as effective
gran. — granulatus [L] granulated

GRAS – generally recognized as
   safe
grav I –
   pregnancy one
   primigravida
GRF –
   gonadotropin-releasing factor
   growth hormone–releasing
      factor
GRH – growth hormone–releasing hormone
gros. – grossus [L] coarse
GRS – β-glucuronidase
GS –
   general surgery
   glomerular sclerosis
G/S – glucose and saline
g/s – gallons per second
GSA –
   general somatic afferent
   Gross (sarcoma) virus antigen
   guanidinosuccinic acid
GSC –
   gas-solid chromatography
   gravity-settling culture
GSD –
   genetically signficant dose
   glycogen storage disease
GSE –
   general somatic efferent
   gluten-sensitive enteropathy
GSH –
   glomerular-stimulating hor-
      mone
   reduced glutathione
GSR –
   galvanic skin response
   generalized Shwartzman reac-
      tion
GSSG – oxidized glutathione
GSSR – generalized Sanarelli-
   Shwartzman reaction

GSW – gunshot wound
GT –
   generation time
   genetic therapy
   gingiva treatment
   glucose tolerance
   glutamyl transpeptidase
   group therapy
G & T – gowns and towels
g/t –
   granulation time
   granulation tissue
gt. – gutta [L] drop
GTD – gestational trophoblastic
   disease
GTF – glucose tolerance factor
GTH – gonadotropic hormone
GTN –
   glomerulo-tubulo-nephritis
   glyceryl trinitrate
GTP –
   glutamyl transpeptidase
   guanosine triphosphate
GTR – granulocyte turnover rate
GTT – glucose tolerance test
gtt. – guttae [L] drops
GU –
   gastric ulcer
   genitourinary
   glycogenic unit
   gonococcal urethritis
   gravitational ulcer
GUS – genitourinary system
guttat. – guttatim [L] drop by
   drop
gutt. quibusd. – guttis quibusdam
   [L] with a few drops
GV – gentian violet
GVA – general visceral afferent
GVE – general visceral efferent
GVH – graft versus host
GVHR – graft-versus-host reaction

GW −
  glycerine in water
  group work
GXT − graded exercise test

Gy. − gray
gyn. − gynecology
GZ − Guilford-Zimmerman personality test

H −
  enthalpy
  haustus [L] a draft
  height
  henry
  heroin
  high
  Holzknecht unit
  homosexual
  hora [L] hour
  horizontal
  hormone
  Hounsfield unit
  human
  hydrogen
  hyoscine
  hypermetropia
  hypodermic
  magnetic field strength
H^+ − hydrogen ion
$[H^+]$ − hydrogen ion concentration
H_1 − alternative hypothesis
^1H, H1, H^1 or hydrogen-1 − protium (ordinary, or light, hydrogen)
^2H, H2, H^2 or hydrogen-2 − deuterium (heavy hydrogen)
^3H, H3, H^3 or hydrogen-3 − tritium
H −
  Hauch [Ger] (motile microorganism)

H (continued)
  oersted (unit of magnetizing force)
H. − Hemophilus
h −
  hecto-
  height
  hora [L] hour
  horizontal
  Planck's constant
  quantum constant
HA −
  headache
  height age
  hemadsorbent
  hemagglutinating antibody
  hemagglutination
  hemolytic anemia
  hepatic artery
  hepatitis-associated (virus)
  high anxiety
  hospital admission
  Hounsfield unit
  hydroxyapatite
Ha − hahnium
HAA −
  hemolytic anemia antigen
  hepatitis-associated antigen
HABA − hydroxybenzeneazobenzoic acid
HABF − hepatic artery blood flow
HAD − hemadsorption

HAE — hereditary angioedema
HAGG — hyperimmune antivariola gamma globulin
HAHTG — horse antihuman thymus globulin
HAI —
  hemagglutination inhibition
  hemagglutinin inhibition
hal. — halothane
H and E staining — hematoxylin and eosin staining
H and P — history and physical
H and V — hemigastrectomy and vagotomy
HANE — hereditary angioneurotic edema
HAP —
  heredopathia atactica polyneuritiformis
  histamine phosphate acid
HAPA — hemagglutinating antipenicillin antibody
HAPC — hospital-acquired penetration contact
HASCVD — hypertensive arteriosclerotic cardiovascular disease
HASHD — hypertensive arteriosclerotic heart disease
haust. — haustus [L] a draft
HAV — hepatitis A virus
HB —
  heart block
  hepatitis B
  housebound
Hb — hemoglobin
Hb A — normal adult hemoglobin
Hb A_2 — minor fraction of adult hemoglobin
HBABA — hydroxybenzeneazobenzoic acid
HB Ag — hepatitis B antigen
HBB — hydroxybenzyl benzimidazole

Hb Barts — Bart's hemoglobin
HB_c — hepatitis B core
HB_cAb — hepatitis B core antibody
HB_cAg — hepatitis B core antigen
Hb CO — carboxyhemoglobin
HBD or HBDH — hydroxybutyrate dehydrogenase
HBE — His bundle electrogram
HB_eAb — hepatitis B e antibody
HB_eAg — hepatitis B e antigen
HBF — hepatic blood flow
Hb F — fetal hemoglobin
HBI — high serum-bound iron
HBIG — hepatitis B immune globulin
Hb M — hemoglobin M
HBO — hyperbaric oxygen
H_3BO_3 — boric acid
HbO_2 — oxyhemoglobin
HBP — high blood pressure
HbP — primitive hemoglobin
HBr — hydrobromic acid
Hb S — sickle cell hemoglobin
HB_s — hepatitis B surface
HB_sAb — hepatitis B surface antibody
HB_sAg — hepatitis B surface antigen
HBSS — Hank's balanced salt solution
HBV — hepatitis B virus
HBW — high birth weight
HC —
  hair cell
  handicapped
  head circumference
  head compression
  heart cycle
  hepatic catalase
  hospital corps
  house call
  Huntington's chorea

HC (*continued*)
   hyaline casts
   hydrocarbon
   hydrocortisone
   hydroxycorticoid
HCC — hydroxycholecalciferol
HCD — heavy chain disease
HCF — highest common factor
hCG — human chorionic gonadotropin
hCG-α subunit — chorionic gonadotropin–alpha subunit
hCG-β subunit — chorionic gonadotropin–beta subunit
HCH — 1,2,3,4,5,6-hexachlorocyclohexane
HCHO — formaldehyde
HCl —
   hydrochloric acid
   hydrogen chloride
HCN — hydrocyanic acid
HCO_3 — the bicarbonate radical
H_2CO_3 — carbonic acid
HCP —
   hepatocatalase peroxidase
   hereditary coproporphyria
HCR — hydrochloric acid
H.C.S. — Harvey Cushing Society
17-HCS — 17-hydroxycorticosteroids
hCS or hCSM — human chorionic somatomammotropin
HCT —
   homocytotropic
   human chorionic placental thyrotropin
   hydrochlorothiazide
Hct. — hematocrit
HCTZ — hydrochlorothiazide
HCU — homocystinuria
HCVD — hypertensive cardiovascular disease

HD —
   Hansen's disease
   hearing distance
   heart disease
   hemodialysis
   herniated disc
   high density
   high dosage
   hip disarticulation
   Hodgkin's disease
   hydatid disease
HD_{50} — hemolyzing dose of complement that lyses 50 per cent of a suspension of sensitized red blood cells
h.d. — hora decubitus [L] at bedtime
HDA — hydroxy dopamine
HDBD — hydroxybutyric dehydrogenase
HDC — histidine decarboxylase
HDH — heart disease history
HDL — high density lipoprotein
HDLW — distance at which a watch is heard by the left ear
HDN —
   hemolytic disease of the newborn
   high density nebulizer
HDP —
   hexose diphosphate
   hydroxydimethylpyrimidine
HDRV — human diploid cell strain rabies vaccine
HDRW — distance at which a watch is heard by the right ear
HDS — herniated disk syndrome
HDU — hemodialysis unit
HE —
   hereditary elliptocytosis
   human enteric
H & E — hematoxylin and eosin (stain)

He – helium
HEAT – human erythrocyte agglutination test
hebdom. – hebdomada [L] a week
HEC – hydroxyergocalciferol
HED – Haut-Einheits-Dosis [Ger] roentgen-ray dosage
HEENT – head, eyes, ears, nose and throat
HEK –
    human embryo kidney (cell culture)
    human embryonic kidney
HEL – human embryo lung (cell culture)
hematol. – hematology
hemocyt. – hemocytometer
hemorr. – hemorrhage
HEMPAS – hereditary erythroblastic multinuclearity with a positive acidified serum
HEPA – high-efficiency particulate air (filter)
herb. recent. – herbarium recentium [L] fresh herbs
HES – hydroxyethyl starch
HET – helium equilibration time
HETP –
    height equivalent to a theoretical plate
    hexaethyltetraphosphate
H.E.W. – Health, Education and Welfare
HF –
    Hageman factor (coagulation factor XII)
    hay fever
    heart failure
    hemorrhagic fever
    high flow
    high frequency
Hf – hafnium

HFC – hard filled capsules
HFI – hereditary fructose intolerance
HFP – hexafluoropropylene
Hfr – high frequency of recombination
hFSH – human follicle-stimulating hormone
HFT – high frequency transduction
Hg – hydrargyrum [L] mercury
hg. – hectogram
HGA – homogentisic acid
Hgb. – hemoglobin
$HgCl_2$ – corrosive mercuric chloride
Hg_2Cl_2 – mild mercurous chloride
HGF – hyperglycemic-glycogenolytic factor (glucagon)
Hg F – fetal hemoglobin
hGG – human gammaglobulin
hGH – human growth hormone
HgI_2 – mercuric iodide
Hg_2I_2 – mercurous iodide
$Hg(NO_3)_2$ – mercuric nitrate
HGO – hepatic glucose output
HgO – mercuric oxide
Hg_2O – mercurous oxide
HGPRT – hypoxanthine guanine phosphoribosyl transferase
hgt. – height
HH – hydroxyhexamide
H & H – hemoglobin and hematocrit
HHA – hereditary hemolytic anemia
HHb – un-ionized hemoglobin
HHD – hypertensive heart disease
HHHO – hypotonia-hypomentia-hypogonadism-obesity
H. + Hm. – compound hypermetropic astigmatism

HHNK — hyperglycemic, hyper-osmolar, nonketotic (coma)
HHT —
hereditary hemorrhagic telangiectasia
12-L-hydroxy-5,8,10-hepta-decatrienoic acid
HI —
hemagglutination inhibition
high impulsiveness
hydriodic acid
hydroxyindole
Hi — histidine
HIA — hemagglutination-inhibi-tion antibody
5-HIAA — 5-hydroxyindoleacetic acid
HiCN — cyanmethemoglobin
HID — headache, insomnia, de-pression (syndrome)
HIg — human immunoglobulin
HIHA — high impulsiveness, high anxiety
HiHb — hemiglobin
HILA — high impulsiveness, low anxiety
HIO_3 — iodic acid
HIOMT — hydroxyindole-O-methyl transferase
HIP — hydrostatic indifference point
Hippuran-^{131}I — iodohippurate
His — histidine
hist. — histology
HIT —
hemagglutination-inhibition test
hypertrophic infiltrative tendinitis
HJ — Howell-Jolly (bodies)
HJR — hepatojugular reflex
HK —
heat-killed

HK (continued)
heel-to-knee
hexokinase
HKLM — heat-killed Listeria monocytogenes
HL —
half life
hearing level
hearing loss
histiocytic lymphoma
histocompatibility locus
hypertrichosis lanuginosa
H/L — hydrophile/lipophile
H & L — heart and lungs
Hl — latent hyperopia
HLA —
homologous leukocytic anti-bodies
human leukocyte antigen
human lymphocyte antigen
HLDH — heat-stable lactic dehy-drogenase
hLH — human luteinizing hor-mone
HLK — heart, liver, kidney
HLP — hyperlipoproteinemia
HLR — heart-lung resuscitator
hLT — human lymphocyte trans-formation
hlth. — health
HLV — herpes-like virus
HM —
hand movement(s)
heart murmur
human milk
hydatidiform mole
Hm. — manifest hyperopia
hm — hectometer
HMB — homatropine methyl bro-mide
HMC —
heroin, morphine, cocaine
hydroxymethyl cytosine

HMD − hyaline membrane disease

HME − heat and moisture exchanger

HMF − hydroxymethylfurfural

HMG − hydroxymethylglutaryl

hMG − human menopausal gonadotropin

hML − human milk lysozyme

HMM − hexamethylolmelamine

HMMA − 4-hydroxy-3-methoxymandelic acid

HMO −
Health Maintenance Organization
heart minute output

HMP −
hexose monophosphate
hexose monophosphate pathway
hot moist packs

HMPA − hexamethylphosphoramide

HMPG − 4-hydroxy-3-methoxyphenylethylene glycol

HMPS − hexose monophosphate shunt

HMSAS − hypertrophic muscular subaortic stenosis

hMT − human molar thyrotropin

HMU − hydroxymethyl uracil

HMW − high molecular weight

HMX − heat-massage-exercise

HN −
hereditary nephritis
hilar node

HN_2 − nitrogen mustard, mechlorethamine

h.n. − hoc nocte [L] tonight

HNB − hydroxynitrobenzylbromide

HNC − hypothalamic-neurohypophyseal complex

HNO_2 − nitrous acid

HNO_3 − nitric acid

HNP − herniated nucleus pulposus

hnRNA − heterogeneous nuclear RNA

HNSHA − hereditary nonspherocytic hemolytic anemia

HNV − has not voided

HO −
high oxygen
hyperbaric oxygen

H/O − history of

H_2O − water

H_2O_2 − hydrogen peroxide

Ho − holmium

H_o − null hypothesis

HOB − head of bed

HOC − hydroxycorticoid

HOCM − hypertrophic obstructive cardiomyopathy

hoc vesp. − hoc vespere [L] this evening

HOD − hyperbaric oxygen drenching

HOH − hard of hearing

Homeo. − homeopathy

homo. − homosexual

HOOD − hereditary osteo-onychodysplasia

HOP − high oxygen pressure

hor. decub. − hora decubitus [L] at bedtime

hor. interm. − horis intermediis [L] at the intermediate hours

hor. som. − hora somni [L] at bedtime

hor. un. spatio. − horae unius spatio [L] at the end of one hour

HOS − human osteosarcoma

H_2OsO_4 − osmic acid

hosp. − hospital

HOT — human old tuberculin
HP —
  high potency
  high power
  high pressure
  high protein
  House Physician
  human pituitary
  hydrostatic pressure
  hyperphoria
H & P — history and physical
Hp. — haptoglobin
HPA —
  human papilloma virus
  hypothalamic-pituitary-
    adrenal
HPAA — hydroxyphenylacetic
  acid
HPC — hydroxyphenyl-cincho-
  ninic acid
HPE — history and physical examination
HPF — heparin-precipitable fraction
hpf — high-power field
HPFH — hereditary persistence of
  fetal hemoglobin
hPFSH — human pituitary follicle-
  stimulating hormone
hPG — human pituitary gonadotropin
HPI — history of present illness
hPL — human placental lactogen
HPLA — hydroxyphenyllactic
  acid
HPLC — high-pressure liquid
  chromatography
HPO — high-pressure oxygen
HPO_3 — metaphosphoric acid
H_3PO_2 — hypophosphorous acid
H_3PO_3 — phosphorous acid
H_3PO_4 —
  orthophosphoric acid

H_3PO_4 (*continued*)
  phosphoric acid
$H_4P_2O_6$ — hypophosphoric acid
$H_4P_2O_7$ — pyrophosphoric acid
HPP — hydroxypyrazolopyrimi-
  dine
HPPA — hydroxyphenylpyruvic
  acid
HPPH — hydroxyphenyl-phenyl-
  hydantoin
hPr — human prolactin
HPS —
  hematoxylin-phloxine-saffron
  high protein supplement
  hypertrophic pyloric stenosis
HPT — hyperparathyroidism
hPT — human placental thyrotropin
HPV — *Hemophilus pertussis* vaccine
HPVD — hypertensive pulmonary
  vascular disease
HPVG — hepatic portal venous gas
HR —
  heart rate
  hospital record
  hospital report
H & R — hysterectomy and radiation
Hr. — blood type factor
hr. — hour
HRBC — horse red blood cells
HRE — high-resolution electrocardiogram
HRIG — human rabies immune
  globulin
HRL — head rotated left
HRR — head rotated right
HRS — Hamilton Rating Scale
HRT — heart rate
HS —
  half strength
  heart sounds

HS (*continued*)
    heat-stable
    heme synthetase
    hereditary spherocytosis
    herpes simplex
    homologous serum
    horse serum
    House Surgeon
    Hurler's syndrome
H & S — hysterectomy and sterilization
H_2S — hydrogen sulfide
h.s. — hora somni [L] at bedtime
HSA —
    human serum albumin
    hypersomnia-sleep apnea syndrome
HS-Co A — reduced coenzyme A
HSD — hydroxysteroid dehydrogenase
HSG —
    herpes simplex genitalis
    hysterosalpingogram
H_2SiO_3 — metasilicic acid
H_4SiO_4 — orthosilicic acid
HSL — herpes simplex labialis
H_2SO_3 — sulfurous acid
H_2SO_4 — sulfuric acid
HSR — Harleco synthetic resin
HSV — herpes simplex virus
HSV I — herpes simplex virus I
HSV II — herpes simplex virus II
HT —
    hemagglutination titer
    histologic technician
    hydroxytryptamine
    hypermetropia, total
    hypertension
    hyperthyroidism
    hypodermic tablet
3-HT — hydroxytyramine
^{3}HT — tritiated thymidine
5-HT — 5-hydroxytryptamine (serotonin)

Ht. —
    heart
    total hyperopia
ht —
    heart tones
    height
    high tension
HTA — hydroxytryptamine
HTC — hepatoma cells
HTF — heterothyrotropic factors
HTH — homeostatic thymus hormone
HTHD — hypertensive heart disease
HTLV — human T cell leukemia-lymphoma virus
htn. — hypertension
HTOH — hydroxytryptophol
HTP — hydroxytryptophan
hTSH — human thyroid-stimulating hormone
HTV — herpes-type virus
HU —
    heat unit
    hemagglutinating unit
    hydroxyurea
    hyperemia unit
HUS —
    hemolytic-uremic syndrome
    hyaluronidase unit for semen
HUTHAS — human thymus antiserum
HV —
    hepatic vein
    herpes virus
    hospital visit
    hyperventilation
H & V — hemigastrectomy and vagotomy
HVA — homovanillic acid
HVD — hypertensive vascular disease

HVE — high-voltage electrophoresis
HVG — host versus graft
HVH — herpes virus hominis
HVL — half-value layer
HVM — high-velocity missile
HVSD — hydrogen-detected ventricular septal defect
HWS — hot water–soluble
Hx. — history
Hy. —
    hypermetropia
    hyperopia

hy. — hysteria
Hyp — hydroxyproline
hyper. T & A — hypertrophy of tonsils and adenoids
hypo. —
    hypochromia
    hypodermic (injection)
    under
hys. — hysteria
hyster. — hysterectomy
HZ — herpes zoster
Hz. — hertz

I

I —
    electric current
    inosine
    intensity of magnetism
    iodine
    ionic strength
    moment of inertia
    permanent incisor
^{125}I, ^{130}I, ^{131}I, ^{132}I — radioactive iodine
i — isochromosome
i. —
    deciduous incisor
    insoluble
    optically inactive
I, ι — iota (ninth letter of the Greek alphabet)
IA —
    impedance angle
    internal auditory
    intra-aortic
    intra-arterial
    intra-atrial
IAA — indole-3-acetic acid

Ia antigen — immune response gene-associated antigen
IABP — intra-aortic balloon pump
IAC — internal auditory canal
IADH — inappropriate antidiuretic hormone
IADHS — inappropriate antidiuretic hormone syndrome
IAE — intra-atrial electrocardiogram
I.A.E.A. — International Atomic Energy Agency
IAFI — infantile amaurotic familial idiocy
I.A.G.P. — International Association of Geographic Pathology
I.A.G.U.S. — International Association of Genito-Urinary Surgeons
IAHD — idiopathic acquired hemolytic disease
IAM —
    internal acoustic meatus
    internal auditory meatus

IAO –
    immediately after onset
    intermittent aortic occlusion
I.A.P. – International Academy
    of Pathology
I.A.P.B. – International Association for Prevention of Blindness
I.A.P.P. – International Association for Preventive Pediatrics
I.A.R.C. – International Agency for Research on Cancer
IAS –
    interatrial septum
    intra-amniotic saline (infusion)
IASD – interatrial septal defect
IAT –
    invasive activity test
    iodine-azide test
IB –
    immune body
    inclusion body
ib. – ibidem [L] in the same place
IBB – intestinal brush border
IBC – iron-binding capacity
IBF – immunoglobulin-binding factor
IBI – intermittent bladder irrigation
IBP – iron-binding protein
IBR – infectious bovine rhinotracheitis
IBS – irritable bowel syndrome
IBT – isatin-beta-thiosemicarbasone
IBU – international benzoate unit
IBV – infectious bronchitis vaccine
IBW – ideal body weight
IC –
    inspiratory capacity
    integrated circuit
    intensive care

IC (*continued*)
    intercostal
    intermediate care
    intermittent claudication
    internal capsule
    International Classification
    interstitial cells
    intracardiac
    intracarotid
    intracavitary
    intracellular
    intracerebral
    intracranial
    intracutaneous
    irritable colon
    isovolumic contraction
i.c. – inter cibos [L] between meals
ICA –
    internal carotid artery
    intracranial aneurysm
ICAO – internal carotid artery occlusion
ICBP – intracellular binding proteins
ICC –
    immunocompetent cells
    Indian childhood cirrhosis
    intensive coronary care
ICCU – intensive coronary care unit
ICD –
    intrauterine contraceptive device
    isocitrate dehydrogenase
I.C.D. – International Classification of Diseases (of the World Health Organization)
I.C.D.A. – International Classification of Diseases, Adapted
ICDH – isocitric dehydrogenase
ICF –
    intensive care facility

ICF (*continued*)
    intracellular fluid
ICG —indocyanine green
ICH — infectious canine hepatitis
ICM — intercostal margin
I.C.N. — International Council of Nurses
I.C.N.N.D. — Interdepartmental Committee on Nutrition in National Defense
ICP — intracranial pressure (catheter)
I.C.R.P. — International Commission on Radiological Protection
I.C.R.U. — International Commission on Radiological Units and Measurements
ICS —
    impulse-conducting system
    intensive care, surgical
    intercostal space
I.C.S. — International College of Surgeons
ICSH — interstitial cell-stimulating hormone
I.C.S.H. — International Committee for Standardization in Hematology
I.C.S.P. — International Council of Societies of Pathology
ICT —
    indirect Coombs' test
    inflammation of connective tissue
    insulin coma therapy
    isovolumic contraction time
ict. ind. — icterus index
ICU — intensive care unit
ICW — intracellular water
ID —
    identification
    iditol dehydrogenase

ID (*continued*)
    immunodiffusion
    inclusion disease
    index of discrimination
    infant deaths
    infectious disease
    infective dose
    inhibitory dose
    inside diameter
    internal diameter
    intradermal
    intraduodenal
I & D — incision and drainage
ID_{50} — median infectious dose
id. — idem [L] the same
IDA —
    image display and analysis
    iron deficiency anemia
IDD — insulin-dependent diabetes mellitus
IDDM — insulin-dependent diabetes mellitus
IDI — induction-delivery interval
IDL — intermediate-density lipoprotein
IDM —
    idiopathic disease of the myocardium
    infant of diabetic mother
ID-MS — isotope dilution–mass spectrometry
IDP —
    immunodiffusion procedures
    initial dose period
    inosine diphosphate
    instantaneous diastolic pressure
IDPN — β-iminodipropionitrile
IDR — intradermal reaction
IDS — immunity deficiency state
IDU —
    idoxuridine
    iododeoxyuridine

IDV — intermittent demand ventilation

IDVC — indwelling venous catheter

IE — immunoelectrophoresis

I/E — inspiratory-expiratory ratio

I.E. — Immunitäts Einheit [Ger] immunizing unit

i.e. — id est [L] that is

IEA — intravascular erythrocyte aggregation

IEC —
  injection electrode catheter
  intraepothelial carcinoma

IEM — inborn error of metabolism

IEMG — integrated electromyogram

IEOP — immunoelectro-osmophoresis

IEP —
  immunoelectrophoresis
  isoelectric point

IF —
  immunofluorescence
  inhibiting factor
  interstitial fluid
  intrinsic factor

IFA — indirect fluorescent antibody (test)

IFC — intrinsic factor concentrate

I.F.C.C. — International Federation of Clinical Chemistry

IFR — inspiratory flow rate

IFRA — indirect fluorescent rabies antibody (test)

IFV — intracellular fluid volume

IG —
  immune globulin
  intragastric

Ig — immunoglobulin

IgA — gamma A immunoglobulin

IgD — gamma D immunoglobulin

IGDM — infant of gestational diabetic mother

IgE — gamma E immunoglobulin

IGFET — insulated gate field effect transistor

IgG — gamma G immunoglobulin

IGH —
  idiopathic growth hormone
  immunoreactive growth hormone

IgM — gamma M immunoglobulin

IGP — intestinal glycoprotein

IGV — intrathoracic gas volume

IH —
  infectious hepatitis
  inhibiting hormone
  inner half
  iron hematoxylin

IHA — indirect hemagglutination

IHBTD — incompatible hemolytic blood transfusion disease

IHC —
  idiopathic hypercalciuria
  inner hair cell

IHD — ischemic heart disease

IHO — idiopathic hypertrophic osteoarthropathy

IHP — idiopathic hypoparathyroidism

IHPH — intrahepatic portal hypertension

IHR —
  intrahepatic resistance
  intrinsic heart rate

I.H.S. — Indian Health Service

IHSA — iodinated human serum albumin

IHSS — idiopathic hypertrophic subaortic stenosis

IHT — intravenous histamine test

IID — insulin-independent diabetes mellitus

IIF − indirect immunofluorescent

III-para − tertipara

II-para − secundipara

IJP −
    inhibitory junction potential
    internal jugular pressure

IK − immunoconglutinin

I.K. − Immunekörper [Ger] immune body

IL − incisolingual

IL 1 − interleukin 1

IL 2 − interleukin 2

Il − illinium

ILA − insulin-like activity

I.L.A. − International Leprosy Association

ILa − incisolabial

ILB or ILBW − infant low birth weight

ILD −
    ischemic leg disease
    ischemic limb disease

Ileu. − isoleucine

IM −
    Index Medicus
    infectious mononucleosis
    Internal Medicine
    intramedullary
    intramuscularly

im- − (indicates presence of) NH group

IMA − internal mammary artery

I.M.A. − Industrial Medical Association

IMAA − iodinated macroaggregated albumin

IMB − intermenstrual bleeding

IMBC − indirect maximum breathing capacity

I.M.B.I. − Institute of Medical and Biological Illustrators

IMF − intermaxillary fixation

IMH − idiopathic myocardial hypertrophy

IMHP − 1-iodomercuri-2-hydroxypropane

IMI − intramuscular injection

IMP − inosine-5′-monophosphate

imp. −
    impression
    improved

IMPA − incisal mandibular plane angle

IMPS − Inpatient Multidimensional Psychiatric Scale

IMR − infant mortality rate

IMRAD − introduction, methods, results and discussion

IMS − incurred in military service

IMV − intermittent mandatory ventilation

IMViC tests − indole, methyl red, Voges-Proskauer, and citrate tests

IN −
    icterus neonatorum
    intranasal

In − indium

in. − inch

I.N.A. − International Neurological Association

INAD − infantile neuroaxonal dystrophy

INAH − isonicotinic acid hydrazide

inc. −
    increase
    incurred

incl. − including

incr. − increase

IND − Investigational New Drug

in d. − in dies [L] daily

ind. − independent

INDM − infant of nondiabetic mother

Ind. Med. – Index Medicus
INE – infantile necrotizing encephalomyelopathy
inf. –
  infant
  infected
  inferior
  infunde [L] pour in
  infusum [L] infusion
inf. mono. – infectious mononucleosis
info. – information
ing. – inguinal
InGP – indolglycerophosphate
INH –
  isoniazid
  isonicotinic acid hydrazide
  isonicotinoylhydrazine
inj. –
  inject
  injury
inj. enem. – injiciatur enema [L] let an enema be injected
inl. – inlay
I.N.N. – International Nonproprietary Names
INO – intranuclear ophthalmoplegia
inoc. – inoculate
INPH – iproniazid phosphate
INPV – intermittent negative-pressure assisted ventilation
INS – idiopathic nephrotic syndrome
inspir. –
  inspiration
  inspiratory
int. –
  intermediate
  intermittent
  internal
int. cib. – inter cibos [L] between meals

int. med. – internal medicine
int. noct. –inter noctem [L] during the night
int. obst. – intestinal obstruction
inv. –
  inversion
  involuntary
IO –
  incisal opening
  inferior oblique
  internal os
  intestinal obstruction
  intraocular
I/O – input/output
I & O –
  in and out
  intake and output
Io – ionium
IOFB – intraocular foreign body
IOL – intraocular lenses
IOP – intraocular pressure
IOU – intensive therapy observation unit
IP –
  incisoproximal
  incubation period
  inosine phosphorylase
  instantaneous pressure
  interphalangeal
  intraperitoneal
  isoelectric point
I.P.A.A.– International Psychoanalytical Association
I-para – primipara
IPC – isopropyl chlorophenyl
IPD – inflammatory pelvic disease
IPG – impedance plethysmograph
IPH – idiopathic pulmonary hemosiderosis
IPL – intrapleural
IPP –
  intermittent positive pressure
  intrapleural pressure

IPPB — intermittent positive-pressure breathing

IPPI — interruption of pregnancy for psychiatric indication

IPPO — intermittent positive-pressure inflation with oxygen

IPPR — intermittent positive-pressure respiration

IPPV — intermittent positive-pressure ventilation

IPQ — intimacy potential quotient

IPRT — interpersonal reaction test

IPS — initial prognostic score

IPSID — immunoproliferative small intestinal disease

IPSP — inhibitory postsynaptic potential

IPTG — isopropyl thiogalactoside

IPU — inpatient unit

IPV —
    inactivated poliovaccine
    infectious pustular vaginitis

IQ — intelligence quotient

IR —
    immunoreactive
    index of response
    inferior rectus
    infrared
    intelligence ratio
    internal resistance

Ir — iridium

IRBBB — incomplete right bundle branch block

IRC — inspiratory reserve capacity

IRDS —
    idiopathic respiratory distress syndrome
    infant respiratory distress syndrome

IRG — immunoreactive glucagon

IRHCS — immunoradioassayable human chorionic somatomammotropin

IRhGH — immunoreactive human growth hormone

IRI — immunoreactive insulin

I.R.I.S. — International Research Information Service

IRM — innate releasing mechanism

IRMA —
    immunoradiometric assay
    intraretinal microangiopathy
    intraretinal microvascular abnormalities

irr. — irradiation

irrig. — irrigation

IRS — infrared spectrophotometry

IRSA — idiopathic refractory sideroblastic anemia

IRV — inspiratory reserve volume

IS —
    immune serum
    intercostal space
    interspace
    intraspinal

ISA — iodinated serum albumin

ISA_5 — internal surface area of lung at volume of 5 liters

ISADH — inappropriate secretion of antidiuretic hormone

IS and R — information storage and retrieval

ISC — irreversibly sickled cell

I.S.C.L.T. — International Society for Clinical Laboratory Technology

I.S.C.P. — International Society of Comparative Pathology

ISD or ISDN — isosorbide dinitrate

ISE — ion-selective electrode

ISF — interstitial fluid

ISG — immune serum globulin

I.S.G.E. — International Society of Gastroenterology

ISH — icteric serum hepatitis

I.S.H. – International Society of Hematology

I.S.M. – International Society of Microbiologists

I.S.O. – International Standards Organization

iso. – isoproterenol

ISP –
interspace
interspinal

i.s.q. – in status quo [L] unchanged

IST –
insulin sensitivity test
insulin shock therapy

I.S.U. – International Society of Urology

ISW – interstitial water

IT –
implantation test
inhalation test
inhalation therapy
intensive therapy
intradermal test
intrathecal
intrathoracic
intratracheal
intratracheal tube
intratumoral
isomeric transition

I.T.A. – International Tuberculosis Association

ITC – imidazolyl-thioguanine chemotherapy

ITLC – instant thin-layer chromatography

ITP –
idiopathic thrombocytopenic purpura
inosine triphosphate

ITPA – Illinois Test of Psycholinguistic Abilities

ITT – insulin tolerance test

ITU – intensive therapy unit

IU –
immunizing unit
International Unit (of hormone activity)
intrauterine
in utero

I.U.B. – International Union of Biochemistry

IUCD – intrauterine contraceptive device

IUD –
intrauterine death
intrauterine device

IUDR – 5-iododeoxyuridine

IUFB – intrauterine foreign body

IUGR – intrauterine growth rate

IUM – intrauterine fetally malnourished

I.U.P.A.C. – International Union of Pure and Applied Chemistry

IUT – intrauterine transfusion

IV –
interventricular
intervertebral
intravascular
intravenous
intraventricular
intravertebral
invasive
in vitro
in vivo

i.v. – iodine value

IVag – intravaginal

IVAP – in vivo adhesive platelet

IVC –
inferior vena cava
intravenous cholangiogram
isovolumic contraction

IVCC – intravascular consumption coagulopathy

IVCD — intraventricular conduction defect
IVCP — inferior vena cava pressure
IVCV — inferior venacavography
IVD — intervertebral disk
IVF — intravascular fluid
IVGTT — intravenous glucose tolerance test
IVH — intraventricular hemorrhage
IVJC — intervertebral joint complex
IVM — intravascular mass
IVP —
 intravenous push
 intravenous pyelogram
 intravenous pyelography
IVPB — intravenous piggyback

IVPF — isovolume pressure flow curve
IVR — isovolumic relaxation time
IVS — interventricular septum
IVSD — interventricular septal defect
IVT — intravenous transfusion
IVTTT — intravenous tolbutamide tolerance test
IVU —
 intravenous urogram
 intravenous urography
IWL — insensible water loss
IWMI — inferior wall myocardial infarction
IYS — inverted Y-suspensor
IZS — insulin zinc suspension

J

J — Joule's equivalent
J. —
 Jewish
 joint
 journal
 juice
JAI — juvenile amaurotic idiocy
J.A.M.A. — Journal of the American Medical Association
jaund. — jaundice
JBE — Japanese B encephalitis
J.C.A.E. — Joint Committee on Atomic Energy
J.C.A.H. — Joint Commission on Accreditation of Hospitals
jct. — junction
JEE — Japanese equine encephalitis
jej. — jejunum

JEMBEC — agar plates used for transportation of cultures of gonococci
JFET — junction field effect transistor
J.F.S. — Jewish Family Service
JG — juxtaglomerular
JGA — juxtaglomerular apparatus
JGC — juxtaglomerular cell
JGI —
 juxtaglomerular granulation index
 juxtaglomerular index
JJ — jaw jerk
JND — just noticeable difference
jnt. — joint
JODM — juvenile onset diabetes mellitus
JPC — junctional premature contraction

JPS — joint position sense
J.P.S.A. — Joint Program for the Study of Abortions
JRA — juvenile rheumatoid arthritis
JS unit — Junkman-Schoeller unit

jt. — joint
juv. — juvenile
JV —
    jugular vein
    jugular venous
JVP — jugular venous pulse

K —
    absolute zero
    calix
    capsular antigen
    electrostatic capacity
    equilibrium constant
    ionization constant
    kalium [L] potassium
    kathode (cathode)
    Kell blood system
    Kelvin
    kidney
    lysine
    potassium (kalium)
    1000, 1024 (in computer technology)
$K\Omega$ — kilohm
K-10 — gastric tube
17-K — 17-ketosteroids
k —
    Boltzmann constant
    constant
    kilo- [Gr] thousand
k — magnetic susceptibility
K, κ — kappa (tenth letter of the Greek alphabet)
κ —
    magnetic susceptibility
    one of the two immunoglobulin light chains
KA —
    ketoacidosis

KA (*continued*)
    King-Armstrong (units)
K_a — acid ionization constant
Ka. — kathode (cathode)
Kal. — kalium [L] potassium
KAP — knowledge, attitudes and practice
K/A ratio — ratio of ketogenic to antiketogenic substances
kat. — katal
KAU — King-Armstrong units
KB — ketone bodies
K_b — base ionization constant
kb — kilobase
kbp — kilobase pair
KBr — potassium bromide
KC — kathodal (cathodal) closing
kc. — kilocycle
kcal. — kilocalorie
KCC — kathodal (cathodal) closing contraction
KCG — kinetocardiogram
$KC_2H_3O_2$ — potassium acetate
KCl — potassium chloride
$KClO_3$ — potassium chlorate
KCNS — potassium thiocyanate
K_2CO_3 — potassium carbonate
kc.p.s. — kilocycles per second
KCS — keratoconjunctivitis sicca
KCT — kathodal (cathodal) closing tetanus

KD — kathodal (cathodal) duration

K_d — dissociation constant

KDT — kathodal (cathodal) duration tetanus

KE —
Kensall's compound E
kinetic energy

K_e — exchangeable body potassium

keto — 17-ketosteroid test

keV. — kilo electron volt

kf. — flocculation speed in antigen-antibody reactions

KFAB — kidney-fixing antibody

KFD — Kyasanur Forest disease

KFS — Klippel-Feil syndrome

αKG — alpha-ketoglutarate

kg. — kilogram

kg.-cal. — kilogram-calorie

kg.-m. — kilogram-meter

kg.p.s. — kilogram per second

KGS — ketogenic steroid

$KHCO_3$ — potassium bicarbonate

kHz. — kilohertz

KI —
karyopyknotic index
Krönig's isthmus
potassium iodide

KIA — Kliger iron agar

kilo. — a thousand

KIU — kallikrein-inhibiting unit

kJ — kilojoule

k.j. — knee jerk

k.k. — knee kick

kl. —
kiloliter
Klang [Ger] musical overtone

KL bac. — Klebs-Löffler bacillus

Kleb. — *Klebsiella*

KLH — keyhole-limpet hemocyanin

KLS — kidney, liver, spleen

KM — kanamycin

K_m — Michaelis constant

km. — kilometer

kMc. — kilomegacycle

kMc.p.s. — kilomegacycles per second

KMEF — keratin, myosin, epidermin, fibrin

$KMnO_4$ — potassium permanganate

km.p.s. — kilometers per second

KMV — killed measles virus vaccine

kn. — knee

KNO_3 — potassium nitrate

KO — knocked out

KOC — kathodal (cathodal) opening contraction

KOH — potassium hydroxide

KP —
keratitic precipitates
keratitis punctata

K-P — Kaiser-Permanente (diet)

kPa. — kilopascal

KPI — karyopyknotic index

K_3PO_3 — normal ortho- or tribasic potassium phosphate

KPTI — Kunitz pancreatic trypsin inhibitor

KPTT — kaolin partial thromboplastin time

Kr — krypton

KRB — Krebs-Ringer bicarbonate buffer

KRP —
Kolmer's test with Reiter protein
Krebs-Ringer phosphate

KRPS — Krebs-Ringer phosphate buffer solution

KS —
ketosteroid
Klinefelter's syndrome

KS (*continued*)
    Kveim-Siltzbach (test)
K_2SO_4 – potassium sulfate
K_{sp} – potassium solubility product
KTSA – Kahn Test of Symbol
    Arrangement
KU – Karmen units
KUB – kidney, ureter and bladder
KUS – kidney, ureter and spleen
KV – killed vaccine
kV. – kilovolt
kVA – kilovolt-ampere

kV.c.p. – kilovolt constant potential
KVO – keep vein open
kVp. – kilovolt peak
KW –
    Keith-Wagener (test)
    Kimmelstiel-Wilson (syndrome)
kW. – kilowatt
KWB – Keith, Wagener, Barker
    (classification)
kW.-hr. – kilowatt-hour

L

L –
    angular momentum
    coefficient of induction
    inductance
    Lambert
    Latin
    left
    length
    lethal
    leucine
    lewisite
    liber [L] book
    libra [L] pound
    ligament
    light sense
    lilac
    limes (boundary)
    lingual
    liter
    liver
    low
    lower
    lumbar
L_o – limes nul (neutralized toxin-antitoxin mixture)
L+ – limes tod (fatal dose toxin-antitoxin mixture)

L_1, L_2 – first lumbar vertebra or
    nerve, second, etc.
L. –
    Lactobacillus
    Leishmania
L – chemical prefix
l- – levo
l. –
    length
    liter
Λ, λ – lambda (11th letter of the
    Greek alphabet)
λ – decay constant
LA –
    lactic acid
    latex agglutination
    left atrial
    left atrium
    left auricle
    leucine aminopeptidase
    linguoaxial
    local anesthesia
    long-acting
    low anxiety
L & A – light and accommodation
La –
    labial

La (*continued*)
lanthanum
l.a. — lege artis [L] according to
the art
LAA — leukocyte ascorbic acid
LAAO — L-amino acid oxidase
lab. — laboratory
LAC — linguoaxiocervical
LaC — labiocervical
lac. — laceration
lact. — lactating
LAD —
lactic acid dehydrogenase
left anterior descending
left axis deviation
LADA — left acromio-dorso-
anterior
LADP — left acromio-dorso-
posterior
LAE — left atrial enlargement
laev. — laevus [L] left
LAF — laminar air flow
LAG —
labiogingival
linguoaxiogingival
lymphangiogram
LaG — labiogingival
lag. — lagena [L] a flask
LAH —
lactalbumin hydrolysate
left atrial hypertrophy
LaI — labioincisal
LAIT — latex agglutination-
inhibition test
LaL — labiolingual
lam. —
laminectomy
laminogram
LAO — left anterior oblique
L.A.O. — Licentiate in Obstetric
Science
LAP —
left atrial pressure

LAP (*continued*)
leucine aminopeptidase
leukocyte alkaline phosphatase
lyophilized anterior pituitary
lap. — laparotomy
lapid. — lapideum [L] stony
LAR — left arm recumbent
LARC — leucocyte automatic
recognition computer
LAS —
linear alkylate sulfonate
local adaptation syndrome
LASER — light amplification by
stimulated emission of radiation
lat. — lateral
lat. admov. — lateri admoveatum
[L] let it be applied to the
side
lat. dol. — lateri dolenti [L] to
the painful side
LATS — long-acting thyroid stimulator
LATS-p — long-acting thyroid
stimulator protector
lax. — laxative
LB —
laboratory
lipid body
live births
loose body
low back
lb. — libra [L] pound
LBB — left bundle branch
LBBB — left bundle branch block
LBCD — left border of cardiac
dullness
LBD — left border of dullness
LBF — *Lactobacillus bulgaricus*
factor
LBH — length, breadth, height
LBI — low serum-bound iron
LBM — lean body mass

LBNP — lower-body negative pressure

LBP —
low back pain
low blood pressure

LBW — low birth weight

LBWI — low birth weight infant

LBWR — lung-body weight ratio

LC —
Laennec's cirrhosis
lethal concentration
linguocervical
lipid cytosomes
living children
long-chain (triglycerides)

LCA — left coronary artery

LCAT — lecithin-cholesterol acyltransferase

LCCS — low cervical cesarean section

LCD — liquor carbonis detergens

LCFA — long-chain fatty acid

L.Ch. — Licentiate in Surgery

LCL —
Levinthal-Coles-Lillie (bodies)
lymphocytic leukemia
lymphocytic lymphosarcoma

LCM —
left costal margin
lowest common multiple
lymphatic choriomeningitis
lymphocytic choriomeningitis

L.C.M.E. — Liaison Committee on Medical Education

LCMG — long-chain monoglyceride

LCP — long-chain polysaturated (fatty acids)

L.C.P.S. — Licentiate of the College of Physicians and Surgeons

LCT — long-chain triglyceride

LD —
laboratory data

LD (continued)
labyrinthine defect
lactate dehydrogenase
lactic dehydrogenase
left deltoid
legionnaires' disease
lethal dose
light difference
linguodistal
living donor
low density
low dosage
lymphocyte-defined

L-D — Leishman-Donovan (bodies)

L/D — light-dark ratio

LD_{50} — median lethal dose

LDA —
left dorsoanterior
linear displacement analysis

LDD — light-dark discrimination

LDDS — local dentist

LDE — lauric diethamide

LDH — lactate dehydrogenase

LDL —
loudness discomfort level
low-density lipoprotein

LDLP — low-density lipoprotein

LDP — left dorsoposterior

LDUB — long double upright brace

LDV — lactic dehydrogenase virus

LE —
left eye
leukoerythrogenetic
lower extremity
lupus erythematosus

Le — Leonard (unit for cathode rays)

LE cell — lupus erythematosus cell

LED —
light-emitting diode
lupus erythematosus disseminatus

LEM — Leibovitz-Emory (median)

lenit. – leniter [L] gently
LEP – low egg passage
LES –
    Locke egg serum
    lower esophageal sphincter
    systemic lupus erythematosus
l.e.s. – local excitatory state
LET – linear energy transfer
leu. – leucine
leuk. – leukemia
lev. – levis [L] light
LF –
    laryngofissure
    low forceps
Lf – limit flocculation
lf. – low frequency
LFA – left femoral artery
L.F.A. – left frontoanterior
LFD –
    lactose-free diet
    least fatal dose
    low fat diet
    low forceps delivery
LFH – left femoral hernia
LFN – lactoferrin
L.F.P. – left frontoposterior
LFT –
    latex flocculation test
    liver function test
    low frequency transduction
L.F.T. – left frontotransverse
LG –
    laryngectomy
    left gluteal
    linguogingival
lg. – large
LGA – large for gestational age
LGB – Landry-Guillain-Barré
    (syndrome)
LGH – lactogenic hormone
LGN –
    lateral geniculate nucleus
    lobular glomerulonephritis

LGV – lymphogranuloma ven-
    ereum
LH –
    left hand
    left hyperphoria
    lower half
    lues hereditaria
    luteinizing hormone
LHC – left hypochondrium
LHF – left heart failure
LHL – left hepatic lobe
LHRF – luteinizing hormone–re-
    leasing factor
LH-RH – luteinizing hormone–re-
    leasing hormone
LHT – left hypertropia
LI –
    labeling index
    linguoincisal
    low impulsiveness
Li – lithium
LIA –
    leukemia-associated inhibitory
        activity
    lock-in amplifier
LIAFI – late infantile amaurotic
    familial idiocy
LIB – left in bottle
lib. – libra [L] a pound
LIBC – latent iron-binding capa-
    city
LiBr. – lithium bromide
LIC – limiting isorrheic concen-
    tration
LICM – left intercostal margin
Lic. Med. – Licentiate in Medicine
Li_2CO_3 – lithium carbonate
LICS – left intercostal space
LIF –
    left iliac fossa
    leukocyte inhibitory factor
lig. –
    ligament

lig. (*continued*)
    ligamentum
    ligation
ligg. –
    ligamenta
    ligaments
LIH – left inguinal hernia
LIHA – low impulsiveness, high anxiety
LILA – low impulsiveness, low anxiety
Li_2O – lithium oxide
LiOH – lithium hydroxide
LIQ – lower inner quadrant
liq. –
    liquid
    liquor
LIR – left iliac region
LIRBM – liver, iron, red bone marrow
LIS –
    left intercostal space
    lobular in situ
LISP – *List P*rocessing Language
LISS – low-ionic-strength medium test
LIV –
    law of initial value
    left innominate vein
LJM – Löwenstein-Jensen medium
LK – left kidney
LKS – liver, kidneys and spleen
LL –
    left leg
    left lower
    left lung
    lower lid
    lower lobe
    lysolecithin
LLB – long leg brace
LLBCD – left lower border of cardiac dullness

LLC –
    long leg cast
    lymphocytic leukemia, chronic
LLE – left lower extremity
LLF –
    Laki-Lorand factor
    left lateral femoral
LLL – left lower lobe
LLM – localized leukocyte mobilization
LLQ – left lower quadrant
LLR – left lumbar region
LM –
    legal medicine
    light microscopy
    light minimum
    linguomesial
    lipid-mobilizing (hormone)
    longitudinal muscle
    lower motor
L.M. –
    Licentiate in Medicine
    Licentiate in Midwifery
lm. – lumen
L.M.A. – left mentoanterior
LMCA – left middle cerebral artery
LMD –
    local medical doctor
    low molecular weight dextran
LMDX – low molecular weight dextran
LME – left mediolateral episiotomy
LMF – leukocyte mitogenic factor
LMM – light meromyosin
LMN – lower motor neuron
LMNL – lower motor neuron lesion
LMP – last menstrual period
L.M.P. – left mentoposterior

L.M.S. − Licentiate in Medicine and Surgery

L.M.S.S.A. − Licentiate in Medicine and Surgery of the Society of Apothecaries

L.M.T. − left mentotransverse

LMW − low molecular weight

LMWD − low molecular weight dextran

LN −
lipoid nephrosis
lupus nephritis
lymph node

L/N − letter-numerical (system)

ln − logarithm, natural

LNMP − last normal menstrual period

LNPF − lymph node permeability factor

LO −
linguo-occlusal
low

LOA − leave of absence

L.O.A. − left occipitoanterior

LOC −
level of consciousness
loss of consciousness

lo. cal. − low calorie

loc. cit. − loco citato [L] in the place quoted

loc. dol. − loco dolenti [L] to the painful spot

LOD − line of duty

log. − logarithm

L.O.L. − left occipitolateral

LOM −
limitation of motion
loss of motion

LOMSA − left otitis media suppurative acute

LOMSCh − left otitis media suppurative chronic

long. − longitudinal

L.O.P. − left occipitoposterior

LOPS − length of patient stay

LOQ − lower outer quadrant

LOS −
length of stay
low output syndrome

L.O.T. − left occipitotransverse

lot. − lotio [L] lotion

LOWBI − low birth weight infant

LP −
latency period
leukocyte-poor
light perception
linear programming
linguopulpal
lipoprotein
low power
low pressure
low protein
lumbar puncture
lymphoid plasma

L/P −
lactate-pyruvate ratio
liver to plasma concentration ratio
lymphocyte/polymorph ratio
lymph-plasma ratio

LPA − left pulmonary artery

LPC − late positive component

LPE − lipoprotein electrophoresis

LPF −
leukocytosis-promoting factor
localized plaque formation
lymphocytosis-promoting factor

lpf − low-power field

LPL − lipoprotein lipase

lpm − liters per minute

LPN − Licensed Practical Nurse

LPO −
left posterior oblique
light perception only

LPR − lactate-pyruvate ratio

LPS –
   lipase
   lipopolysaccharide
lps – liters per second
LPV –
   left pulmonary vein
   lymphopathia venereum
lpw – lumens per watt
Lp.-X – lipoprotein-X
LQ – lowest quadrant
LR –
   laboratory references
   labor room
   lactated Ringer's (solution)
   latency relaxation
   lateral rectus (muscle)
   light reaction
L/R – left to right ratio
L & R – left and right
L→R – left to right
Lr – lawrencium
LRF –
   latex and resorcinol formaldehyde
   liver residue factor
   luteinizing hormone–releasing factor
LRH – luteinizing hormone–releasing hormone
LRM – left radical mastectomy
LRQ – lower right quadrant
LRR – labyrinthine righting reflex
LRS – lactated Ringer's solution
LRT – lower respiratory tract
LS –
   left side
   legally separated
   liminal sensitivity
   liver and spleen
   lumbosacral
   lymphosarcoma
L.S. – Licentiate in Surgery

LSA – lymphosarcoma
L.S.A. – left sacroanterior
LSA/RCS – lymphosarcoma–reticulum cell sarcoma
LSB – left sternal border
LSC – liquid scintillation counting
L.Sc.A. – left scapuloanterior
L.Sc.P. – left scapuloposterior
LSCS – lower segment cesarean section
LSD –
   least significant digit
   lysergic acid diethylamide
LSD 25 – D-lysergic acid diethylamine tartrate 25
LSH – lymphocyte-stimulating hormone
LSI – large-scale integration
LSK – liver, spleen and kidneys
LSL – left sacrolateral
LSM –
   late systolic murmur
   lysergic acid morpholide
L.S.P. – left sacroposterior
L-sp. – lumbar spine
L.Sp. – left span
L/S ratio – lecithin-sphingomyelin ratio
L.S.T. – left sacrotransverse
LSU – lactose-saccharose-urea (agar)
LSV – left subclavian vein
LT –
   left thigh
   Levine tube
   levothyroxine
   long-term
   low temperature
   lymphotoxin
lt. – left
LTAS – lead tetra-acetate Schiff
LTB – laryngotracheobronchitis

LTC — long-term care
ltd. — limited
LTF —
    lipotrophic factor (or hormone)
    lymphocyte transforming factor
LTH —
    lactogenic hormone
    low temperature holding
    luteotropic hormone
lt. lat. — left lateral
LTPP — lipothiamide pyrophosphate
LTT — lymphoblastic transformation test
LU — left upper
L & U — lower and upper
Lu — lutetium
LUE — left upper extremity
Lues I — primary syphilis
Lues II — secondary syphilis
Lues III — tertiary syphilis
LUL — left upper lobe
lumb. — lumbar
LUO — left ureteral orifice
LUOQ — left upper outer quadrant
LUQ — left upper quadrant
lut. — luteum [L] yellow
LV —
    left ventricle
    leukemia virus
    live vaccine
    live virus
    lung volume
LV_D — left ventricular end-diastolic pressure
LVDP — left ventricular diastolic pressure
LVDV — left ventricular diastolic volume
LVE — left ventricular enlargement

LVED — left ventricular end-diastolic
LVEDC — left ventricular end-diastolic circumference
LVEDP — left ventricular end-diastolic pressure
LVEDV — left ventricular end-diastolic volume
LVEP — left ventricular end-diastolic pressure
LVET — left ventricular ejection time
LVF —
    left ventricular failure
    low-voltage fast
    low-voltage foci
LVH —
    large vessel hematocrit
    left ventricular hypertrophy
LVI — left ventricular insufficiency
LVN —
    Licensed Visiting Nurse
    Licensed Vocational Nurse
LVP —
    left ventricular pressure
    lysine-vasopressin
LVS — left ventricular strain
LV_S — mean left ventricular systolic pressure
LVSP — left ventricular systolic pressure
LVSV — left ventricular stroke volume
LVSW — left ventricular stroke work
LVT —
    left ventricular tension
    lysine vasotonin
LVW — left ventricular work
LVWI — left ventricular work index
LW —
    lacerating wound

LW (*continued*)
    Lee-White (method)
L & W – living and well
LX – local irradiation

lx. – lux
lymphs. – lymphocytes
Lys – lysine
lzm – lysozyme

M –
    mega-
    molar
    thousand
α_2M – alpha$_2$-macroglobulin
M_1 – mitral first heart sound
M_2 – mitral second heart sound
M. –
    male
    malignant
    married
    mature
    maximal
    meter
    methionine
    minim
    minute
    mix
    monocyte
    month
    morphine
    mother
    mucoid
    mucoid colony
    multipara
    murmur
    muscle
    myopia
    permanent molar
    strength of pole
M. –
    Micrococcus
    Microsporum
    Mycobacterium

M. (*continued*)
    Mycoplasma
m- – meta-
m. –
    deciduous molar
    macerare [L] macerate
    magnetic moment
    manipulus [L] a handful
    mass
    mean
    median
    mentum [L] chin
    mesial
    meter
    mil, milli [L] thousand
    milli-
    misce [L] mix
    mistura [L] mixture
    mitte [L] send
    motile
    sample mean
M, μ – mu (12th letter of the
    Greek alphabet)
μ –
    micro-
    micron
MA –
    mandelic acid
    mean arterial (blood pressure)
    medical audit
    menstrual age
    mental age
    meter angle
    Miller-Abbott (tube)

MA (*continued*)
  moderately advanced
  muscle activity
M.A. – Master of Arts
Ma – masurium
mA. –
  milliamperage
  milliampere
μA. – microampere
ma. –
  meter-angle
  milliampere
MAA – macroaggregated albumin
M.A.A.C. – Medical Assistants
  Advisory Council
M.A.B. – Metropolitan Asylums
  Board (British)
MABP – mean arterial blood pressure
MAC –
  malignancy-associated changes
  maximum allowable concentration
  minimum alveolar concentration
mac. – macerare [L] macerate
MAD –
  maximal acid output
  methylandrostenediol
  mind-altering drug
MAE – moves all extremities
MAF –
  macrophage activation factor
  minimum audible field
MAFH – macroaggregated ferrous
  hydroxide
mag. –
  magnification
  magnus [L] large
mag. cit. – magnesium citrate
MAggF – macrophage agglutination factor
magn. – magnus [L] large

MAL – midaxillary line
mal. – malum [L] ill
malig. – malignant
MAM – methylazomethanol
M+Am – myopic astigmatism
mam. – milliampere-minute
MAN-6-P – mannose-6-phosphate
man. –
  mane [L] morning
  manipulate
  manipulus [L] a handful
manip. –
  manipulation
  manipulus [L] a handful
MANOVA – multivariate analysis
  of variance
man. pr. – mane primo [L] early
  in the morning
MAO –
  maximal acid output
  monoamine oxidase
MAOI – monoamine oxidase inhibitor
MAP –
  mean aortic pressure
  mean arterial pressure
  megaloblastic anemia of pregnancy
  methylacetoxyprogesterone
  methylaminopurine
  minimum audible pressure
  muscle-action potential
MAPF – microatomized protein
  food
MAR – minimal angle resolution
MAS – Manifest Anxiety Scale
mAs. – milliampere-second
masc. – mass concentration
MASER –
  microwave amplification by
  stimulated emission of radiation

MASER (*continued*)
  molecular application by stimulated emission of radiation
M.A.S.H. – Mobile Army Surgical Hospital
mas. pil. – massa pilularum [L] pill mass
MAST – Military Anti-Shock Trousers
matut. – matutinus [L] in the morning
max. –
  maxilla
  maximum
max. EP – maximal esophageal pressure
MB –
  buccal margin
  mesiobuccal
  methyl bromide
  methylene blue
  microbiological assay
M. B. – Medicinae Baccalaureus [L] Bachelor of Medicine
Mb – myoglobin
m.b. – misce bene [L] mix well
MBA – methylbovine albumin
mbar. – millibar
μbar – microbar
MBAS – methylene blue active substance
MBC –
  maximal breathing capacity
  minimal bactericidal concentration
MBD –
  methylene blue dye
  minimal brain damage
  minimal brain dysfunction
  Morquio-Brailsford disease
MBF – myocardial blood flow
MBFLB – monaural bifrequency loudness balance

MBK – methyl butyl ketone
MBL –
  menstrual blood loss
  minimal bactericidal level
MBO – mesiobucco-occlusal
MBP –
  antigen prepared from *Brucella melitensis*, *B. bovis* and *B. suis*
  mean blood pressure
  mesiobuccopulpal
  myelin basic protein
MBRT – methylene blue reduction time
MBSA – methylated bovine serum albumin
MC –
  mast cell
  maximum concentration
  medium-chain (triglycerides)
  mesiocervical
  metacarpal
  mineralocorticoid
  monkey cells
  myocarditis
  mitomycin-C
M & C – morphine and cocaine
M.C. –
  Magister Chirurgiae [L] Master of Surgery
  Medical Corps
Mc. –
  megacurie
  megacycle
mC. – millicoulomb
μC. – microcoulomb
mc., mCi. or MCU – millicurie
μc. – microcurie
MCA –
  methylcholanthrene
  middle cerebral artery
  multichannel analyzer

MCB — membranous cytoplasmic body

MCBR — minimum concentration of bilirubin

MCC —
mean corpuscular hemoglobin concentration
minimum complete-killing concentration

MCCU — mobile coronary care unit

MCD —
mean cell diameter
mean corpuscular diameter
mean of consecutive differences
medullary cystic disease

MCF —
macrophage chemotactic factor
medium corpuscular fragility
myocardial contractile force

MCFA — medium-chain fatty acid

mcg. — microgram

MCH — mean corpuscular hemoglobin and red cell indices

M. Ch. — Magister Chirurgiae [L] Master of Surgery

mc.h. — millicurie-hour

μc.h. — microcurie-hour

MCHb — mean corpuscular hemoglobin

MCHC — mean corpuscular hemoglobin concentration and red cell indices

M.C.H.R. — Medical Committee on Human Rights

mc.hr. — millicurie-hour

μC.hr. — microcurie-hour

MCI — mean cardiac index

MCi. — megacurie

mCi. — millicurie

μCi. — microcurie

mCi.-hr. — millicurie-hour

μCi.-hr. — microcurie-hour

MCL —
midclavicular line
midcostal line
modified chest lead
most comfortable loudness level

M colony — mucoid colony

mcoul. — millicoulomb

μcoul. — microcoulomb

MCP —
metacarpophalangeal
mitotic-control protein

MCPH — metacarpophalangeal

mc. p. s. — megacycles per second

MCQ — multiple choice question

MCR —
message competition ratio
metabolic clearance rate

MCS — myocardial contractile state

M.C.S.P. — Member of the Chartered Society of Physiotherapists (British)

MCT —
mean cell threshold
mean circulation time
mean corpuscular thickness
medium-chain triglyceride

MCTD — mixed connective tissue disease

MCV —
mean cell volume
mean clinical value
mean corpuscular volume and red cell indices

MD —
malic dehydrogenase
manic-depressive
Mantoux diameter
Marek's disease
maternal deprivation

MD (*continued*)
  mean deviation
  medium dosage
  mentally deficient
  mesiodistal
  mitral disease
  movement disorder
  muscular dystrophy
  myocardial damage
  myocardial disease
M.D. – Medicinae Doctor [L]
  Doctor of Medicine
Md – mendelevium
MDA –
  3-4-methylenedioxyampheta-
    mine
  monodehydroascorbate
  motor discriminative acuity
M.D.A. –
  mento-dextra anterior [L]
    right mentoanterior; a pre-
    sentation of the fetus
  Muscular Dystrophy Associa-
    tion
MDC – minimum detectable concentration
MDD – mean daily dose
MDF –
  mean dominant frequency
  myocardial depressant factor
MDH – malic dehydrogenase
MDI – manic-depressive illness
m. dict. – moro dicto [L] as
  directed
M.D.L. – Master Drug List
MDM – minor determinant mix-
  ture
MDNB – metadinitrobenzene
M.D.P. – mento-dextra posterior
  [L] right mentoposterior; a
  presentation of the fetus
MDQ – minimum detectable
  quantity

MDR – minimum daily require-
  ment
MDT – median detection threshold
M.D.T. – mento-dextra transversa
  [L] right mentotransverse; a
  presentation of the fetus
MDTR – mean diameter-thickness
  ratio
MDUO – myocardial disease of
  unknown origin
MDY – month, date, year
ME –
  maximum effort
  median eminence
  medical education
  mercaptoethanol
  metabolizable energy
  middle ear
M/E – myeloid-erythroid (ratio)
2 ME – 2-mercaptoethanol
M.E. – Medical Examiner
Me. – methyl
MEA –
  mercaptoethylamine
  multiple endocrine adeno-
    matosis
MEC – minimum effective concentration
mec. – meconium
MED –
  median erythrocyte diameter
  minimal effective dose
  minimal erythema dose
med. –
  median
  medical
  medication
  medicine
  medium
MEDAC syndrome – multiple endocrine deficiency–Addison's
  disease–candidiasis

MEDICO — Medical Internation Cooperation
MEDLARS — Medical Literature Analysis and Retrieval System
MEDLINE — MEDLARS on-line
meds. —
    medications
    medicines
MEE — methylethyl ether
MEF — maximal expiratory flow
MEFR — maximal expiratory flow rate
MEFSR — maximal expiratory flow—static recoil curve
MEFV — maximal expiratory flow volume
MEG —
    magnetoencephalograph
    mercaptoethylguanidine
meg. —
    megacycle
    megakaryocytes
mega- — one million
megalo- — great size
MEK — methyl ethyl ketone
MEM —
    macrophage electrophoretic mobility (test)
    minimum essential medium
MEN — multiple endocrine neo-plasia
MeOH — methyl alcohol
MEP —
    mean effective pressure
    motor end-plate
mep. — meperidine
MEPP — miniature end-plate po-tential
mEq. or meq. — milliequivalent
mEq/L — milliequivalents per liter
MER —
    mean ejection rate

MER (continued)
    methanol-extruded residue
MER-29 — triparanol
M/E ratio — myeloid/erythroid ratio
MES — maintenance electrolyte solution
Mesc. — mescaline
MeSH — Medical Subject Headings
Met. — methionine
Meth. — methedrine
MetHb — methemoglobin
m. et n. — mane et nocte [L] morning and night
Mets. — metastases
m. et sig. — misce et signa [L] mix and label
MeV. — megaelectron volt
mev — million electron volts
MF —
    medium frequency
    5-methyltetrahydrofolate
    microscopic factor
    mitotic figure
    multiplying factor
    mycosis fungoides
    myelin figures
M/F — male-female (ratio)
M & F —mother and father
Mf. — Microfilaria
mF. — millifarad
μF. — microfarad
mf. — microfilaria
MFA — methyl fluoracetate
MFB — metallic foreign body
MFD —
    midforceps delivery
    minimal fatal dose
m. flac. — membrana flaccida [L] pars flaccida membranae tympani (Shrapnell's mem-brane)
MFP — monofluorophosphate

MFR — mucus flow rate
MFT — muscle function test
m. ft. — mistura fiat [L] make a
mixture
MFW — multiple fragment wounds
MG —
menopausal gonadotropin
mesiogingival
methyl glucoside
Michaelis-Gutmann (bodies)
monoglyceride
muscle group
myasthenia gravis
Mg — magnesium
mg. — milligram
mg.% —
milligrams percent
milligrams per deciliter
milligrams per 100 milliliters
μg. — microgram
mγ. — milligamma (millimicrogram, micromilligram or nanogram)
$\mu\gamma$. — microgamma (micromicrogram or picogram)
MGA — melengestrol acetate
MgCL$_2$ — magnesium chloride
MGD — mixed gonadal dysgenesis
mg-el. — milligram-element
MGF — mother's grandfather
MGGH — methylglyoxal guanyl-
hydrazone
MGH — monoglyceride hydrolase
mgh. — milligram-hour
MGM — mother's grandmother
mgm. — milligram
MGN — membranous glomerulonephritis
MgO — magnesium oxide
MGP — marginal granulocyte pool
MGR — modified gain ratio
MgSO$_4$ — magnesium sulfate
mgtis. — meningitis

MGW — magnesium sulfate, glycerine, water
MH —
mammotropic hormone
marital history
medical history
melanophore hormone
menstrual history
mental health
mH. — millihenry
μH. — microhenry
MHA —
methemalbumin
microangiopathic hemolytic
anemia
mixed hemadsorption
MHA-TP — micro-hemagglutina-
tion-*Treponema pallidum*
MHB — maximum hospital benefit
MHb. — methemoglobin
MHC — major histocompatibility
complex
m.h.c.p. — mean horizontal candle
power
MHD —
magnetohydrodynamics
mean hemolytic dose
minimum hemolytic dose
mHg. — millimeters of mercury
MHN — massive hepatic necrosis
MHP — 1-mercuri-2-hydroxypro-
pane
MHPE — 3-methoxy-4-hydroxy-
phenylethanol
MHPG — methoxyhydroxyphen-
ylglycol
MHR — maximal heart rate
MHVD — Marek's herpesvirus
disease
MH virus — murine hepatitis
virus
M. Hx. — medical history
MHz. — megahertz

MI –
  maturation index
  mercaptoimidazole
  mesioincisal
  metabolic index
  mitotic index
  mitral incompetence
  mitral insufficiency
  myocardial infarction
MIBK – methyl isobutyl ketone
MIBT – methyl isatin-betathio-
  semicarbasone
MIC –
  minimal isorrheic concentration
  minimal inhibitory concentration
M.I.C. – Maternity and Infant
  Care
mic. pan. – mica panis [L] bread
  crumb
micro- – one-millionth
microbiol. –
  microbiological
  microbiology
MICU –
  medical intensive care unit
  mobile intensive care unit
MID –
  maximum inhibiting dilution
  mesioincisodistal
  minimal inhibiting dose
  minimum infective dose
midnoc. – midnight
MIF –
  macrophage-inhibiting factor
  melanocyte-stimulating hormone–inhibiting factor
  Merthiolate-iodine-formalde-
  hyde
  migration inhibition factor
  mixed immunofluorescence

MIFR – maximal inspiratory flow
  rate
mil. – 0.001
milli- – one-thousandth
min. –
  mineral
  minimal
  minimum [L] a minim
  minimum
  minor
  minute
MINA – monoisonitrosoacetone
MINIA – monkey intranuclear
  inclusion agent
MIO – minimal identifiable odor
MIP –
  maximum inspiratory pressure
  mean intravascular pressure
MIRD – Medical Internal Radiation Dose
MIRU – myocardial infarction research unit
misc. –
  miscarriage
  miscellaneous
misce. – mix
mist. – mistura [L] a mixture
MIT –
  miracidial immobilization test
  monoiodotyrosine
mit. – mitte [L] send
mit. sang. – mitte sanguinem [L]
  bleed
mIU – milli-International Unit
μIU – micro-International Unit
mixt. – mixture [L] mixture
MJ – marijuana
MK – monkey kidney
mkg. – meter kilogram
mks. – meter-kilogram-second
MKV – killed-measles vaccine
ML –
  mesiolingual

ML (*continued*)
  middle lobe
  midline
M:L — monocyte-lymphocyte
  ratio
M.L. — Licentiate in Medicine
mL. — millilambert
ml. — milliliter
μl. — microliter
MLA —
  mesiolabial
  monocytic leukemia, acute
M.L.A. — mento-laeva anterior
  [L] left mentoanterior; a
  presentation of the fetus
MLAI —mesiolabioincisal
MLAP —
  mean left atrial pressure
  mesiolabiopulpal
MLC —
  minimal lethal concentration
  mixed leukocyte culture
  mixed lymphocyte culture
  multilamellar cytosome
  myelomonocytic leukemia,
    chronic
MLD —
  median lethal dose
  metachromatic leukodys-
    trophy
  minimal lethal dose
MLD_{50} — median lethal dose
MLI — mesiolinguoincisal
MLNS — mucocutaneous lymph
  node syndrome
MLO — mesiolinguo-occlusal
MLP — mesiolinguopulpal
M.L.P. — mento-laeva posterior
  [L] left mentoposterior; a
  presentation of the fetus
MLR — mixed lymphocyte reaction

MLS —
  mean life span
  median longitudinal section
  myelomonocytic leukemia,
    subacute
MLT — median lethal time
M.L.T. — mento-laeva transversa
  [L] left mentotransverse; a
  presentation of the fetus
MLV —
  Moloney's leukemogenic
    virus
  mouse leukemia virus
MM —
  malignant melanoma
  Marshall-Marchetti
  medial malleolus
  mucous membranes
  multiple myeloma
  muscles
  muscularis mucosa
  myeloid metaplasia
M & M — milk and molasses
mM. — millimolar
mm or mm. —
  millimeter
  muscles
mm^3 — cubic millimeter
mμ —
  millimicro- (prefix meaning
    one-billionth, replaced by
    nano)
  millimicron
μm. — micrometer
$\mu\mu$ —
  micromicro- (prefix meaning
    one-trillionth, replaced by
    pico-)
  micromicron
MMA — methylmalonic acid
MMC — minimal medullary
  concentration

mμc. − millimicrocurie (nanocurie)

μμc. − micromicrocurie (picocurie)

MMD −
mass median diameter
minimal morbidostatic dose

MMEF − maximal midexpiratory
flow

MMEFR − maximal midexpiratory flow rate

MMF − maximal midexpiratory
flow

MMFR −
maximal midexpiratory flow
rate
maximal midflow rate

mμg. − millimicrogram (nanogram)

μmg. − micromilligram

μμg. − micromicrogram (picogram)

mmHg. − millimeters of mercury

MMM −
myeloid metaplasia with mye-
lofibrosis
myelosclerosis with myeloid
metaplasia

mmm. − millimicron

μmm. − micromillimeter

mmol. − millimole

μmol. − micromole

MMPI − Minnesota Multiphasic
Personality Inventory

mm.p.p. − millimeters partial
pressure

MMPR − methylmercaptopurine
riboside

MMR −
mass miniature radiography
maternal mortality rate
measles, mumps, rubella

MMR (*continued*)
mobile mass x-ray
monomethylolrutin
myocardial metabolic rate

M.M. Sc. − Master of Medical
Science

MMT − manual muscle test

MMTV − mouse mammary tumor
virus

MMU − mercaptomethyl uracil

mmu. − millimass units

MN −
midnight
mononuclear
motor neuron
multinodular
myoneural

M & N − morning and night

Mn − manganese

mN. − millinormal

mn. − midnight

MNA − maximum noise area

MNCV − motor nerve conduction
velocity

MND − minimum necrosing dose

MNJ − myoneural junction

MNU − methylnitrosourea

MO −
manually operated
mesio-occlusal
mineral oil
minute output
molecular orbit
no evidence of distant metastases

MO_2 − myocardial oxygen consumption

M.O. − Medical Officer

Mo − molybdenum

MΩ − megohm

μΩ − microhm

mo. − month(s)

MOD — mesio-occlusodistal
mod. — moderate
MODM — mature-onset diabetes mellitus
mod. praesc. — modo praescripto [L] in the way directed
M.O.H. — Medical Officer of Health
mol. — mole
molc. — molar concentration
moll. — mollis [L] soft
mol/l. — molecules per liter
mol. wt. — molecular weight
MOM — milk of magnesia
MOMA — methoxyhydroxyman-delic acid
mono. — mononucleosis
Monos. — monocytes
MOPP — Mustargen, Oncovin, pro-carbazine and prednisone
MOPV — monovalent oral polio-virus vaccine
M.O.R.C. — Medical Officers Reserve Corps
mor. dict. — more dicto [L] in the manner directed
morph. — morphology
mor. sol. — more solito [L] in the usual way
MOSFET — metal oxide semicon-ductor field effect transistor
mOsm. — milliosmol, milliosmole
MOTT — mycobacteria other than the tubercle bacillus
MP —
    mean pressure
    menstrual period
    mesiopulpal
    metacarpophalangeal
    metatarsophalangeal
    methylprednisolone
    monophosphate
    mucopolysaccharide

MP (continued)
    multiparous
6-MP — 6-mercaptopurine
mp. — modo prescripto [L] as directed
m.p. — melting point
MPA —
    main pulmonary artery
    medroxyprogesterone acetate
    methylprednisolone acetate
mPa — megapascal
MPAP — mean pulmonary arterial pressure
MPC —
    marine protein concentrate
    maximum permissible concen-tration
    meperidine, promethazine, chlorpromazine
    minimum mycoplasmacidal concentration
MPCU — maximum permissible concentration of unidentified radionucleotides
MPD —
    maximum permissible dose
    myofacial pain dysfunction
MPEH — methylphenylethylhy-dantoin
MPGN — membranoproliferative glomerulonephritis
M.P.H. — Master of Public Health
M phase — phase of mitosis
MPHR — maximum predicted heart rate
M. Phys. A. — Member of the Physiotherapists' Association (British)
MPI —
    maximum point of impulse
    Multiphasic Personality In-ventory
MPJ — metacarpophalangeal joint

MPL –
   maximum permissible level
   mesiopulpolingual
MPLa – mesiopulpolabial
MPN – most probable number
MPO – myeloperoxidase
MPP – mercaptopyrazidopyrimi-
   dine
MPR – marrow production rate
MPS –
   mononuclear-phagocyte sys-
      tem
   movement-produced stimuli
   mucopolysaccharide
   multiphasic screening
M.P.U. – Medical Practitioners
   Union (British)
MR –
   medial rectus
   mental retardation
   metabolic rate
   methyl red
   mitral reflux
   mitral regurgitation
   mortality rate
   mortality ratio
   muscle relaxant
M & R – measure and record
mR. – milliroentgen
μR. – microroentgen
M.R.A. – Medical Record Administrator
mrad. – millirad
MRAP – mean right atrial pressure
MRBC – monkey red blood cells
MRC – methylrosaniline chloride
M.R.C. –
   Medical Research Council
      (units)
   Medical Reserve Corps
M.R.C.P. – Member of the Royal
   College of Physicians

M.R.C.P.E. – Member of the
   Royal College of Physicians of
   Edinburgh
M.R.C.P. (Glasg.) – Member of the
   Royal College of Physicians
   and Surgeons of Glasgow
M.R.C.P.I. – Member of the Royal
   College of Physicians of Ireland
M.R.C.S. – Member of the Royal
   College of Surgeons
M.R.C.S.E. – Member of the
   Royal College of Surgeons of
   Edinburgh
M.R.C.S.I. – Member of the Royal
   College of Surgeons of Ireland
M.R.C.V.S. – Member of the
   Royal College of Veterinary
   Surgeons
MRD – minimum reacting dose
mrd. – millirutherford
MR-E – methemoglobin reduc-
   tase
mrem. –
   millirem
   milliroentgen equivalent, man
mrep. – milliroentgen equivalent,
   physical
MRF –
   melanocyte-stimulating hor-
      mone–releasing factor
   mesencephalic reticular forma-
      tion
   mitral regurgitant flow
MRH – melanocyte-stimulating
   hormone–releasing hormone
mrhm. – milliroentgen per hour
   at 1 meter
MRIH – melanocyte-stimulating
   hormone–release-inhibiting
   hormone
M.R.L. – Medical Record Librarian

mRNA – messenger RNA (ribonucleic acid)
MRR – marrow release rate
MRT –
median recognition threshold
milk-ring test
MRU – minimal reproductive units
MRV – mixed respiratory vaccine
MRVP –
mean right ventricular pressure
methyl red, Voges-Proskauer
(medium)
MS –
mass spectrometry
mental status
mitral stenosis
modal sensitivity
molar solution
morphine sulfate
mucosubstance
multiple sclerosis
muscle shortening
muscle strength
musculoskeletal
MS-222 – tricaine methane
sulfonate
M.S. –
Master of Science
Master of Surgery
ms. –
manuscript
millisecond
μs. – microsecond
MSA –
mannitol salt agar
multiplication-stimulating
activity
M.S.A. – Medical Services Administration
MSB – most significant bit
m.s.c.p. – mean spherical candle
power

MSD – most significant digit
mse. – mean square error
msec. – millisecond
μsec. – microsecond
MSER – mean systolic ejection
rate
MSG – monosodium glutamate
MSH –
medical self-help
melanocyte-stimulating hormone
melanophore-stimulating hor-
mone
MSH-IF – melanocyte-stimulating
hormone–inhibiting factor
MSI – medium-scale integration
MSK – medullary sponge kidney
MSL – midsternal line
MSLA – mouse-specific lympho-
cyte antigen
MSN – mildly subnormal
MSRPP – multidimensional scale
for rating psychiatric patients
MSS – mental status schedule
M.S.S.V.D. – Medical Society for
the Study of Venereal Diseases
MST – mean survival time
MSU –
mid-stream urine specimen
monosodium urate
MSUD – maple syrup urine disease
MSV –
Moloney's sarcoma virus
murine sarcoma virus
M.S.W. –
Master of Social Work
Medical Social Worker
MT –
empty
malignant teratoma
maximal therapy
medical technologist

MT (*continued*)
   membrana tympani
   metatarsal
   methoxytyramine
   methyltyrosine
   more than
   muscles and tendons
   music therapy
MTBF − mean time between failures
MTD − maximum tolerated dose
MTDT − modified tone decay test
MTF −
   maximum terminal flow
   modulation transfer function
MTHF − methyltetrahydrofolic acid
MTI −
   malignant teratoma intermediate
   minimum time interval
MTP − metatarsophalangeal
MTR − Meinicke turbidity reaction
MTT −
   malignant trophoblastic teratoma
   mean transit time
   monotetrazolium
MTU − methylthiouracil
MTV − mammary tumor virus
MTX − methotrexate
MU − Montevideo unit
M.u. − Mache unit
mU. − milliunit
μU. − microunit
m.u. − mouse unit
MUC − maximum urinary concentration
muc. − mucilago [L] mucilage
MUGA − multigated angiogram
MU-GAL − methylumbelliferyl-β-galactosidase

multip. − multipara (woman who has borne two or more children)
multivits. − multivitamins
MuLV − murine leukemia virus
MUMPS − Massachusetts General Hospital Utility Multi-Programming System
MUO − myocardiopathy of unknown origin
MUP − motor unit potential
MUST − medical unit, self-contained, transportable
MUU − mouse uterine units
MUWU − mouse uterine weight unit
MV −
   megavolt
   microvilli
   minute volume
   mitral valve
   mixed venous
M.V. − Medicus Veterinarius [L] veterinary physician
Mv −mendelevium
mV. − millivolt
μV. − microvolt
MVA − motor vehicle accident
MVC − myocardial vascular capacity
MVE − Murray Valley encephalitis
MV grad. − mitral valve gradient
MVM − microvillous membrane
MVO_2 − myocardial oxygen ventilation rate
MVP − mitral valve prolapse
MVR − massive vitreous retraction
MVV − maximal voluntary ventilation
MVV_1 − maximal ventilatory volume
M.W. − molecular weight
mW. − milliwatt

μW. − microwatt
mw − microwave
Mx − maxwell
Mx. − Medex
My. − myopia

my. − mayer (unit of heat capacity)
MyG. − myasthenia gravis
MZ − monozygotic

N

N −
asparagine
nasal
negative
neurology
neutron number
newton
nicotinamide
nitrogen
non-malignant
Nonne (test)
normal solution
number of molecules
population size
refractive index
size of sample
unit of neutron dosage
N. −
Neisseria
Nocardia
n −
index of refraction
nano-
naris [L] nostril
nasal
natus [L] born
nerve
neuter
neutron
normal
number density of molecule
number of observations
sample size

N, ν − nu (13th letter of the Greek alphabet)
NA −
neutralizing antibody
nicotinic acid
no abnormality
Nomina Anatomica
noradrenalin
not admitted
not applicable
not available
nucleic acid
N.A. − numerical aperture
Na − natrium [L] sodium
^{24}Na − radioactive sodium
NAA −
naphthaleneacetic acid
neutron activation analysis
nicotinic acid amide
no apparent abnormalities
N.A.A.C.L.S. − National Accrediting Agency for Clinical Laboratory Sciences
NAAP − N-acetyl-4-amino-phenazone
$Na_2B_4O_7 \cdot 10H_2O$ − borax
NaBr − sodium bromide
NAC − N-acetyl-L-cysteine
NAC-EDTA − N-acetyl-L-cysteine ethylenediaminetetra-acetic acid
NaCl − sodium chloride
NaClO − sodium hypochlorite

NaClO$_3$ — sodium chlorate
Na$_2$CO$_3$ — sodium carbonate
Na$_2$C$_2$O$_4$ — sodium oxalate
N.A.C.O.R. — National Advisory Committee on Radiation
NAD —
  nicotinamide-adenine dinucleotide
  no acute distress
  no appreciable disease
  normal axis deviation
  nothing abnormal detected
NAD+ — nicotinamide-adenine dinucleotide (oxidized form)
NADH — nicotinamide-adenine dinucleotide (reduced form)
NADP — nicotinamide-adenine dinucleotide phosphate
NADP+ — nicotinamide-adenine dinucleotide phosphate (oxidized form)
NADPH — nicotinamide-adenine dinucleotide phosphate (reduced form)
Na$_e$ — exchangeable body sodium
NaF — sodium fluoride
NAG — non-agglutinating
NaHCO$_3$ — sodium bicarbonate
NaH$_2$PO$_4$ — monosodium acid phosphate (sodium biphosphate)
Na$_2$HPO$_2$ — disodium acid phosphate (sodium phosphate)
NAI — non-accidental injury
NaI(Tl) crystal — thallium-activated sodium iodide crystal
N.A.M.E. — National Association of Medical Examiners
N.A.M.H. — National Association of Mental Health
NANA — N-acetylneuraminic acid
NaOH — sodium hydroxide

NAP —
  nasion pogonion
  nucleic acid phosphorus
NAPA —
  N-acetylated procainamide
  N-acetyl-p-aminophenol
NaPG — sodium pregnanediol glucuronide
NAPH — naphthyl
N.A.P.N.E.S. — National Association for Practical Nurse Education and Services
NAR — nasal airway resistance
narc. — narcotic
NAS —
  nasal
  no added salt
N.A.S. — National Academy of Sciences
N.A.S.E. — National Association for the Study of Epilepsy
N.A.S.-N.R.C. — National Academy of Sciences–National Research Council
Na$_2$SO$_4$ — sodium sulfate
Na$_2$S$_2$O$_3$ — sodium thiosulfate
nat. —
  national
  native
  natural
NB —
  newborn
  nitrous oxide–barbiturate
Nb — niobium
^{95}Nb — radioactive niobium
nb. — nota bene [L] note well
NBI — no bone injury
NBM — nothing by mouth
N.B.M.E. — National Board of Medical Examiners
NBO — nonbed occupancy
NBS — normal blood serum

N.B.S. – National Bureau of
   Standards
NBT – nitroblue tetrazolium
NBTE – nonbacterial thrombotic
   endocarditis
NBTNF – newborn, term, normal,
   female
NBTNM – newborn, term, normal,
   male
NBT test – nitroblue tetrazolium
   dye test
NBW – normal birth weight
NC –
   nitrocellulose
   no casualty
   no change
   noise criterion
   noncontributory
   not cultured
N/C – no complaints
NCA – neurocirculatory asthenia
N.C.A. – National Council on
   Alcoholism
N.C.A.M.L.P. – National Certifica-
   tion Agency for Medical Lab-
   oratory Personnel
N.C.C.L.S. – National Committee
   for Clinical Laboratory Stan-
   dards
NCD – not considered disabling
NCF – neutrophil chemotactic
   factor
N.C.H.C.A. – National Commis-
   sion for Health Certifying
   Agencies
N.C.H.L.S. – National Council of
   Health Laboratory Services
NCI –
   naphthalene creosote, iodo-
     form
   National Cancer Institute
nCi. – nanocurie

N.C.M.H. – National Committee
   for Mental Hygiene
N.C.N. – National Council of
   Nurses
N:C ratio – nuclear-cytoplasmic
   ratio
N.C.R.N.D. – National Committee
   for Research in Neurological
   Diseases
NCV – nerve conduction velocity
ND –
   natural death
   neonatal death
   neoplastic disease
   neurotic depression
   neutral density
   Newcastle disease
   new drugs
   no data
   no disease
   nondisabling
   normal delivery
   not detectable
   not detected
   not determined
   not done
Nd – neodymium
n_D – refractive index
NDA –
   new drug application
   no data available
   no demonstrable antibodies
N.D.A. – National Dental Association
NDF – new dosage form
NDGA – nordihydroguaiaretic
   acid
NDI – nephrogenic diabetes
   insipidus
NDMA – nitrosodimethylaniline
NDP – net dietary protein
NDT – non-destructive testing

NDV – Newcastle disease virus
Nd. YAG – neodymium-yttrium-aluminum-garnet
NE –
    nerve ending
    nerve excitability
    neurologic examination
    no effect
    nonelastic
    norepinephrine
    not enlarged
    not evaluated
    not examined
Ne – neon
nebul. – nebula [L] a spray
NEC –
    necrotizing enterocolitis
    not elsewhere classifiable
    not elsewhere classified
NED –
    no evidence of disease
    normal equivalent deviation
NEEP – negative end-expiratory pressure
NEFA – nonesterified fatty acid
neg. – negative
NEM – N-ethylmaleimide
nem – Nährungs Einheit Milch [Ger] nutritional unit milk
N.E.M.A. – National Eclectic Medical Association
nema. – nematode
NEP –
    negative expiratory pressure
    nephrology
NER – no evidence of recurrence
NERD – no evidence of recurrent disease
NES – not elsewhere specified
n. et m. – nocte et mane [L] night and morning
neur. – neurology

neuro. or neurol. – neurologic
NF –
    neutral fraction
    none found
    normal flow
    not found
N.F. – National Formulary
nF – nanofarad
N.F.L.P.N. – National Federation for Licensed Practical Nurses
NFTD – normal full-term delivery
NG –
    nasogastric
    new growth
    no good
ng. – nanogram
NGF – nerve growth factor
NGU – nongonococcal urethritis
NH –
    nonhuman
    nursing home
NH_3 – ammonia
NHA – nonspecific hepatocellular abnormality
NH_4Br – ammonium bromide
NHC – nonhistone chromosomal (protein)
N.H.C. – National Health Council
NH_4Cl – ammonium chloride
NH_4CNO – ammonium cyanate
$(NH_2)_2CO$ – urea
$(NH_4)_2CO_3$ – ammonium carbonate
$(NH_4)HS$ – ammonium hydrosulfide
NHI – National Heart Institute
N.H.I. – National Health Insurance
NHLI – National Heart and Lung Institute
N.H.M.R.C. – National Health and Medical Research Council
NH_4NO_3 – ammonium nitrate

$NH_4O \cdot CO \cdot NH_2$ – ammonium carbamate
NHS –
normal horse serum
normal human serum
N.H.S. – National Health Service (British)
$(NH_4)_2 \cdot SO_2$ – ammonium sulfate
NI –
no information
not identified
not isolated
Ni – nickel
NIA –
nephelometric inhibition assay
no information available
NIAID – National Institute of Allergy and Infectious Diseases
NIAMD – National Institute of Arthritis and Metabolic Diseases
Nic. – nicotinyl alcohol
NICHHD – National Institute of Child Health and Human Development
NIDDM – noninsulin-dependent diabetes mellitus
NIDR – National Institute of Dental Research
NIEHS – National Institute of Environmental Health Sciences
NIF – negative inspiratory force
nig. – niger [L] black
NIGMS – National Institute of General Medical Sciences
NIH – National Institute of Health
NIH 204 – an antimalarial drug
NIIP – National Institute of Industrial Psychology

NIMH – National Institute of Mental Health
NIMR – National Institute for Medical Research
NINDB – National Institute of Neurological Diseases and Blindness
NINDS – National Institute of Neurological Diseases and Stroke
NIOSH – National Institute of Occupational Safety and Health
NIP – mono-nitroiodophenyl
NIRNS – National Institute for Research in Nuclear Science
NJ feeding – nasojejunal feeding
NK – not known
NK cell – natural killer cell
NKH – nonketotic hyperosmotic
NL – normal limits
Nl. – normal
nl. –
nanoliter
non licet [L] it is not permitted
non liquet [L] it is not clear
NLA – neuroleptanalgesia
N.L.M. – National Library of Medicine
N.L.N. – National League for Nursing
NLP – no light perception
NLT – normal lymphocyte transfer (test)
NM –
neuromuscular
nitrogen mustard
non-motile
not measurable
not measured
nuclear medicine

Nm. — nux moschata [L] nutmeg
N·m — newton-meter
nm — nonmetallic
nm. — nanometer
NMA — neurogenic muscular atrophy
N.M.A. —
  National Malaria Association
  National Medical Association
NMF — non-migrating fraction
NMI — no middle initial
NMJ — neuromuscular junction
NMN —
  nicotinamide mononucleotide
  normetanephrine
nmol. — nanomole
NMP — normal menstrual period
NMR — nuclear magnetic resonance
NMRI — National Medical Research Institute
N.M.S.S. — National Multiple Sclerosis Society
NMT — neuromuscular tension
N/N — nurses' notes
N:N — (indicates presence of) the azo group
nn. —
  nervi [L] nerves
  nomen novum [L] new name
NND —
  neonatal death
  New and Nonofficial Drugs
NNI — noise and number index
N.N.M.C. — National Naval Medical Center
NNN — Novy, MacNeal and Nicolle's (medium)
NNR — New and Nonofficial Remedies
NO —
  nitric oxide
  none obtained

N_2O — dinitrogen monoxide (nitrous oxide)
No — nobelium
No. —
  number
  numero [L] to the number of
noct. —
  nocte [L] at night
  nocturnal
noct. maneq. — nocte maneque [L] at night and in the morning
non-REM — nonrapid eye movement
non repetat. — non repetatur [L] do not repeat
N.O.P.H.N. — National Organization for Public Health Nursing
NOS — not otherwise specified
N.O.T.B. — National Ophthalmic Treatment Board (British)
nov. — novum [L] new
NP —
  nasopharyngeal
  nasopharynx
  near point
  neuropathology
  neuropsychiatric
  nitrogen-phosphorus
  normal plasma
  not performed
  not practiced
  nucleoplasmic index
  nucleoprotein
  nurse practitioner
  nursing procedure
Np —
  neper
  neptunium
np. — nomen proprium [L] proper name
NPB — nodal premature beat

NPC —
    near-point of convergence
    nodal premature contraction
NPCa — nasopharyngeal car-
    cinoma
NPD —
    natriuretic plasma dialysate
    Niemann-Pick disease
NP detector — nitrogen-phos-
    phorus detector
NPDL — nodular, poorly differ-
    entiated lymphocytes
NPDR — nonproliferative diabetic
    retinopathy
NPH — neutral protamine Hage-
    dorn (insulin)
NPI — Neuropsychiatric Institute
NPN — nonprotein nitrogen
NPO — nulla per os [L] nothing
    by mouth
NPO/HS — nulla per os hora som-
    ni [L] nothing by mouth at
    bedtime
4-NPP — 4-nitrophenylphosphate
NPR — net protein ratio
NPT —
    neoprecipitin test
    normal pressure and tempera-
    ture
NPU — net protein utilization
NR —
    neutral red
    nonreactive
    non-rebreathing
    no radiation
    no refill
    no response
    normal
    normal range
    not readable
    not recorded
    not resolved

NR (continued)
    nutritive ratio
    Reynold's number
NRBC — nucleated red blood
    cell
NRC — normal retinal corres-
    pondence
N.R.C. —
    National Research Council
    Nuclear Regulatory Commis-
    sion
N.R.C.C. — National Registry in
    Clinical Chemistry
NRD — nonrenal death
NREM —nonrapid eye movement
N.R.M. — National Registry of
    Microbiologists
NRS —
    normal rabbit serum
    normal reference serum
N.R.S.C.C. — National Reference
    System in Clinical Chemistry
NS —
    nephrotic syndrome
    nervous system
    neurologic survey
    neurosurgery
    nonspecific
    nonsymptomatic
    normal saline
    normal serum
    no sample
    no specimen
    not significant
    not sufficient
N/S — normal saline
ns. —
    nanosecond
    no sequelae
    no specimen
    not significant
    nylon suture

NSA –
  no serious abnormality
  no significant abnormality
N.S.A. – Neurological Society of
  America
NSAID – nonsteroidal antiinflam-
  matory drug
NSC –
  no significant change
  not service-connected
N.S.C.C. – National Society for
  Crippled Children
NSCD – nonservice-connected
  disability
NSD –
  nominal single dose
  normal spontaneous delivery
  no significant defect
  no significant deviation
  no significant difference
  no significant disease
nsec. – nanosecond
N.S.F. – National Science Foun-
  dation
NSFTD – normal spontaneous
  full-term delivery
NSG – neurosecretory granules
nsg. – nursing
N.S.H. – National Society for
  Histotechnology
NSILA – nonsuppressible insulin-
  like activity
NSM – neurosecretory material
N.S.M.R. – National Society for
  Medical Research
N.S.N.A. – National Student
  Nurse Association
NSND – nonsymptomatic, non-
  disabling
N.S.P.B. – National Society for
  the Prevention of Blindness
NSQ – not sufficient quantity

NSR – normal sinus rhythm
NSS –
  normal saline solution
  not statistically significant
NST – nonstress test
NSU – nonspecific urethritis
NT –
  nasotracheal
  neotetrazolium
  neutralization test
  neutralizing
  nontypable
  not tested
N & T –nose and throat
5'-NT – 5'-nucleotidase
NTA – nitrilotriacetic acid
N.T.A. – National Tuberculosis
  Association
NTAB – nephrotoxic antibody
NTD – 5'-nucleotidase
NTG –
  nitroglycerin
  nontoxic goiter
NTN – nephrotoxic nephritis
NTP –
  normal temperature and pres-
  sure
  5'-nucleotidase
nU. – nanounit
NUG – necrotizing ulcerative
  gingivitis
NV – negative variation
N & V – nausea and vomiting
Nv. – naked vision
NVA – near visual acuity
NVD –
  nausea, vomiting and diarrhea
  neck vein distention
  Newcastle virus disease
  nonvalvular (heart) disease
NW – naked weight
NWB – nonweight-bearing

NYD – not yet diagnosed
nyst. – nystagmus

NZB – New Zealand black mouse
NZW – New Zealand white mouse

O – oxygen
O_2 –
  both eyes
  diatomic form of oxygen
  molecular oxygen
O_3 – ozone
O – nonmotile organism
O. –
  none
  obstetrics
  occiput
  occlusal
  octarius [L] pint
  oculus [L] eye
  opening
  operator
  operon
  opium
  oral
  orange
  orderly
  oxygen
  respirations (anesthesia chart)
  suture size (zero)
o- – ortho
O, *o* – omicron (15th letter of the
  Greek alphabet)
Ω, ω – omega (24th letter of the
  Greek alphabet)
Ω – ohm
OA –
  occipital artery
  occiput anterior
  old age
  osteoarthritis
  oxalic acid

OAA –
  Old Age Assistance
  oxaloacetic acid
OAAD – ovarian ascorbic acid
  depletion
OAD – obstructive airway disease
OADC – oleic acid, albumin, dex-
  trose, catalase
OAF – osteoclast-activating factor
OAP –
  Old Age Pension
  ophthalmic artery pressure
  osteoarthropathy
OAR – other administrative rea-
  sons
OASDHI – Old Age, Survivors,
  Disability and Health Insur-
  ance
OASI – Old Age and Survivors In-
  surance
OASP – organic acid soluble
  phosphorus
OAV – oculoauriculovertebral
  dysplasia
OB –
  objective benefit
  obstetrics
O & B – opium and belladonna
ob. – obiit [L] he died
OBG – obstetrician-gynecologist
OB-GYN – obstetrics-gynecology
obl. – oblique
OBP – ova, blood and parasites
OBS –
  obstetrical service
  obstetrics

OBS (*continued*)
  organic brain syndrome
Obs. —
  observed
  obsolete
obs. or obst. — obstetrics
obst. — obstruction
OC —
  occlusocervical
  office call
  on call
  only child
  oral contraceptive
  original claim
  oxygen consumed
O&C — onset and course
O_2 cap. — oxygen capacity
occ. —
  occasionally
  occipital
  occiput
  occlusion
occup. — occupation, occupational
OCD — ovarian cholesterol depletion
OCG — oral cholecystogram
OCR — optical character recognition
OCT —
  optimal cutting temperature
  ornithine-carbamoyltransferase
  oxytocin challenge test
octup. — octuplus [L] eightfold
OCV — ordinary conversational voice
OD —
  drug overdose
  occupational disease
  open drop
  optical density
  originally derived
  out-of-date

OD (*continued*)
  outside diameter
  overdose
O.D. —
  Doctor of Optometry
  oculus dexter [L] right eye
od. — omni die [L] every day, daily, once daily
O.D.A. — occipito-dextra anterior [L] right occipitoanterior; a presentation of the fetus
ODD — oculodentodigital dysplasia
ODM — ophthalmodynamometry
odoram. — odoramentum [L] a perfume
odorat. — odoratus [L] odorous, smelling, perfuming
O.D.P. — occipito-dextra posterior [L] right occipitoposterior; a presentation of the fetus
O.D.T. — occipito-dextra transversa [L] right occipitotransverse; a presentation of the fetus
OE —
  on examination
  otitis externa
O & E — observation and examination
Oe — oersted (the unit of magnetizing force)
OEE — outer enamel epithelium
OEM — open-end marriage
OER — oxygen enhancement ratio
OF —
  occipital frontal
  osteitis fibrosa
  Ovenstone factor
O/F — oxidation/fermentation
OFC — occipitofrontal circumference

OFD –
    object-film distance
    oral-facial-digital
Off. – official
OG –
    obstetrics and gynecology
    occlusogingival
    orange green (stain)
OGS – oxogenic steroid
OGTT – oral glucose tolerance
    test
OH –
    hydroxycorticosteroids
    hydroxyl group
    occupational history
OHC –
    hydroxycholecalciferol
    outer hair cell
17-OHCS – 17-hydroxycortico-
    steroid
OHD – organic heart disease
OH-DOC – hydroxydeoxycorti-
    costerone
OHFA – hydroxy fatty acid
OHI – ocular hypertension in-
    dicator
OH-IAA – hydroxyindoleacetic
    acid
OHP – oxygen under high pres-
    sure
17-OHP – 17-hydroxyprogester-
    one
OI –
    opsonic index
    orgasmic impairment
    oxygen intake
OIF – oil immersion field
OIH –
    orthoiodohippurate
    ovulation-inducing hormone
oint. – ointment
OIT – organic integrity test
OJ – orange juice

OKN – optokinetic nystagmus
O.L. – oculus laevus [L] left
    eye
Ol. – oleum [L] oil
O.L.A. – occipito-laeva anterior
    [L] left occipitoanterior; a
    presentation of the fetus
OLH – ovine lactogenic hormone
Ol. oliv. – oleum olivea [L] olive
    oil
O.L.P. – occipito-laeva posterior
    [L] left occipitoposterior; a
    presentation of the fetus
ol. res. – oleoresin
O.L.T. – occipito-laeva transversa
    [L] left occipitotransverse; a
    presentation of the fetus
OM –
    obtuse marginal
    occipitomental
    Occupational Medicine
    osteomalacia
    osteomyelitis
    otitis media
o.m. – omni mane [L] every
    morning
OMCA – otitis media, catarrhal,
    acute
OMD – ocular muscle dystrophy
OMI – old myocardial infarction
Omn. bih. – omni bihora [L]
    every two hours
Omn. hor. – omni hora [L] every
    hour
Omn. 2 hor. – omni secunda hora
    [L] every two hours
Omn. man. – omni mane [L]
    every morning
Omn. noct. – omni nocte [L]
    every night
Omn. quad. hor. – omni quad-
    rante hora [L] every quarter
    of an hour

OMPA —
 octamethyl pyrophosphora-
  mide
 otitis media, purulent, acute
OM & S — Osteopathic Medicine
 and Surgery
o.n. — omni nocte [L] every night
ONP — ortho-nitrophenyl
ONPG — o-nitrophenyl-β-galacto-
 side
ONP-GAL — ortho-nitrophenyl-
 β-galactosidase
OOB — out of bed
OOLR — ophthalmology, otology,
 laryngology, rhinology
OP —
 occiput posterior
 opening pressure
 operation
 operative procedure
 osmotic pressure
 outpatient
 overproof
 ovine prolactin
O & P — ova and parasites
op. —
 operation
 opposite
 opus [L] work
OPC — Outpatient Clinic
op. cit. — opus citatum [L] in the
 work cited
OP code — operation code
OPD —
 optical path difference
 Outpatient Department
OPG —
 ocular plethysmography
 oxypolygelatin
oph. or ophth. — ophthalmology
OPK — optokinetic
OPS — Outpatient Service

OPT —
 outpatient
 outpatient treatment
opt. —
 optical
 optician
 optimum
 optional
OPV —
 oral poliovaccine
 oral poliovirus vaccine
OR — operating room
O-R — oxidation-reduction
ORD — optical rotary dispersion
O.R.E.F. — Orthopedic Research
 and Education Foundation
OR enema — oil retention enema
ORIF — open reduction, internal
 fixation
orl. — otorhinolaryngology
Orn. — ornithine
ORS — orthopedic surgery
O.R.S. — Orthopedic Research
 Society
ORT — operating room technician
orth. or ortho. — orthopedics
OS —
 opening snap
 oral surgery
 Osgood-Schlatter (disease)
 osteogenic sarcoma
 osteosclerosis
O.S. — oculus sinister [L] left eye
Os — osmium
O.S.A. — Optical Society of
 America
O_2 sat. — oxygen saturation
OSHA — Occupational Safety and
 Health Administration
OSM — oxygen saturation meter
Osm or osmol — osmole
osm. — osmotic

O.S.R.D. – Office of Scientific Research and Development
OST – object sorting test
osteo. –
    osteomyelitis
    osteopathy
O.S.U.K. – Ophthalmological Society of the United Kingdom
OT –
    objective test
    occlusion time
    occupational therapist
    occupational therapy
    old term
    old terminology
    old tuberculin
    orotracheal
    otolaryngology
    otology
OTA – orthotoluidine arsenite
OTC –
    ornithine transcarbamylase
    over the counter
    oxytetracycline

OTD – organ tolerance dose
OTM – orthotoluidine manganese sulfate
oto. or otol. – otology
oto. or otolar. – otolaryngology
OTR – Ovarian Tumor Registry
OU – observation unit
O.U. –
    oculi unitas [L] both eyes
    oculus uterque [L] each eye
OURQ – outer upper right quadrant
OV – office visit
Ov. – ovary
ov. – ovum [L] egg
OVD – occlusal vertical dimension
OVLT – organum vasculosum of the lamina terminalis
OW – out of wedlock
O/W –
    oil in water
    oil-water ratio
ox – oxymel
oz. – ounce

P

P – phosphorus
~ P - high-energy phosphate bond
P_1 – parental generation
P_2 – pulmonic second sound
^{32}P – radioactive phosphorus
P-50 – oxygen half-saturation pressure of hemoglobin
P-55 – hydroxypregnanedione
P. –
    near point
    partial pressure
    percentile
    percussion
    peyote

P. (continued)
    pharmacopeia
    plasma
    poise
    polarization
    population
    position
    posterior
    postpartum
    premolar
    presbyopia
    pressure
    primipara
    probability

P. (*continued*)
proline
protein
psychiatry
pulse
pupil

P. −
Pasteurella
Plasmodium
Proteus

p −
atomic orbital with angular momentum quantum number 1
frequency of more common allele of a pair
momentum
para-
pico-
pint
probability
proton
sample proportion
short arm of a chromosome

$\bar{p}$ − after, following

p. −
parte [L] part
pater [L] father
per [L] by
pondere [L] by weight
pondus [L] weight
post [L] after
proximum [L] near
pugillus [L] handful
punctum proximum [L] near point

Π, π − pi (16th letter of the Greek alphabet)

Φ, ϕ − phi (21st letter of the Greek alphabet)

Ψ, ψ − psi (23rd letter of the Greek alphabet)

PA −
paralysis agitans
pathology
pernicious anemia
phakic-aphakic
phosphatidic acid
phosphoarginine
photoallergenic
platelet adhesiveness
posteroanterior
pregnancy-associated
primary amenorrhea
primary anemia
prior to admission
prolonged action
psychogenic aspermia
pulmonary artery
pulpoaxial

P & A − percussion and auscultation

P_A − partial pressure in arterial blood

P.A. − Physician's Assistant

Pa −
pascal
protactinium

p.a. − per annum [L] yearly

3-PAA − 3-pyridineacetic acid

PAB or PABA − para-aminobenzoic acid

PAC −
papular acrodermatitis of childhood
parent-adult-child
phenacetin, aspirin, codeine
premature atrial contraction
premature auricular contraction

PA_{CO_2} − alveolar CO_2 pressure, tension

Pa_{CO_2} − arterial carbon dioxide pressure, tension

PACP — pulmonary artery counter-pulsation

PAD — phenacetin, aspirin, desoxyephedrine

p. ae. — partes aequales [L] equal parts

PAF —
  paroxysmal atrial fibrillation
  platelet-activating factor
  pulmonary arteriovenous fistula

PAFIB — paroxysmal atrial fibrillation

PAGE — polyacrylamide gel electrophoresis

PAGMK — primary African green monkey kidney

PAH —
  para-aminohippurate
  polycyclic aromatic hydrocarbon
  pulmonary artery hypertension

PAHA — para-aminohippuric acid

P.A.H.O. — Pan American Health Organization

PAL — posterior axillary line

palp. —
  palpable
  palpate
  palpated

PAM —
  crystalline penicillin G in 2 per cent aluminum monostearate
  phenylalanine mustard
  pulmonary alveolar macrophage
  pulmonary alveolar microlithiasis
  pyridine aldoxime methiodide

2-PAM — pralidoxime

PAN —
  periarteritis nodosa
  periodic alternating nystagmus
  peroxyacetyl nitrate
  peroxyacylnitrate

PANS — puromycin aminonucleoside

PAO — peak acid output

PA_{O_2} — alveolar O_2 pressure, tensions

Pa_{O_2} — arterial oxygen pressure

PAOD —
  peripheral arterial occlusive disease
  peripheral arteriosclerotic occlusive disease

PAP —
  Papanicolaou (smear, stain, test)
  peroxidase-antiperoxidase
  positive airway pressure
  primary atypical pneumonia
  prostatic acid phosphatase
  pulmonary alveolar proteinosis
  pulmonary artery pressure

PAPP — para-aminopropiophenone

PAPS —
  phosphoadenosine diphosphosulfate
  3'-phosphoadenosine-5'-phosphosulfate
  phosphoadenosyl-phosphosulfate

PAP technique — peroxidase-antiperoxidase technique

Pap test — Papanicolaou test

PAPVC — partial anomalous pulmonary venous connection

PAR —
  postanesthesia room
  pulmonary arteriolar resistance

Para. – number of pregnancies
Para I – primipara
para. – paracentesis
par. aff. – pars affecta [L] the part affected
part. – partim [L] part
part. aeq. – partes aequales [L] equal parts
part. vic. – partitis vicibus [L] in divided doses
parv. – parvus [L] small
PAS –
  para-aminosalicylic acid
  periodic acid–Schiff (method, reaction, stain, technique, test)
  pulmonary artery stenosis
PASA – para-aminosalicylic acid
PAS-C – para-aminosalicylic acid crystallized with ascorbic acid
PASM – periodic acid–silver methenamine
Past. – Pasteurella
PAT –
  paroxysmal atrial tachycardia
  pregnancy at term
path. – pathology
PAW – pulmonary artery wedge pressure
PB –
  phenobarbital
  phonetically balanced
  pressure breathing
  protein binding
P.B. – Pharmacopoeia Britannica
Pb. – plumbum [L] lead
PBA – pulpobuccoaxial
P_{BA} – brachial arterial pressure
PBBs – polybromated biphenyls
PBC –
  point of basal convergence
  prebed care
  primary biliary cirrhosis

$Pb(C_2H_3O_2)_2$ – lead acetate
$PbCO_3$ – lead carbonate
$PbCrO_4$ – lead chromate
PBE – Perlsucht Bacillenemulsion [Ger] a form of tuberculin
PBF – pulmonary blood flow
PB-Fe – protein-bound iron
PBG – porphobilinogen
PBI – protein-bound iodine
PbI_2 – lead iodide
PBK – phosphorylase b kinase
PBN – paralytic brachial neuritis
$Pb(NO_3)_2$ – lead nitrate
PBO –
  penicillin in beeswax
  placebo
PbO – lead monoxide
PbO_2 – lead dioxide
PBS –
  phosphate-buffered saline
  phosphate-buffered sodium
PbS – lead sulfide
$PbSO_4$ – lead sulfate
PBSP – prognostically bad signs during pregnancy
PBT_4 – protein-bound thyroxine
PBV –
  predicted blood volume
  pulmonary blood volume
PBZ –
  phenylbutazone
  pyribenzamine
PC –
  packed cells
  palmitoyl carnitine
  parent cells
  pentose cycle
  phosphate cycle
  phosphatidylcholine
  phosphocreatine
  platelet concentrate
  platelet count
  portacaval

PC (*continued*)
   postcoital
   present complaint
   printed circuit
   pubococcygeus
   pulmonary capillary
   pulmonic closure
   pyruvate carboxylase
pc. – picocurie
p.c. –
   pondus civile [L] avoirdupois
      weight
   post cibum [L] after meals
PCA –
   passive cutaneous anaphylaxis
   perchloric acid
   percutaneous carotid arterio-
      gram
   phenylcarboxylic acid
   porous-coated anatomic (pros-
      thesis)
   posterior cerebral artery
PCB –
   paracervical block
   polychlorinated biphenyl(s)
PcB – near-point of convergence
   to the intercentral base line
PCC –
   pheochromocytoma
   phosphate carrier compound
P.C.C. – Poison Control Center
P.Cc. – periscopic concave
PCD –
   phosphate-citrate-dextrose
   polycystic disease
   posterior corneal deposits
PCF –
   posterior cranial fossa
   prothrombin conversion factor
PCG – phonocardiogram
PCH – paroxysmal cold hemo-
      globinuria
pCi – picocurie

P.C.I.C. – Poison Control Infor-
      mation Center
PCL – persistent corpus luteum
PCM – protein-calorie malnutrition
p-CMB – parachloromercuriben-
   zoate
P.C.M.O. – Principal Colonial
   Medical Officer
PCN – pregnenolone carbonitril
pcn. – penicillin
P_{CO_2}, pco_2 or pCO_2 – carbon
   dioxide partial pressure or
   tension
PCP –
   parachlorophenate
   pentachlorophenol
   phencyclidine piperdine
PCPA – parachlorophenylalanine
pcpt. – perception
PCS – portacaval shunt
pcs. – preconscious
PCT –
   plasmacrit test
   porphyria cutanea tarda
   portacaval transposition
   prothrombin consumption
      time
   proximal convoluted tubule
pct. – percent
PCV –
   packed cell volume
   polycythemia vera
PCV-M – myeloid metaplasia with
   polycythemia vera
P.Cx. – periscopic convex
PD –
   paralyzing dose
   Parkinson's disease
   pars distalis
   patent ductus
   pediatrics
   phosphate dehydrogenase

PD (*continued*)
    plasma defect
    poorly differentiated
    porphobilinogen deaminase
    postural drainage
    potential difference
    pressor dose
    progression of disease
    psychotic depression
    pulmonary disease
    pulpodistal
P.D. – Doctor of Pharmacy
Pd – palladium
p.d. –
    papilla diameter
    per diem [L] by the day
    prism diopter
    pupillary distance
PDA –
    patent ductus arteriosus
    pediatric allergy
    predialyzed human albumin
PDAB – para-dimethylamino-
    benzaldehyde
PDB – paradichlorobenzene
PDC – pediatric cardiology
PDD – pyridoxine-deficient diet
P.D.D.S. – Parasitic Disease Drug
    Service
PDE – paroxysmal dyspnea on
    exertion
PDG – phosphogluconate dehy-
    drogenase
PDGA – pteroyldiglutamic acid
PDH –
    packaged disaster hospital
    past dental history
    phosphate dehydrogenase
pdl – pudendal
PDLL – poorly differentiated
    lymphocytic lymphoma
PDP – piperidino-pyrimidine
PDR – Physician's Desk Reference

PDS –
    paroxysmal depolarizing shift
    predialyzed human serum
PE –
    paper electrophoresis
    pharyngoesophageal
    phenylephrine
    phosphatidylethanolamine
    photographic effect
    physical evaluation
    physical examination
    pleural effusion
    polyethylene
    potential energy
    powdered extract
    probable error
    pulmonary edema
    pulmonary embolism
Pe. – pressure on expiration
P.E.B. – Physical Evaluation Board
PEBG – phenethylbiguanide
ped. or peds. – pediatrics
PEEP – positive end-expiratory
    pressure
PEF – peak expiratory flow
PEFR – peak expiratory flow rate
PEFSR – partial expiratory flow–
    static recoil curve
PEFV – partial expiratory flow
    volume
PEG –
    pneumoencephalography
    polyethylene glycol
PEI –
    phosphate excretion index
    physical efficiency index
pen – penicillin
pent – pentothal
PEO – progressive external oph-
    thalmoplegia
PEP –
    phosphoenolpyruvate
    polyestradiol phosphate

PEP (*continued*)
   pre-ejection period
   Psychiatric Evaluation Profile
PEPP — positive expiratory pressure plateau
PEPR — precision encoder and pattern recognizer
PER — protein efficiency ratio
per. — perineal
PERK — prospective evaluation of radial keratotomy
PERLA — pupils equal, react to light and accommodation
per. op. emet. — peracta operatione emetici [L] when the action of the emetic is over
perpad — perineal pad
PERRLA — pupils equal, round, regular, react to light and accommodation
PERT — program evaluation and review technique
pert. — pertussis (whooping cough)
PET —
   positron-emission tomography
   pre-eclamptic toxemia
PETN — pentaerythritol tetranitrate
PETT — positron emission transverse tomography
PEx — physical examination
PF —
   peak flow
   peritoneal fluid
   permeability factor
   personality factor
   picture frustration (study)
   plantar flexion
   platelet factor
   pulmonary factor
P/F — pass-fail system
pF — picofarad
PFA — parafluorophenylalanine

PFAS — performic acid–Schiff reaction
PFC — plaque-forming cell
PFD — primary flash distillate
PFIB — perfluoroisobutylene
PFK — phosphofructokinase
PFO — patent foramen ovale
PFP — platelet-free plasma
PFQ — personality factor questionnaire
PFR — peak flow rate
PFT —
   posterior fossa tumor
   pulmonary function test
PFU — plaque-forming units
PFV — physiological full value
PG —
   paregoric
   phosphatidylglycerol
   pituitary gonadotropin
   plasma triglyceride
   postgraduate
   pregnanediol glucuronide
   prostaglandin
   pyoderma gangrenosum
6-PG — 6-phosphogluconate
P.G. — Pharmacopoeia Germanica (German pharmacopeia)
Pg. — pregnant
pg. — picogram
PGA —
   prostaglandin A
   pteroylglutamic acid
PGA₁ — prostaglandin A₁
PGA₂ — prostaglandin A₂
PGA₃ — prostaglandin A₃
PGB — prostaglandin B
PGD —
   phosphogluconate dehydrogenase
   phosphoglyceraldehyde dehydrogenase
PGD₂ — prostaglandin D₂

PGDH − phosphogluconate dehydrogenase
PGDR − plasma-glucose disappearance rate
PGE −
  platelet granule extract
  prostaglandin E
PGE_1 − prostaglandin E_1
PGE_2 − prostaglandin E_2
PGF_{1a} − prostaglandin F_{1a}
PGF_{2a} − prostaglandin F_{2a}
PGG_2 − prostaglandin G_2
PGH −
  pituitary growth hormone
  plasma growth hormone
PGH_2 − prostaglandin H_2
PGI −
  phosphoglucoisomerase
  potassium, glucose and insulin
PGI_2 − prostaglandin I_2
PGK − phosphoglycerate kinase
PGM − phosphoglucomutase
PGO − ponto-geniculo-occipital
PGP − postgamma proteinuria
PGR − psychogalvanic response
PgR − progesterone receptor
PGTR − plasma glucose tolerance
  rate
PGU − postgonococcal urethritis
PGUT − phosphogalactose-uridyl
  transferase
PH −
  past history
  personal history
  pharmacopeia
  prostatic hypertrophy
  public health
  pulmonary hypertension
Ph − phenyl
Ph^1 − Philadelphia chromosome
Ph. − Pharmacopeia

pH − hydrogen ion concentration
  (H+)
pH_1 − isoelectric point
PHA −
  passive hemagglutination
  phenylalanine
  phytohemagglutinin
  pulse height analyzer
PHA-M − phytohemagglutinin M
phar., pharm. − pharmacy
Phar. B. − Pharmaciae Baccalaur-
  eus [L] Bachelor of Pharmacy
Phar. C. − Pharmaceutical Chemist
Phar. D. − Pharmaciae Doctor [L]
  Doctor of Pharmacy
Phar. G. − Graduate in Pharmacy
Phar. M. − Pharmaciae Magister
  [L] Master of Pharmacy
Pharm. D. − Doctor of Pharmacy
Ph.B. − British Pharmacopoeia
PHBB − propylhydroxybenzyl
  benzimidazole
PHC − posthospital care
Ph.C. − Pharmaceutical Chemist
Ph.D. − Philosophiae Doctor [L]
  Doctor of Philosophy
PHE − post-heparin esterase
Phe − phenylalanine
Ph.G. −
  Graduate in Pharmacy
  Pharmacopoeia Germanica
    (German Pharmacopeia)
PHI − phosphohexoisomerase
P.H.I. − Public Health Inspector
phial. − phiala [L] bottle
PHK − platelet phosphohexokin-
  ase
PHLA − postheparin lipolytic
  activity
P.H.L.S. − Public Health Labora-
  tory Service (British)
PH_2O − partial pressure of water
  vapor

phos. —
    phosphate
    phosphorus
PHP —
    postheparin phospholipase
    primary hyperparathyroidism
    pseudohypoparathyroidism
PHPV — persistent hyperplastic
    primary vitreous
P.H.S. — Public Health Service
PHx — past history
Phys. —
    physician
    physiology
PI —
    pacing impulse
    performance intensity
    phosphatidylinositol
    present illness
    primary infarction
    proactive inhibition
    protamine insulin
    pulmonary incompetence
    pulmonary infarction
P.I. — Protocol Internationale
    (International Protocol)
P_i — inorganic phosphate
Pi. — pressure of inspiration
pI — isoelectric point
PIA — plasma insulin activity
PIC — postinflammatory corticoid
PICA — posterior inferior cerebel-
    lar artery
pico- — one-trillionth
PICU — pulmonary intensive care
    unit
PID —
    pelvic inflammatory disease
    photoionization detector
    plasma-iron disappearance
    prolapsed intervertebral disk
PIDT — plasma-iron disappearance
    time

PIE —
    pulmonary infiltrate with
      eosinophilia
    pulmonary interstitial emphy-
      sema
PIF —
    peak inspiratory flow
    prolactin-inhibiting factor
    proliferation inhibitory factor
PIFR — peak inspiratory flow rate
PII — plasma inorganic iodine
pil. —
    pilula [L] pill
    pilulae [L] pills
PIP —
    proximal interphalangeal
    Psychotic Inpatient Profile
PIPIDA — N-para-isopropylacetan-
    ilide-iminodiacetic acid
PIPJ — proximal interphalangeal
    joint
P-IRI — plasma immunoreactive
    insulin
PIT —
    patellar inhibition test
    plasma iron turnover
pit. — pitocin
PITR — plasma iron turnover rate
PIV — parainfluenza virus
pixel — picture element
PK —
    Prausnitz-Küstner (reaction)
    psychokinesis
    pyruvate kinase
pK — dissociation constant
PKA — prokininogenase
pKa — negative log of dissociation
    constant
PK reaction — Prausnitz-Küstner
    reaction
PKU — phenylketonuria
PKV — killed poliomyelitis vac-
    cine

pkV, kVp — peak kilovoltage
PL —
  perception of light
  phospholipid
  placebo
  placental lactogen
  pulpolingual
P_L —
  pulmonary venous pressure
  transpulmonary pressure
PL/1 — programming language one
pl. —
  picoliter
  platelets
  pleural
PLA —
  pulpolabial
  pulpolinguoaxial
PLD —
  platelet defect
  potentially lethal damage
PLED — periodic lateralized epileptiform discharge
Pleur. Fl. — pleural fluid
PLEVA — pityriasis lichenoides et
  varioliformis acuta
PLGV — psittacosis–lymphogranuloma venereum
PLP — pyridoxal phosphate
PLS — prostaglandin-like substance
pls. — please
PLT — psittacosis–lymphogranuloma venereum–trachoma
plumb. — plumbum [L] lead
PLV —
  live poliomyelitis vaccine
  panleukopenia virus
  phenylalanine-lysine-vasopres-
  sin
  posterior left ventricle
PM —
  petit mal

PM (continued)
  photomultiplier tube
  physical medicine
  polymorph
  polymyositis
  post meridiem [L] after noon
  post mortem [L] after death
  premolar
  presystolic murmur
  preventive medicine
  prostatic massage
  pulpomesial
Pm — promethium
pm — picometer
PMA —
  p-methoxyamphetamine
  prevalence of gingivitis (pap-
    illary, marginal, attached)
  Primary Mental Abilities (test)
  progressive muscular atrophy
  pyridylmercuric acetate
P.M.A. — Pharmaceutical Manu-
  facturers Association
PMB —
  para-hydroxymercuribenzoate
  polychrome methylene blue
  polymorphonuclear basophils
  postmenopausal bleeding
PMC —
  phenylmercuric chloride
  pseudomembranous colitis
PMD —
  primary myocardial disease
  progressive muscular dystro-
    phy
PME — polymorphonuclear eo-
  sinophils
PMF — progressive massive fibrosis
PMH — past medical history
PMI —
  phosphomannose isomerase
  point of maximal impulse
  point of maximal intensity

PMI (*continued*)
   posterior myocardial infarction
PML –
   polymorphonuclear leukocytes
   progressive multifocal leukoencephalopathy
PMN – polymorphonuclear neutrophils
PMNR – periadenitis mucosa necrotica recurrens
PMP –
   past menstrual period
   previous menstrual period
PMR –
   perinatal mortality rate
   physical medicine and rehabilitation
   proportionate morbidity ratio
   proportionate mortality ratio
   protein magnetic resonance
PMS –
   phenazine methosulfate
   postmenopausal syndrome
   postmitochondrial supernatant
   pregnant mare serum
   premenstrual syndrome
PMSC – pluripotent myeloid stem cell
PMSG – pregnant mare serum gonadotropin
PMT –
   Porteus maze test
   premenstrual tension
PMTT – pulmonary mean transit time
PN –
   perceived noise
   percussion note
   periarteritis nodosa
   peripheral nerve

PN (*continued*)
   peripheral neuropathy
   pneumonia
   positional nystagmus
   postnatal
   psychoneurotic
   pyelonephritis
P & N – psychiatry and neurology
P_{N_2} – partial pressure of nitrogen
P.N. – Practical Nurse
PNA – pentosenucleic acid
P_{NA} – plasma sodium
PNAvQ – positive-negative ambivalent quotient
PNBT – para-nitroblue tetrazolium
PNC – penicillin
PND –
   paroxysmal nocturnal dyspnea
   postnasal drainage
   postnasal drip
pnd. – pound
pneu. – pneumonia
PNF – proprioceptive neuromuscular facilitation
PNH – paroxysmal nocturnal hemoglobinuria
PNI –
   peripheral nerve injury
   postnatal infection
PNMT – phenylethanolamine-N-methyltransferase
PNP – para-nitrophenol
P.N.P. – Pediatric Nurse Practitioner
PNPG – p-nitrophenyl-β-galactoside
PNPP – para-nitrophenylphosphate
PNPR – positive-negative pressure respiration
P-NPS – p-nitrophenylsulfate

PNS —
    parasympathetic nervous system
    peripheral nerve stimulator
    peripheral nervous system
PNU — protein nitrogen unit
Pnx. — pneumothorax
PO —
    parieto-occipital
    period of onset
    posterior
    postoperative
Po — polonium
P_{O_2} — partial pressure of oxygen
PO_4 — phosphate
p.o. — per os [L] by mouth
POA —
    point of application
    primary optic atrophy
POB —
    phenoxybenzamine
    place of birth
    prevention of blindness
POC — postoperative care
pocill. — pocillum [L] a small cup
pocul. — poculum [L] cup
POD —
    place of death
    postoperative day
Pod. D. — Doctor of Podiatry
PODx — preoperative diagnosis
POF — pyruvate oxidation factor
pOH — hydroxyl concentration
poik. —
    poikilocyte
    poikilocytosis
polio — poliomyelitis
poly. — polymorphonuclear leukocyte
poly(A) — polyadenylic acid
poly(U) — polyuridylic acid
POMP — prednisone, Oncovin, methotrexate, 6-mercaptopurine

POMR — problem-oriented medical record
pond. — pondere [L] by weight
POP —
    plasma oncotic pressure
    plaster of Paris
P.O.P. — paroxypropione
pop. — popliteal
POPOP — 1,4-bis-(5-phenoxazole) benzene
POR — problem-oriented record
pos. —
    position
    positive
pos. pr. — positive pressure
POSS — proximal over-shoulder strap
poss. — possible
post. —
    posterior
    postmortem
post-op. — postoperative
post. sag. D — posterior sagittal diameter
post sing. sed. liq. — post singulas sedes liquidas [L] after every loose stool
pot. —
    potassa
    potion
POU — placenta, ovary, uterus
PP —
    pancreatic polypeptide
    partial pressure
    pellagra preventive
    permanent partial
    pink puffers (emphysema)
    pinpoint
    posterior pituitary
    postpartum
    postprandial
    private practice
    prothrombin-proconvertin
    protoporphyrin

PP (*continued*)
  proximal phalanx
  pulse pressure
  pyrophosphate
P & P − prothrombin and proconvertin test
PP_1 − inorganic pyrophosphate
P-5'-P − pyridoxal-5'-phosphate
p.p. − punctum proximum [L]
  near-point of accommodation
PPA − phenylpyruvic acid
P_{Pa} − pulmonary artery pressure
p.p.a. − phiala prius agitata [L]
  after shaking
p.p. & a. − palpation, percussion and auscultation
PPB −
  platelet-poor blood
  positive pressure breathing
ppb − parts per billion
PPBS − postprandial blood sugar
PPC − progressive patient care
PPCA − plasma prothrombin conversion accelerator
PPCF − plasma prothrombin conversion factor
PPD −
  paraphenylenediamine
  permanent partial disability
  phenyldiphenyloxadiazole
  progressive perceptive deafness
  purified protein derivative
ppd − prepared
PPD-S − purified protein derivative−standard
PPF −
  pellagra preventive factor
  plasma protein fraction
ppg. − picopicogram
PPH −
  postpartum hemorrhage
  primary pulmonary hypertension

PPH (*continued*)
  protocollagen proline hydroxylase
PPHP − pseudopseudohypoparathyroidism
PPL −
  penicilloyl polylysine
  proteinpolysaccharide
Ppl − intrapleural pressure
PPLO − pleuropneumonia-like organism
PPM − permanent pacemaker
PPO −
  2, 5 diphenyloxazole
  pleuropneumonia organisms
ppm − parts per million
PPNG − penicillinase-producing *Neisseria gonorrhoeae*
PPP −
  pentose phosphate pathway
  platelet-poor plasma
PPPI − primary private practice income
PPR − Price precipitation reaction
PPS −
  pepsin A
  postpartum sterilization
  postperfusion syndrome
  postpump syndrome
PPT −
  partial prothrombin time
  plant protease test
ppt. − precipitate
PPTL − postpartum tubal ligation
PPV − positive-pressure ventilation
PQ −
  permeability quotient
  pyrimethamine-quinine
PR −
  partial remission
  peer review
  percentile rank
  peripheral resistance

PR (*continued*)
    phenol red
    pityriasis rosea
    pregnancy rate
    proctologist
    progressive resistance
    prosthion
    protein
    public relations
    pulse rate
Pr. −
    praseodymium
    presbyopia
    prism
    prolactin
    propyl
p.r. −
    per rectum [L] through the rectum
    punctum remotum [L] far-point of accommodation
PRA − plasma renin activity
prand. − prandium [L] dinner
PRAS − prereduced anaerobically sterilized (media)
p. rat. aetat. − pro ratione aetatis [L] in proportion to age
P.R.B. −
    Population Reference Bureau
    Prosthetics Research Board
PRBV − placental residual blood volume
PRC −
    packed red cells
    plasma renin concentration
PRCA −
    pure red cell agenesis
    pure red cell aplasia
PRD −
    partial reaction of degeneration
    postradiation dysplasia
PRE − progressive resistive exercise

pre. − preliminary
preg. − pregnant
preop. − preoperative
prep. −
    preparation
    preparatory
    prepare
PRERLA − pupils round, equal, react to light and accommodation
PRF − prolactin-releasing factor
PRFM − prolonged rupture of fetal membranes
PRH − prolactin-releasing hormone
PRHBF − peak reactive hyperemia blood flow
PRI − phosphoribose isomerase
PRIH − prolactin release−inhibiting hormone
primip. − woman bearing first child
PRL − prolactin
PRM −
    phosphoribomutase
    premature rupture of membranes
    preventive medicine
    Primary Reference Material
p.r.n. − pro re nata [L] as the occasion arises, as necessary
Pro −
    proline
    prothrombin
proct. − proctology
procto. − proctoscopy
prog. − prognosis
prolong. − prolongatus [L] prolonged
PROM −
    premature rupture of membranes
    prolonged rupture of membranes

pro rect. — pro recto [L] by rectum

prot. — protein

pro-time — prothrombin time

prox. — proximal

prox. luc. — proxima luce [L] the day before

PRP —
pityriasis rubra pilaris
platelet-rich plasma
polymer of ribose phosphate
proliferative retinopathy photocoagulation
Psychotic Reaction Profile

PRPP — phosphoribosylpyrophosphate

PRRE — pupils round, regular and equal

PRT — phosphoribosyltransferase

PRU — peripheral resistance unit

PS —
performing scale
periodic syndrome
phosphatidylserine
physical status
plastic surgery
point of symmetry
population sample
Porter-Silber (chromogen)
prescription
psychiatric
pulmonary stenosis
pyloric stenosis

P/S — polyunsaturated-to-saturated fatty acids ratio

P & S — paracentesis and suction

Ps. — *Pseudomonas*

ps — picosecond

p.s. — per second

PSA — polyethylene sulfonic acid

PSC —
Porter-Silber chromogen

PSC (*continued*)
posterior subcapsular cataract

PSD — peptone-starch-dextrose

PSE —
point of subjective equality
portal-systemic encephalopathy

psec — picosecond

PSG —
peak systolic gradient
polysomnogram
presystolic gallop

PSGN — poststreptococcal glomerulonephritis

PSI —
posterior sagittal index
Problem-Solving Information

psi — pounds per square inch

psia — pounds per square inch absolute

psig — pounds per square inch gauge

PSIL — preferred-frequency speech interference level

PSL — parasternal line

PSMA — progressive spinal muscular atrophy

PSP —
periodic short pulse
phenolsulfonphthalein
positive spike pattern
postsynaptic potential
progressive supranuclear palsy

psp. — postsynaptic potential

PSR — extrahepatic portal-systemic resistance

PSRO — Professional Standards Review Organization

PSS —
physiological saline solution
progressive systemic sclerosis

PST — penicillin, streptomycin and tetracycline

P.S.W. – Psychiatric Social Worker
Psy. – psychiatry
psych. – psychology
PT –
  parathyroid
  paroxysmal tachycardia
  permanent and total
  pharmacy and therapeutics
  phototoxicity
  physical therapy
  physical training
  physiotherapy
  pneumothorax
  posterior tibial
  propylthiouracil
  prothrombin time
  pulmonary tuberculosis
Pt – platinum
pt. –
  part
  patient
  perstetur [L] let it be contin-
    ued
  pint
  point
PTA –
  percutaneous transluminal
    angioplasty
  persistent truncus arteriosus
  phosphotungstic acid
  plasma thromboplastin ante-
    cedent
  post-traumatic amnesia
  prior to admission
  prior to arrival
PTAH – phosphotungstic acid
  hematoxylin
PTAP – purified diphtheria toxoid precipitated by aluminum
  phosphate
PTB –
  patellar tendon–bearing
  prior to birth

PTC –
  percutaneous transhepatic
    cholangiogram
  phenylthiocarbamide
  phenylthiocarbamoyl
  pheochromocytoma, thyroid
    carcinoma syndrome
  plasma thromboplastin com-
    ponent
PTCA – percutaneous transluminal coronary angioplasty
PTC peptide – phenylthiocarbamoyl peptide
PTD –
  permanent and total disability
  prior to discharge
PTE –
  parathyroid extract
  pulmonary thromboembolism
PTED – pulmonary thromboembolic disease
PTEN – pentaerythritol tetranitrate
PTF – plasma thromboplastin
  factor
PTFE – polytetrafluoroethylene
PTH –
  parathormone
  parathyroid hormone
  phenylthiohydantoin
  post-transfusion hepatitis
PTHS – parathyroid hormone secretion (rate)
PTI – persistent tolerant infection
PTM – post-transfusion mononucleosis
PTMA – phenyltrimethylammo-
  nium
PTO – Perlsucht Tuberculin
  Original
PTP –
  post-tetanic potentiation
  prior to program

P_{TP} — transpulmonary pressure
PTR —
    peripheral total resistance
    Perlsucht Tuberculin Rest
PTS — para-toluenesulfonic acid
PTT —
    partial thromboplastin time
    particle transport time
PTU — propylthiouracil
PTX — parathyroidectomy
PTZ — pentylenetetrazol
PU —
    peptic ulcer
    pregnancy urine
Pu — plutonium
PUD —
    peptic ulcer disease
    pulmonary disease
PUE — pyrexia of unknown
    etiology
PUFA — polyunsaturated fatty
    acid
PUH — pregnancy urine hormone
pul. — pulmonary
pulm. —
    pulmentum [L] gruel
    pulmonary
pulv. — pulvis [L] powder
pulv. gros. — pulvis grossus [L] a
    coarse powder
pulv. subtil. — pulvis subtilis [L] a
    smooth powder
PUO — pyrexia of unknown origin
purg. — purgativus [L] cathartic,
    purgative
PV —
    paraventricular
    peripheral vascular
    peripheral vein
    peripheral vessels
    plasma volume
    polycythemia vera

PV (*continued*)
    portal vein
    postvoiding
    pressure/volume
P & V — pyloroplasty and vagot-
    omy
p.v. — per vaginam [L] through
    the vagina
PVA — polyvinyl alcohol
PVC —
    polyvinyl chloride
    postvoiding cystogram
    premature ventricular contrac-
    tion
    pulmonary venous congestion
Pv_{CO_2} — venous carbon dioxide
    pressure
PVD — peripheral vascular disease
PVF — portal venous flow
PVM — pneumonia virus of mice
PVP —
    penicillin V potassium
    peripheral vein plasma
    polyvinylpyrrolidone
    portal venous pressure
PVP-I — povidone-iodine
PVR —
    peripheral vascular resistance
    pulmonary vascular resistance
PVS — premature ventricular sys-
    tole
PVT —
    paroxysmal ventricular tachy-
    cardia
    portal vein thrombosis
    pressure, volume, temperature
pvt. — private
PW — posterior wall
PWB — partial weight-bearing
PWC — physical work capacity
pwd. — powder
PWI — posterior wall infarct

PWM – pokeweed mitogen
PWP – pulmonary wedge pressure
PX – physical examination
Px. – pneumothorax
PXE – pseudoxanthoma elasticum
PYC – proteose-yeast castione (medium)
PyC – pyogenic culture

PYGM – peptone-yeast glucose maltose (agar)
Pyr. – pyridine
PZ – pancreozymin
PZA – pyrazinamide
PZ-CCK – pancreozymin-cholecystokinin
PZI – protamine zinc insulin

Q

Q –
    glutamine
    quantity of electric charge
    quantity of heat
    quartile
    quinacrine
    quotient
    volume of blood
Q_{10} – temperature coefficient
Q. – coulomb (electric quantity)
q –
    electric charge
    the long arm of a chromosome
q. –
    quaque [L] each, every
    quart
QAC – quaternary ammonium compound
q.AM – every morning
QAP – quinine, Atabrine, Plasmoquine
Q_B – total body clearance
QC –
    quality control
    quinine-colchicine
QCIM – Quarterly Cumulative Index Medicus
q.d. – quaque die [L] every day
QEW – quick early warning (test)

QF – quality factor
Q fever – query fever
q.h. – quaque hora [L] every hour
q.2h – quaque secunda hora [L] every two hours
q.3h – quaque tertia hora [L] every three hours
q.4h – quaque quarta hora [L] every four hours
q.h.s. – quaque hora somni [L] every hour of sleep
q.i.d. – quater in die [L] four times a day
q.l. – quantum libet [L] as much as desired
q.m. – quaque mane [L] every morning
QMT – quantitative muscle testing
q.n. – quaque nocte [L] every night
q.n.s. – quantity not sufficient
QO_2 or qO_2 – oxygen quotient
QP –
    Qualified Psychiatrist
    quanti-Pirquet reaction
q.p. – quantum placeat [L] as much as desired
q.q. – quaque [L] each

q.q.h. – quaque quarta hora [L] every four hours
Qq.hor. – quaque hora [L] every hour
q.r. – quantitum rectum [L] the quantity is correct
QRZ – Quaddel Reaktion Zeit [Ger] wheal reaction time
q.s. – quantum satis [L] sufficient quantity
q.suff. – quantum sufficit [L] as much as will suffice
QT – qualification test
qt. –
    quart
    quiet

quadrupl. – quadruplicato [L] four times as much
qual. – quality
quant. – quantity
quat. – quattuor [L] four
QUICHA – quantitative inhalation challenge apparatus
quinq. – quinque [L] five
quint. – quintus [L] fifth
quor. – quorum [L] of which
quot. – quoties [L] as often as necessary
quotid. – quotidie [L] daily
q.v. – quantum vis [L] as much as you please

R

R –
    arginine
    gas constant
    organic radical
    radioactive mineral
    radiology
    rectal
    regression coefficient
    Reiz [Ger] stimulus
    remote
    repressor
    resistance
    respiration
    response
    right
    Rinne test
    roentgen
    rub
R. –
    Behnken's unit
    Rankine (scale)

R. (*continued*)
    Réaumur (scale)
    rectus
    remotum [L] far
    respiration
    right
    rough colony
R. – *Rickettsia*
r –
    radius (of a circle)
    ribose
    ring chromosome
    sample correlation coefficient
P, ρ – rho (17th letter of the Greek alphabet)
RA –
    radioactive
    renal artery
    repeat action
    residual air
    rheumatoid arthritis

RA (*continued*)
   right angle
   right arm
   right atrial
   right atrium
   right auricle
R_A — airway resistance
Ra — radium
RABBI — Rapid Access Blood Bank Information
RA cell — rheumatoid arthritis cell
RAD —
   reactive airway disease
   right axis deviation
Rad. — radiotherapist
rad —
   radial
   radian
   radiation absorbed dose
   radical
   radius
   radix [L] root
RADA — right acromiodorso-anterior
RADP — right acromiodorso-posterior
RADTS — rabbit antidog thymus serum
Rad. Ul. — radius-ulna
RAE — right atrial enlargement
RAEM — refractory anemia with excess myeloblasts
RAF — rheumatoid arthritis factor
RAH — right atrial hypertrophy
RAI — radioactive iodine
RAIU — radioactive iodine uptake
RAM —
   random-access memory
   rapid alternating movements
RAMT — rabbit antimouse thymo-cyte
RAO — right anterior oblique

RAP — right atrial pressure
RAR — right arm recumbent
RARLS — rabbit antirat lympho-cyte serum
RAS —
   renal artery stenosis
   reticular activating system
ras. — rasurae [L] scrapings or filings
RAST — radioallergosorbent test
RATHAS — rat thymus antiserum
RATx — radiation therapy
RAV — Rous-associated virus
RAW — airway resistance
RB —
   Rating Board
   respiratory bronchiole
Rb — rubidium
RBA — rose bengal antigen
RBB — right bundle branch
RBBB — right bundle branch block
RBC —
   red blood cell
   red blood corpuscle
   red blood (cell) count
RBC/hpf — red blood cells per high power field
RBCM — red blood cell mass
RBCV — red blood cell volume
RBD — right border of dullness
RBE — relative biological effective-ness
RBF — renal blood flow
RBL — Reid's base line
RBP — retinol-binding protein
RBS — random blood sugar
RC —
   red cell
   red cell casts
   respiratory center
   retention catheter
   retrograde cystogram
   root canal

RCA –
  red cell agglutination
  right coronary artery
RCBV – regional cerebral blood
  volume
RCC – red cell count
RCD – relative cardiac dullness
RCF –
  red cell folate
  relative centrifugal force
RCITR – red cell iron turnover
  rate
RCM –
  red cell mass
  reinforced clostridial medium
  right costal margin
R colony – rough colony
RCR – respiratory control ratio
R.C.R.A. – Resource Conservation
  and Recovery Act
RCS –
  rabbit aorta-contracting substance
  reticulum cell sarcoma
R.C.S. – Royal College of Surgeons
R/CS – repeat cesarean section
RCU – respiratory care unit
RCV – red cell volume
RD –
  Raynaud's disease
  reaction of degeneration
  resistance determinant
  respiratory disease
  retinal detachment
  right deltoid
  right dorsoanterior
  rubber dam
rd. – rutherford
RDA –
  recommended daily allowance
  recommended dietary allowance

RDA (*continued*)
  right dorsoanterior
RDDA – recommended daily
  dietary allowance
RDE – receptor-destroying enzyme
R determinant – resistance deter-
  minant
R.D.H. – Registered Dental
  Hygienist
RDI – rupture-delivery interval
rDNA – ribosomal DNA
RDP – right dorsoposterior
RdQ – reading quotient
RDRV – Rhesus diploid cell
  strain rabies vaccine
RDS – respiratory distress syndrome
RDW – red cell distribution width
RE –
  radium emanation
  rectal examination
  regional enteritis
  resting energy
  reticuloendothelial
  right eye
R & E – research and education
R_E – respiratory exchange ratio
Re – rhenium
R_e – Reynold's number
REA – radioenzymatic assay
rec. –
  recens [L] fresh
  recent
  record
  recreation
  recurrent
RECG – radioelectrocardiog-
  raphy
rect. –
  rectificatus [L] rectified
  rectum
  rectus muscle

redig. in pulv. — redigatur in pulverem [L] let it be reduced to powder

red. in pulv. — reductus in pulverem [L] reduced to a powder

redox — reduction oxidation

REF — renal erythropoietic factor

REG —
Radiation Exposure Guide
radioencephalogram

reg. — regular

reg. umb. — regio umbilici [L] umbilical region

rehab. — rehabilitation

REL — rate of energy loss

reliq. — reliquus [L] remainder

REM —
rapid eye movement
roentgen-equivalent—man

rem. — removal

REMAB — radiation-equivalent manikin absorption

REMCAL — radiation-equivalent manikin calibration

REMP — roentgen-equivalent — man period

ren. —
renal
renovetur [L] renew

ren. sem. — renovetum semel [L] shall be renewed only once

REO virus — respiratory and enteric orphan virus

REP —
retrograde pyelogram
roentgen-equivalent—physical

rep. —
repetatur [L] let it be repeated
report

req. — requested

RER —
renal excretion rate

RER (*continued*)
rough endoplasmic reticulum

RES — reticuloendothelial system

res. —
research
reserve
resident

resp. —
respectively
respiration
respiratory
responsible

resus. — resuscitation

retic. — reticulocyte

reverse T_3 — reverse triiodothyronine

RF —
Reitland-Franklin (unit)
relative flow (rate)
relative fluorescence
releasing factor
replicative form
resistance factor
respiratory failure
rheumatic fever
rheumatoid factor
root canal, filling of

Rf — rutherfordium

R_f — rate of flow

RFA — right femoral artery

R.F.A. — right frontoanterior

RFB — retained foreign body

RFC — rosette-forming cells

RFL — right frontolateral

RFLA — rheumatoid factor-like activity

RFLS — rheumatoid factor-like substance

R.F.P. — right frontoposterior

RFS — renal function study

R.F.T. — right frontotransverse

RFT — rod-and-frame test

RFW — rapid-filling wave

RG — right gluteal
RGE — relative gas expansion
RH —
　radiant heat
　reactive hyperemia
　relative humidity
　releasing hormone
　right hand
　right hyperphoria
Rh —
　rhesus (factor)
　rhodium
^{106}Rh — radioactive rhodium
Rh- — Rhesus negative
Rh+ — Rhesus positive
rh. —
　rheumatic
　rhonchi [L] rales
RHB — right heart bypass
RHBF — reactive hyperemia
　blood flow
RHC —
　resin hemoperfusion column
　right hypochondrium
RHD —
　relative hepatic dullness
　rheumatic heart disease
rheum. — rheumatic
RHF — right heart failure
RHL — right hepatic lobe
RHLN — right hilar lymph node
rhm — roentgen (per) hour (at 1)
　meter
Rh neg. — Rhesus factor negative
Rh$_{null}$ — rare blood type in which
　all Rh factors are lacking
Rh pos. — Rhesus factor positive
RHS — right hand side
RI —
　radiation intensity
　radioisotope
　refractive index
　regional ileitis

RI (*continued*)
　release-inhibiting
　replicative intermediate
　respiratory illness
　retroactive inhibition
RIA — radioimmunoassay
RIA-DA — radio-immunoassay
　double antibody (test)
RICM — right intercostal margin
RICU — respiratory intensive care
　unit
RID — radial immunodiffusion
RIF — right iliac fossa
RIFA — radioiodinated fatty acid
RIFC — rat intrinsic factor con-
　centrate
RIGH — rabies immune globulin,
　human
RIH — right inguinal hernia
RIHSA — radioactive iodinated
　human serum albumin
R.I.M.R. — Rockefeller Institute
　for Medical Research
RIOJ — recurrent intrahepatic ob-
　structive jaundice
RIR — right iliac region
RIRB — radioiodinated rose ben-
　gal
RISA — radioactive iodinated
　serum albumin
RIST — radioimmunosorbent test
RIT — radio-iodinated triolein
RITC — rhodamine isothiocyanate
RIU — radioactive iodine uptake
RK —
　rabbit kidney
　right kidney
RKW — renal potassium wasting
RKY — roentgenkymography
RL —
　reduction level
　right leg
　right lower

RL (*continued*)
   right lung
   Ringer's lactate
R-L, R→L — right-to-left
RLBCD — right lower border of cardiac dullness
RLC — residual lung capacity
RLD —
   related living donor
   ruptured lumbar disc
RLE — right lower extremity
RLF —
   retrolental fibroplasia
   right lateral femoral
RLL — right lower lobe
RLMD — rat liver mitochondria
RLN — recurrent laryngeal nerve
RLP — radiation-leukemia-protection
RLQ — right lower quadrant
RLS — Ringer's lactate solution
RM —
   radical mastectomy
   reference materials
   respiratory movement
R.M.A. — right mentoanterior
RMCA — right middle cerebral artery
RMD — right manubrial dullness
RMK — rhesus monkey kidney
RML —
   right mediolateral
   right middle lobe
RMP — rapidly miscible pool
R.M.P. — right mentoposterior
RMS — root-mean-square
RMSF — Rocky Mountain spotted fever
RMT — retromolar trigone
R.M.T. — right mentotransverse
RMV — respiratory minute volume
R.N. — Registered Nurse
Rn — radon

RNA —
   ribonucleic acid
   rough, non-capsulated, avirulent
RNase — ribonuclease
RND — radical neck dissection
R.N.M.S. — Registered Nurse for the Mentally Sub-Normal
RNP — ribonucleoprotein
RNP complex — ribonucleoprotein complex
RO —
   Ritter-Oleson (technique)
   routine order
R/O — rule out
R.O.A. — right occipitoanterior
ROC — receiver operating characteristic
roent. — roentgenology
ROH — rat ovarian hyperemia (test)
ROI — region of interest
ROL — right occipitolateral
ROM —
   range of motion
   read-only memory
   rupture of membranes
R.O.P. — right occipitoposterior
ROS — review of systems
ROT — remedial occupational therapy
R.O.T. — right occipitotransverse
rot. —
   rotate
   rotating
RP —
   radial pulse
   reactive protein
   refractory period
   resting pressure
   rest pain
   retrograde pyelogram
R-5-P — ribose-5-phosphate

R_P — pulmonary resistance
RPA — right pulmonary artery
RPCF — Reiter protein complement-fixation
RPCFT — Reiter protein complement-fixation test
RPE — retinal pigment epithelium
RPF —
    relaxed pelvic floor
    renal plasma flow
RP film — rapid processing film
RPG —
    radiation protection guide
    retrograde pyelogram
RPGN — rapidly progressive glomerulonephritis
R.Ph. — Registered Pharmacist
RPI — reticulocytic production index
RPM — rapid processing mode
rpm — revolutions per minute
RPO — right posterior oblique
RPP — retropubic prostatectomy
RPR — rapid plasma reagin (test)
RPS — renal pressor substance
rps — revolutions per second
RPV — right pulmonary vein
RQ — respiratory quotient
RR —
    radiation reaction
    radiation response
    recovery room
    renin release
    respiratory rate
    response rate
R & R —
    rate and rhythm
    rest and recuperation
RRA — radioreceptor assay
RR & E — round, regular and equal
RR-HPO — rapid recompression—high pressure oxygen

R.R.L. — Registered Record Librarian
rRNA — ribosomal ribonucleic acid
RRP — relative refractory period
RRR — renin-release rate
RRT —
    relative retention time
    resazurin reduction time
RS —
    rating schedule
    Rauwolfia serpentina
    reading of standard
    recipient's serum
    Reed-Sternberg (cell)
    reinforcing stimulus
    Reiter's syndrome
    resorcinol-sulfur
    respiratory syncytial (virus)
    response to stimulus
    Reye's syndrome
    right side
    Ringer's solution
RSA —
    rabbit serum albumin
    relative specific activity
R.S.A. — right sacroanterior
RSB — right sternal border
R.S.B. — Regimental Stretcher Bearer
RSC — rested-state contraction
R.Sc.A. — right scapuloanterior
R.S.C.N. — Registered Sick Children's Nurse
R.Sc.P. — right scapuloposterior
RSD — relative standard deviation
RSIVP — rapid sequence intravenous pyelogram
RSL — right sacrolateral
R.S.M. — Royal Society of Medicine
R.S.N.A. — Radiological Society of North America

R.S.P. – right sacroposterior
RSPK – recurrent spontaneous psychokinesis
RSR – regular sinus rhythm
RSS – Russian spring-summer (encephalitis)
RST – radiosensitivity test
R.S.T. – right sacrotransverse
RSTL – relaxed skin tension lines
RSV –
    respiratory syncytial virus
    right subclavian vein
    Rous sarcoma virus
R-S variation – rough-smooth variation
RT –
    radiation therapy
    radiotherapy
    radium therapy
    reaction time
    reading test
    recreational therapy
    respiratory therapy
    right thigh
    room temperature
R.T. – Registered Technician
rT$_3$ – reverse triiodothyronine
rt. – right
RTA – renal tubular acidosis
RTD – routine test dilution
rtd. – retarded
RTF –
    replication and transfer
    resistance transfer factor
    respiratory tract fluid
rt. lat. – right lateral
rtn. – return
RT N(ARRT) – Registered Technologist in Nuclear Medicine Technology under American Registry of Radiologic Technologists

RT R(ARRT) – Registered Technologist in Radiography under American Registry of Radiologic Technologists
RT T(ARRT) – Registered Technologist in Radiation Therapy Technology under American Registry of Radiologic Technologists
RU –
    rat unit
    resistance unit
    retrograde urogram
    right upper
    roentgen unit
Ru – ruthenium
rub. – ruber [L] red
RUE – right upper extremity
RUG – retrograde ureterogram
RUL –
    right upper lobe
    right upper lung
RUO – right ureteral orifice
RUOQ – right upper outer quadrant
RUQ – right upper quadrant
RUR – resin-uptake ratio
RURTI – recurrent upper respiratory tract infection
RV –
    rat virus
    residual volume
    respiratory volume
    retroversion
    right ventricle
    rubella virus
RVB – red venous blood
RVD – relative vertebral density
RVDV – right ventricular diastolic volume
RVE – right ventricular enlargement

RVEDP — right ventricular end-diastolic pressure
RVH — right ventricular hypertrophy
RVI — relative value index
RVLG — right ventrolateral gluteal
RVO — relaxed vaginal outlet
RVP — red veterinary petrolatum
RVR —
    renal vascular resistance
    resistance to venous return
RVRA —
    renal vein renin activity
    renal venous renin assay
RVRC — renal vein renin concentration

RVS —
    relative value schedule
    relative value study
    reported visual sensation
RVT — renal vein thrombosis
RV time — Russell viper time
RV/TLC — residual volume-total lung capacity (ratio)
RW —
    radiological warfare
    ragweed
R-W — Rideal-Walker (coefficient)
R_x —
    prescription
    recipe [L] take
    therapy
    treatment

S

S —
    entropy
    mean dose per unit cumulated activity
    sacral
    saline
    saturation
    screen-containing cassette
    serine
    serum
    siemens
    silicate
    single
    smooth (colony)
    soluble
    spherical lens
    standard normal deviate
    stimulus
    subject
    substrate
    sulfur

S (*continued*)
    sum
    supravergence
    surgery
    Svedberg unit of sedimentation coefficient (10^{-13} sec.)
S_1 —
    first heart sound
    first sacral vertebra or nerve
S_2 —
    second heart sound
    second sacral vertebra or nerve
S_3 —
    third heart sound
    ventricular gallop sound
S. —
    Salmonella
    Schistosoma
    Spirillum
    Staphylococcus
    Streptococcus

s —
  atomic orbital with angular
    momentum quantum num-
    ber 0
  distance
  sample standard deviation
  satellite (chromosomal)
  second
s̄ — sine [L] without
s. —
  semis [L] half
  signa [L] label, mark, sign,
    write
  sinister [L] left
Σ, σ — sigma (18th letter of the
  Greek alphabet)
σ —
  one-thousandth part of a
    second
  standard deviation
SA —
  salicylic acid
  sarcoma
  secondary amenorrhea
  secondary anemia
  serum albumin
  sinus arrhythmia
  slightly active
  soluble in alkaline solution
  specific activity
  Stokes-Adams (disease)
  surface area
  sustained action
  sympathetic activity
S-A —
  sinoatrial
  sinoauricular
S/A — sugar/acetone (urine)
S & A — sugar and acetone
s.a. — secundum artem [L] according to art
SAA — Stokes-Adams attacks

SAB —
  significant asymptomatic bac-
    teriuria
  subarachnoid block
S.A.B. — Society of American
  Bacteriologists
SACD — subacute combined
  degeneration
SAD —
  source to axis distance
  sugar, acetone, diacetic acid
    (test)
SAFA — soluble antigen fluorescent antibody (test)
SAG — Swiss agammaglobulinemia
SAH —
  S-adenosyl-L-homocysteine
  subarachnoid hemorrhage
SAI — Social Adequacy Index
sal. —
  salicylate
  saline
  saliva
  salt
  secundum artis leges [L]
    according to the rules of
    art
SAM —
  S-adenosyl-L-methionine
  sulfated acid mucopolysac-
    charide
  systolic anterior motion
S.A.M.A. — Student American
  Medical Association
S-A node — sinoatrial node
SaO_2 — oxygen per cent saturation
  (arterial)
SAP —
  serum alkaline phosphatase
  systemic arterial pressure
sarc. — sarcoma
SAS —
  sterile aqueous suspension

SAS (*continued*)
    supravalvular aortic stenosis
SAT — Scholastic Aptitude Test
sat. — saturated
SAU — statistical analysis unit
SB —
    serum bilirubin
    single breath
    sinus bradycardia
    small bowel
    Stanford-Binet (test)
    sternal border
    stillbirth
Sb — stibium [L] antimony
$SbCl_3$ — antimony trichloride
SBD — straight bag drainage
SBE —
    shortness of breath on exertion
    subacute bacterial endocarditis
SBF — splanchnic blood flow
SBFT — small bowel follow-
    through
SBG — selenite brilliant green
S.B.H. — State Board of Health
SBN — single-breath nitrogen
    (test)
SBN_2 — single-breath nitrogen
    (test)
SBO — small bowel obstruction
Sb_2O_3 — antimony trioxide
Sb_2O_5 — antimony pentoxide
Sb_4O_6 — antimony trioxide
SBOM — soybean oil meal
SBP —
    scleral buckling procedure
    spontaneous bacterial peri-
      tonitis
    steroid-binding plasma
    systemic blood pressure
    systolic blood pressure
SBS — social-breakdown syn-
    drome
SBT — single-breath test

SBTI — soybean trypsin inhibitor
SC —
    closure of the semilunar valves
    sacrococcygeal
    self care
    semicircular
    semiclosed
    service connected
    sex chromatin
    sick call
    sickle cell
    single chemical
    special care
    sternoclavicular
    subcutaneous
    succinylcholine
    sugar-coated
Sc — scandium
sc. — scilicet [L] one may know
    (certainly, evidently, of
    course)
SCA — sperm-coating antigen
SCAT — sheep cell agglutination
    test
SCBA — self-contained breathing
    apparatus
SCC — squamous cell carcinoma
S.C.C. — Services for Crippled
    Children
SCD —
    service-connected disability
    subacute combined degenera-
      tion (of spinal cord)
    sudden cardiac death
    sudden coronary death
Sc.D. — Doctor of Science
Sc.D.A. — scapulodextra anterior
    [L] right scapuloanterior; a
    presentation of the fetus
Sc.D.P. — scapulodextra posterior
    [L] right scapuloposterior; a
    presentation of the fetus
SCFA — short-chain fatty acid

SCG —
  serum chemistry graft
  sodium cromoglycate
SCH — succinylcholine
SChE — serum cholinesterase
sched. — schedule
schiz. — schizophrenia
SCI — structured clinical interview
SCID — severe combined immunodeficiency disease
SCIPP — sacrococcygeal to inferior pubic point
SCJ — squamocolumnar junction
SCK — serum creatine kinase
Sc.L.A. — scapulolaeva anterior [L] left scapuloanterior; a presentation of the fetus
Sc.L.P. — scapulolaeva posterior [L] left scapuloposterior; a presentation of the fetus
SCM — sternocleidomastoid muscle
S.C.M. —
  Society of Computer Medicine
  State-Certified Midwife
S colony — smooth colony
scop. — scopolamine
SCP — single-celled protein
s.c.p. — spherical candle power
SCPK — serum creatine phosphokinase
SCR — silicon-controlled rectifier
scr. — scruple
SCRAP — Simple Complex Reaction-Time Apparatus
SCS — silicon-controlled switch
S.C.S. — Society of Clinical Surgery
SCT —
  sex chromatin test
  staphylococcal clumping test
SCU — special care unit

SCUBA — self-contained underwater breathing apparatus
SCV — smooth, capsulated, virulent
SD —
  septal defect
  serologically defined
  serum defect
  shoulder disarticulation
  skin dose
  spontaneous delivery
  standard deviation
  streptodornase
  sudden death
  systolic discharge
S/D — systolic to diastolic
Sd — stimulus drive
S^d — stimulus, discriminative
SDA — specific dynamic action
S.D.A. — sacrodextra anterior [L] right sacroanterior; a presentation of the fetus
SD antigen — serologically defined antigen
SDC — succinyldicholine
SDCL — symptom distress check list
S-D curve — strength-duration curve
SDE — specific dynamic effect
SDF — slow death factor
SDH —
  serine dehydrase
  sorbitol dehydrogenase
  subdural hematoma
  succinate dehydrogenase
SDM — standard deviation of the mean
S.D.P. — sacrodextra posterior [L] right sacroposterior; a presentation of the fetus
SDS —
  Self-Rating Depression Scale

SDS (*continued*)
  sensory deprivation syndrome
  sodium dodecyl sulfate
  sudden death syndrome
S.D.T. − sacrodextra transversa
  [L] right sacrotransverse; a
  presentation of the fetus
S.D.U. − Standard Deviation Unit
SE −
  saline enema
  sphenoethmoidal suture
  standard error
  Starr-Edwards (prosthesis)
Se − selenium
SEA − spontaneous electrical
  activity
SEA test − sheep erythrocyte
  agglutination test
S.E.B.M. − Society for Experimental Biology and Medicine
sec. − second
SED −
  skin erythema dose
  spondyloepiphyseal dysplasia
sed. −
  sedes [L] stool
  sedimentation
sed rate − sedimentation rate
SEE − standard error of the esti-
  mate
SEG − sonoencephalogram
seg. − segmented (leukocyte)
segs. − segmented neutrophils
SEM −
  scanning electron microscope
  standard error of the mean
sem. −
  semen
  seminal
SEMI −
  subendocardial myocardial
  infarction

SEMI (*continued*)
  subendocardial myocardial
  injury
semi. − semis [L] one-half
semid. − semidrachma [L] half a
  drachm (dram)
semih. − semihora [L] half an
  hour
SEP −
  sensory evoked potential
  somatosensory evoked potential
  systolic ejection period
separ. − separatum [L] separately
sept. − septem [L] seven
seq. −
  sequela [L] that which follows
  sequestrum
seq. luce − sequenti luce [L] the
  next day
SER −
  smooth endoplasmic reticulum
  somatosensory evoked response
  systolic ejection rate
Ser. − serine
serv. −
  serva [L] keep, preserve
  services
SES − socioeconomic status
sesquih. − sesquihora [L] an hour
  and a half
sesunc. − sesuncia [L] an ounce
  and a half
SET − systolic ejection time
sev. −
  severe
  severed
s. expr. − sine expressione [L]
  without expressing or pressing
SF −
  scarlet fever

SF (*continued*)
seminal fluid
serum fibrinogen
shell fragment
shrapnel fragment
spinal fluid
Streptococcus faecalis
stress formula
synovial fluid
S_f — Svedberg flotation unit
SFC — spinal fluid count
SFD — skin-film distance
SFEMG — single-fiber electromyography
SFP —
screen filtration pressure
spinal fluid pressure
SFS — split function study
SFT —skinfold thickness
SFW —
shell fragment wound
shrapnel fragment wound
SG —
serum globulin
signs
skin graft
specific gravity
Surgeon General
S-G — Sachs-Georgi (test)
SGA — small for gestational age
SGAW — specific airway conduc-
tance
SGFR — single-nephron glomeru-
lar filtration rate
S.G.O. —
Surgeon-General's Office
Surgery, Gynecology and Ob-
stetrics
SGOT — serum glutamic-oxaloacetic transaminase
SGP —
serine glycerophosphatide
soluble glycoprotein

S.G.P. — Society of General
Physiologists
SGPT — serum glutamic-pyruvic
transaminase
SGV — salivary gland virus
SH —
serum hepatitis
sex hormone
sinus histiocytosis
social history
somatotropic hormone
sulfhydryl
surgical history
S & H — speech and hearing
S.H. —
State Hospital
Student Health
sh. — shoulder
S Hb — sulfhemoglobin
SHBD — serum hydroxybutyrate
dehydrogenase
SHBG — sex hormone–binding
globulin
SHCO — sulfated hydrogenated
castor oil
SHDI — supraoptical hypophysial
diabetes insipidus
SHG — synthetic human gastrin
SHHP — semihorizontal heart
position
SHO — secondary hypertrophic
osteoarthropathy
S.H.O. — Student Health Organization
SHP — surgical hypoparathyroidism
SHT — subcutaneous histamine
test
SI —
sacroiliac
saline injection
saturation index
self-inflicted

SI (*continued*)
  seriously ill
  serum iron
  soluble insulin
  stroke index
S.I. – Système International d'Unités (International System of Units)
Si – silicon
SIA – synalbumin-insulin antagonism
SIADH – syndrome of inappropriate antidiuretic hormone
sic. – siccus [L] dry
SICD – serum isocitric dehydrogenase
SICSVA – sequential impaction cascade sieve volumetric air
SID – sudden infant death
S.I.D. – Society for Investigative Dermatology
SIDS – sudden infant death syndrome
S.I.E.C.U.S. – Sex Information and Education Council of the United States
sig. –
  signa, signetur [L] let it be labeled
  significant
sigmoid. – sigmoidoscopy
sig. n. pro. – signa nomine proprio [L] label with the proper name
SIJ – sacroiliac joint
SIM – sulfide, indole, motility (medium)
S.I.M. – Society of Industrial Microbiology
simp. – simplex [L] simple
simul. – at the same time
sing. –
  singular

sing. (*continued*)
  singulorum [L] of each
si non val. – si non valeat [L] if it is not enough
SiO_2 – silicon dioxide (silica)
si op. sit – si opus sit [L] if necessary
SIRS – soluble immune response suppressor
SIS – sterile injectable suspension
SISI – short-increment sensitivity index
si vir. perm. – si vires permittant [L] if the strength will permit
SIW – self-inflicted wound
606 – arsphenamine
SJR – Shinowara-Jones-Reinhard (unit)
SK –
  Sloan-Kettering (used with numbers to designate various experimental compounds in treating cancer)
  streptokinase
SK-SD – streptokinase-streptodornase
SL –
  satellite-like
  sensation level
  Sibley-Lehninger (unit)
  sodium lactate
  solidified liquid
  streptolysin
sl. –
  slight
  sublingual
s.l. – secundum legum [L] according to law
SLA – slide latex agglutination
S.L.A. – sacrolaeva anterior [L] left sacroanterior; a presentation of the fetus

SLAP — serum leucine aminopeptidase

SLB — short leg brace

SLD — serum lactic dehydrogenase

SLE —
St. Louis encephalitis
systemic lupus erythematosus

SLEV — St. Louis encephalitis virus

SLI — splenic localization index

SLKC — superior limbic keratoconjunctivitis

SLN — superior laryngeal nerve

SLO — streptolysin-O

S.L.P. — sacrolaeva posterior [L]
left sacroposterior; a presentation of the fetus

SLR —
straight leg raising
Streptococcus lactis–resistant

SLRT —
straight leg raising tenderness
straight leg raising test

SLS — segment long-spacing (collagen)

S.L.T. — sacrolaeva transversa [L]
left sacrotransverse; a presentation of the fetus

SM —
simple mastectomy
skim milk
streptomycin
submucous
suction method
sustained medication
symptoms
systolic mean
systolic murmur

Sm — samarium

sm. — small

SMA —
sequential multiple analysis
superior mesenteric artery

SMA 6/60 — Sequential Multiple Analyzer (6 tests on serum in 60 minutes)

SMA 12/60 — Sequential Multiple Analyzer (12-test serum profile)

SMAC-23 — laboratory tests

SMAF —
smooth muscle–activating factor
specific macrophage-arming factor

SMC —
special monthly compensation
succinylmonocholine

SMD — submanubrial dullness

S.M.I. — Senior Medical Investigator

SMO — slip made out

S.M.O. — Senior Medical Officer

SMON — subacute myelo-optical neuropathy

SMP —
slow-moving protease
special monthly pension

SMR —
somnolent metabolic rate
standard morbidity ratio
standard mortality ratio
submucous resection

SMRR — submucous resection and rhinoplasty

S.M.S. — State Medical Society

SN —
serum-neutralizing
subnormal
suprasternal notch

S/N — signal-to-noise ratio

S.N. —
Standard Nomenclature
Student Nurse

Sn. — stannum [L] tin

s.n. – secundum naturam [L] according to nature

S.N.A.I. – Standard Nomenclature of Athletic Injuries

SNB – scalene node biopsy

S.N.D.O. – Standard Nomenclature of Diseases and Operations

SNHL – sensorineural hearing loss

S.N.M. – Society of Nuclear Medicine

S.N.O.P. – Systematized Nomenclature of Pathology

SNR – signal-to-noise ratio

SNS – sympathetic nervous system

S.N.S. – Society of Neurological Surgeons

SO –
   salpingo-oophorectomy
   spheno-occipital synchondrosis
   superior oblique (muscle)

SO_2 – sulfur dioxide

SOA-MCA – superficial occipital artery to middle cerebral artery

SOAP – subjective data, objective data, assessment, and plan

SOB –
   shortness of breath
   suboccipitobregmatic

SOC – sequential-type oral contraceptive

sod. bicarb. – sodium bicarbonate

SOL – space-occupying lesion

sol. –
   soluble
   solutio [L] solution

soln. – solution

solv. –
   solve [L] dissolve
   solvent

SOM –
   secretory otitis media
   serous otitis media
   sulformethoxine

S.O.M.O.S. – Society of Military Orthopedic Surgeons

SOP – standard operating procedure

s. op. s. – si opus sit [L] if necessary

s.o.s. – si opus sit [L] if it is necessary

SOTT – synthetic medium old tuberculin trichloroacetic acid (precipitated)

SP –
   sacrum to pubis
   shunt procedure
   skin potential
   spine
   status post
   steady potential
   stool preservative
   suicide precautions
   summating potential
   suprapubic
   symphysis pubis
   systolic pressure

S/P – status post

2-S P – transport medium used for mycoplasma isolation

Sp. –
   spine
   Spirillum

sp. –
   space
   species
   spinal
   spiritus [L] spirit

SPA – suprapubic aspiration

SPAI – steroid protein activity index

SPBI — serum protein-bound iodine

SPC — salicylamide, phenacetin and caffeine

SPCA — serum prothrombin conversion accelerator

sp. cd. — spinal cord

SPE — serum protein electrophoresis

spec. — specimen

SPF —
  specific pathogen free
  spectrophotofluorometer
  split products of fibrin

sp. fl. — spinal fluid

sp. gr. — specific gravity

SPH — secondary pulmonary hemosiderosis

sph. —
  spherical
  spherical lens

SPI — serum precipitable iodine

sp. indet. — species indeterminata [L] species indeterminate

sp. inquir. — species inquirendae [L] species of doubtful status

spir. — spiritus [L] spirit

spiss. — spissus [L] dried

SPL —
  sound pressure level
  spontaneous lesion

spont. — spontaneous (delivery)

spont. Ab. — spontaneous abortion

SPOOL — simultaneous peripheral operation on-line

SPP — suprapubic prostatectomy

spp. — species

SPPS — stable plasma protein solution

SPS —
  sodium polyanetholesulfonate
  sulfite polymyxin sulfadiazine (agar)

spt. — spiritus [L] spirit

SQ —
  social quotient
  subcutaneous

sq. — square

sq. cell ca. — squamous cell carcinoma

sq. cm. — square centimeter

sq. m. — square meter

sq. mm. — square millimeter

sqq. — sequentia [L] and following

SQUID — superconducting quantum-interference-device

SR —
  sarcoplasmic reticulum
  secretion rate
  sedimentation rate
  sensitivity response
  service record
  sex ratio
  side rails
  sigma reaction
  sinus rhythm
  skin resistance
  soluble repository
  stage of resistance
  stimulus response
  stomach rumble
  stretch reflex
  superior rectus
  systemic resistance
  systems review

Sr — strontium

^{85}Sr — radioactive strontium

sr — steradian

SRaw — specific airway resistance

SRBC — sheep red blood cells

SRC —
  sedimented red cells
  sheep red cells

SRF —
  skin reactive factor

SRF (*continued*)
    somatotropin-releasing factor
    split renal function
    subretinal fluid
SRFS — split renal function study
SRH — somatotropin-releasing
    hormone
SRM —
    standard reference materials
    superior rectus muscle
S.R.M. — Standard Reference
    Material
S.R.N. —
    State Registered Nurse (Eng-
    land and Wales)
    Student Registered Nurse
sRNA — soluble ribonucleic acid
SRR — slow rotation room
SRS — slow-reacting substance
S.R.S. — Social and Rehabilitation
    Service
SRS-A — slow-reacting substance
    of anaphylaxis
SRT —
    sedimentation rate test
    speech reception test
    speech reception threshold
S.R.T. — Stroke Rehabilitation
    Technician
S-R variation — smooth-rough var-
    iation
SS —
    saline soak
    saliva sample
    Salmonella and Shigella (agar)
    saturated solution
    serum sickness
    side-to-side
    signs and symptoms
    single-stranded (DNA)
    Sjögren's syndrome
    soapsuds

SS (*continued*)
    standard score
    statistically significant
    sterile solution
    subaortic stenosis
    suction socket
    sum of squares
    supersaturated
ss. — semis [L] one-half
SSA —
    salicylsalicylic acid
    skin-sensitizing antibody
    sulfosalicylic acid (test)
S.S.A. — Social Security Adminis-
    tration
SSD —
    source to skin distance
    sum of square deviations
SSE — soapsuds enema
SSEP — somatosensory evoked
    potential
SSKI — saturated solution of
    potassium iodide
SSN — severely subnormal
SSP —
    Sanarelli-Shwartzman phe-
    nomenon
    subacute sclerosing panen-
    cephalitis
    supersensitivity perception
SSPE — subacute sclerosing pan-
    encephalitis
SSS —
    scalded skin syndrome
    sick sinus syndrome
    specific soluble substance
    sterile saline soak
s.s.s. — stratum super stratum [L]
    layer upon layer
s. str. — sensu stricto [L] in the
    strict sense
SSU — sterile supply unit

SSV — simian sarcoma virus
s.s.v. — sub signo veneni [L]
    under a poison label
ST —
    esotropia
    sedimentation time
    sinus tachycardia
    skin test
    slight trace
    sphincter tone
    standardized test
    sternothyroid
    subtalar
    subtotal
    surface tension
    survival time
S.T.37 — hexylresorcinol
St —
    stoke
    stomach
    subtype
st. —
    stage (of disease)
    stent [L] let them stand
    stet [L] let it stand
    straight
STA — serum thrombotic ac-
    celerator
STA-MCA — superficial temporal
    artery to middle cerebral
    artery
Staph. — Staphylococcus
stat. —
    German unit of radium
      emanation
    statim [L] immediately
STC — soft tissue calcification
STD —
    sexually transmitted diseases
    skin test dose
    skin to tumor distance
std. —
    saturated

std. (*continued*)
    standard
STH — somatotropic hormone
STI —
    serum trypsin inhibitor
    systolic time interval
stillat. — stillatim [L] by drops
still B. — stillborn
STK — streptokinase
STL — swelling, tenderness,
    limitation
STM — streptomycin
STP —
    2,5-dimethoxy-4-methylam-
      phetamine
    scientifically treated petro-
      leum
    standard temperature and
      pressure
STPD — standard temperature and
    pressure, dry ($0°$ C., 760 mm.
    Hg)
Strep. — *Streptococcus*
STS —
    serologic test for syphilis
    standard test for syphilis
STSG — split-thickness skin graft
STT —
    sensitization test
    serial thrombin time
STU — skin test unit
STVA — subtotal villose atrophy
S.T.Y.C.A.R. — Screening Tests
    for Young Children and Re-
    tardates
SU —
    sensation unit
    strontium unit
su. — sumat [L] let the person
    take
SUA —
    serum uric acid
    single umbilical artery

subcu., subcut. or subq. – subcutaneous

sub fin. coct. – sub finem coctionis [L] toward the end of boiling

subling. – sublingual

sub-q. – subcutaneous

suc. – succus [L] juice

SUD –
sudden unexpected death
sudden unexplained death

SUID – sudden unexplained infant death

sum. –
sumat [L] let the person take
sumendum [L] to be taken

sum. tal. – sumat talem [L] let the person take one like this

SUN – serum urea nitrogen

sup. –
superficial
superior
supra [L] above, superior

supp. – suppository

surg. –
surgery
surgical

SUS – stained urinary sediment

SUUD – sudden unexpected, unexplained death

SV –
sarcoma virus
severe
sinus venosus
snake venom
stroke volume
subclavian vein
supravital

SV 40 – simian virus 40

Sv – sievert

s.v. – spiritus vini [L] alcoholic spirit

SVAS – supravalvular aortic stenosis

SVC –
slow vital capacity
superior vena cava

SVCG – spatial vectorcardiogram

SVC-RPA shunt – superior vena cava-right pulmonary artery shunt

SVCS – superior vena cava syndrome

SVD –
spontaneous vaginal delivery
spontaneous vertex delivery

SVG – saphenous vein graft

SVI – stroke volume index

SVM – syncytiovascular membrane

SVR – systemic vascular resistance

svr. – spiritus vini rectificatus [L] rectified spirit of wine

SVT –
supraventricular tachyarrhythmia
supraventricular tachycardia

s.v.t. – spiritus vini tenuis [L] proof spirit

SW –
Schwartz-Watson (test)
spiral wound
stab wound
stroke work

S.W. – Social Worker

SWD – short wave diathermy

SWI – stroke work index

SWR – serum Wassermann reaction

SWS – slow-wave sleep

Sx. –
signs
symptoms

sym. –
symmetrical

sym. (*continued*)
   symptoms
symp. — symptoms
syn. — synovial
syn. fl. — synovial fluid

syph. — syphilis
syr. — syrupus [L] syrup
Sz —
   schizophrenia
   seizure

T

T —
   absolute temperature
   period (time)
   temperature
   tension (intraocular)
   tera-
   tetra-
   thoracic
   thorax
   threonine
   thymidine
   thyroid
   tidal gas
   topical
   torque
   total
   toxicity
   transmittance
   transverse
   tritium
   tumor
   type
T+ — increased tension
T- — decreased tension
T_3 — triiodothyronine
T_4 — thyroxine
T-1824 — Evans Blue (dye)
T. — tesla
T. —
   Taenia
   Treponema
   Trichophyton
   Trypanosoma

t. —
   temporal
   ter [L] three times
   terminal
   tertiary
   test of significance
   translocation
Θ, θ — theta (eighth letter of the
   Greek alphabet)
T, τ — tau (19th letter of the
   Greek alphabet)
τ — life (time)
$\tau\frac{1}{2}$ — half-life (time)
TA —
   alkaline tuberculin
   axillary temperature
   therapeutic abortion
   titratable acid
   toxin-antitoxin
   transaldolase
   tryptophan (acid)
   tube agglutination
T & A —
   tonsillectomy and adenoidec-
      tomy
   tonsils and adenoids
TA_4 — tetraiodothyroacetic acid
Ta — tantalum
TAB — typhoid, paratyphoid A
   and paratyphoid B
tab. — tabella [L] tablet
TACE — tripara-anisylchloroethyl-
   ene

TAD — thoracic asphyxiant dystrophy

TADAC — therapeutic abortion, dilation, aspiration, curettage

TAF —
toxoid-antitoxin floccules
trypsin-aldehyde-fuchsin
Tuberculin Albumose-frei [Ger] albumose-free tuberculin
tumor angiogenesis factor

TAH —
total abdominal hysterectomy
transabdominal hysterectomy

TAL —
tendo Achillis lengthening
thymic alymphoplasia

tal. — talis [L] of such

TAM — toxoid-antitoxin mixture

TAME — toluene-sulfo-trypsin arginine methyl ester

TAN — total ammonia nitrogen

tan. — tangent

TAO —
thromboangiitis obliterans
triacetyloleandomycin

TAPVD — total anomalous pulmonary venous drainage

TAR — thrombocytopenia with absence of the radius

TARA — tumor-associated rejection antigen

TAT —
tetanus antitoxin
Thematic Apperception Test
thromboplastin activation test
total antitryptic activity
toxin-antitoxin
turn-around time
tyrosine aminotransferase

TATST — tetanus antitoxin skin test

TB —
terminal bronchiole
thymol blue
toluidine blue
total base
total body
tracheobronchitis
tubercle bacillus
tuberculin
tuberculosis

Tb —
terbium
tubercle bacillus
tuberculosis

TBA —
tertiary butylacetate
testosterone-binding affinity
thiobarbituric acid
thyroxine-binding albumin

T banding — telomere or terminal banding

TBC — thyroxine-binding coagulin

tbc. — tuberculosis

TBD — total body density

TBE — tuberculin bacillary emulsion

TBF — total body fat

TBG — thyroxine-binding globulin

TBG cap — T_4-binding capacity of thyroxine-binding globulin assays

TBGP — total blood granulocyte pool

TBH —total body hematocrit

TBI —
thyroxine-binding index
total-body irradiation

TBII — TSH-binding inhibitory immunoglobulin

T bili. — total bilirubin

TBK — total body potassium

TBLC — term birth, living child

TBM –
   tuberculous meningitis
   tubular basement membrane
TBP –
   bithionol
   testosterone-binding protein
   thyroxine-binding protein
   tributyl phosphate
TBPA – thyroxine-binding pre-
   albumin
TB-RD – tuberculosis–respiratory
   disease
TBS –
   total body solute
   tribromosalicylanilide
   triethanolamine-buffered
   saline
tbsp. – tablespoonful
TBT –
   tolbutamide test
   tracheobronchial toilet
TBV – total blood volume
TBW –
   total body water
   total body weight
TBX – whole body irradiation
TC –
   taurocholate
   temperature compensation
   tetracycline
   thermal conductivity
   thoracic cage
   throat culture
   thyrocalcitonin
   tissue culture
   to contain
   total capacity
   total cholesterol
   tuberculin contagious
   tubocurarine
T & C –
   turn and cough
   type and crossmatch

Tc – technetium
$T_4(C)$ – serum thyroxine
   measured by the column
   chromatographic technique
^{99m}Tc – radioactive technetium
TCA –
   tricalcium aluminate
   tricarboxylic acid
   trichloroacetate
   trichloroacetic acid
   tricyclic antidepressant
TCAP – trimethylcetylammonium
   pentachlorophenate
TCB – total cardiopulmonary
   bypass
TCBS agar – thiosulfate-citrate-
   bile salts agar
TCC –
   thromboplastic cell compo-
      nent
   trichlorocarbanilide
TCD – tissue culture dose
TCD_{50} – median tissue culture
   dose
TCDB – turn, cough and deep
   breathe
TCDC – taurochenodeoxycholate
TCDD – tetrachlorodibenzodioxin
TC detector – thermal conductivity detector
TCE – trichloroethylene
TCF – total coronary flow
TCH –
   total circulating hemoglobin
   turn, cough, hyperventilate
TCI –
   to come in
   transient cerebral ischemia
TCID – tissue culture infective
   dose
$TCID_{50}$ – median tissue culture
   infective dose

TCIE – transient cerebral ischemic episode
TCM – tissue culture medium
TCNS – transcutaneous nerve stimulator
TCP –
  therapeutic continuous penicillin
  tricresyl phosphate
tcRNA – translation control RNA
TCSA – tetrachlorosalicylanilide
TCT –
  thrombin-clotting time
  thyrocalcitonin
TCu – copper T
TCV – thoracic cage volume
TD –
  tetanus-diphtheria
  therapy discontinued
  thoracic duct
  three times a day
  threshold of discomfort
  thymus-dependent
  time disintegration
  to deliver
  tone decay
  torsion dystonia
  total disability
  transverse diameter
  treatment discontinued
  typhoid-dysentery
$T_4(D)$ – serum thyroxine measured by displacement analysis
TD_{50} – median toxic dose
t.d. –ter die [L] three times daily
TDA – TSH-displacing antibody
TDC – taurodeoxycholate
TDF –
  thoracic duct fistula
  thoracic duct flow
TDI –
  toluene 2,4-diisocyanate

TDI (continued)
  total-dose infusion
TDL – thoracic duct lymph
TDN – total digestible nutrients
TDP –
  thoracic duct pressure
  thymidine diphosphate
t.d.s. – ter die sumendum [L] to be taken three times a day
TDT –
  terminal deoxynucleotidyl transferase
  tone decay test
TDZ – thymus-dependent zone
TE –
  threshold energy
  tissue-equivalent
  tooth extracted
  total estrogen (excretion)
  tracheoesophageal
Te –
  tellurium
  tetanus
TEA – tetraethylammonium
TEAB – tetraethylammonium bromide
TEAC – tetraethylammonium chloride
TEB – tris-ethylenediaminetetraacetate borate
TeBG – testosterone-estradiol–binding globulin
T & EC – Trauma and Emergency Center
TED –
  threshold erythema dose
  thromboembolic disease
TEE – tyrosine ethyl ester
TEF – tracheoesophageal fistula
TEG – thromboelastogram
TEIB – triethyleneiminobenzoquinone
TEL – tetraethyl lead

TEM –
    transmission electron micro-
      scope
    triethylenemelamine
temp. – temperature
temp. dext. – tempori dextro [L]
    to the right temple
temp. sinist. – tempori sinistro
    [L] to the left temple
TEN –
    total excretory nitrogen
    toxic epidermal necrolysis
tenac. – tenaculum
TENS – transcutaneous electrical
    nerve stimulator
TEP – thromboendophlebectomy
TEPA – triethylenephosphora-
    mide
TEPP – tetraethyl pyrophosphate
ter. –
    tere [L] rub
    threefold
    three times
ter. sim. – tere simul [L] rub
    together
TES – trimethylaminoethane-
    sulfonic acid
TET – tetralogy of Fallot
tet. – tetanus
TETD – tetraethylthiuram disul-
    fide
TETRAC – tetraiodothyroacetic
    acid
TEV – talipes equinovarus
TF –
    tactile fremitus
    tetralogy of Fallot
    thymol flocculation
    tissue-damaging factor
    to follow
    total flow
    transfer factor
    tuberculin filtrate

TF (continued)
    tubular fluid
    tuning fork
Tf – transferrin
TFA – total fatty acids
TFE –
    polytetrafluoroethylene
    Teflon
    tetrafluoroethylene
Tf-Fe – transferrin-bound iron
TFL – tensor fascia lata
Tfm – testicular feminization
    syndrome
TFN – total fecal nitrogen
TF/P – tubular fluid plasma
TFR – total fertility rate
TFS – testicular feminization
    syndrome
TG –
    testosterone glucuronide
    thioguanine
    thyroglobulin
    toxic goiter
    triglyceride
TGA – transposition of the great
    arteries
TGAR – total graft area rejected
TGE –
    transmissible gastroenteritis
    tryptone glucose extract
TGFA – triglyceride fatty acid
TGL –
    triglyceride
    triglyceride lipase
T-group – training group
TGT –
    thromboplastin generation test
    thromboplastin generation
      time
TGV –
    thoracic gas volume
    transposition of the great
      vessels

TGY − tryptone glucose yeast (agar)

TH −
tetrahydrocortisol
thyrohyoid
thyroid hormone (thyroxine)

Th − thorium

th. − thoracic

THA −
tetrahydroaminoacridine
total hydroxyapatite

THAM − tris(hydroxymethyl) aminomethane

THC −
tetrahydrocannabinol
thiocarbanidin

THDOC − tetrahydrodeoxycorticosterone

THE − tetrahydrocortisone

ther. − therapy

therap. − therapeutic

THF −
tetrahydrofluorenone
tetrahydrofolic acid
tetrahydrofuran
thymic humoral factor

THFA −
tetrahydrofolic acid
tetrahydrofurfuryl alcohol

THI − trihydroxyindole

thiotepa, thio-TEPA − triethylene thiophosphoramide

THM − total heme mass

TH_2O − titrated water

THP − total hydroxyproline

THPA − tetrahydropteric acid

THR − total hip replacement

Thr − threonine

THRF − thyrotropic hormone–releasing factor

thromb. − thrombosis

THS − tetrahydro-compound S

THSC − totipotent hematopoietic stem cell

THz − terahertz

TI −
thoracic index
thymus-independent
time interval
transverse inlet
tricuspid incompetence
tricuspid insufficiency

Ti − titanium

TIA − transient ischemic attack

TIBC − total iron-binding capacity

Tib.-Fib. − tibula-fibula

TIC − trypsin-inhibitory capacity

TID − titrated initial dose

t.i.d. − ter in die [L] three times a day

TIE − transient ischemic episode

TIF − tumor-inducing factor

TIG − tetanus immune globulin

TIN − tubulointerstitial nephropathy

t.i.n. − ter in nocte [L] three times a night

tinct. − tinctura, tincture

TIP − translation-inhibiting protein

TIS − tumor in situ

TIT −
Treponema immobilization test
triiodothyronine

TIVC − thoracic inferior vena cava

TJ − triceps jerk

TK −
thymidine kinase
transketolase

TKA − transketolase activity

TKD − tokodynamometer

TKG − tokodynagraph

TKO − to keep open

TKR — total knee replacement
TL —
 terminal limen
 time lapse
 time-limited
 total lipids
 tubal ligation
T-L — thymus-dependent lymphocyte
Tl — thallium
TLA — translumbar aortogram
TLC —
 tender loving care
 thin-layer chromatography
 total L-chain concentration
 total lung capacity
 total lung compliance
TLD —
 thermoluminescent dosimeter
 thoracic lymph duct
 tumor lethal dose
T/LD_{100} — minimum dose causing
 death or malformation of 100
 per cent of fetuses
TLE — thin-layer electrophoresis
TLQ — total living quotient
TLV —
 threshold limit value
 total lung volume
TM —
 temporomandibular
 time motion
 trademark
 transmetatarsal
 tympanic membrane
Tm — thulium
T_m — maximal tubular excretory
 capacity of the kidneys
TMA —
 tetramethylammonium
 trimethoxyamphetamine
 trimethoxyphenyl amino-
 propane

TMAS — Taylor Manifest Anxiety
 Scale
T_{max} — time of maximum concentration
TMCA — trimethyl colchicinic
 acid
TMG — 3,3-tetramethyleneglutaric
 acid
TmG — maximal tubular reabsorp-
 tion of glucose
TMJ — temporomandibular joint
TML — tetramethyl lead
TMP —
 thymidine monophosphate
 thymine ribonucleoside-5'-
 phosphate
 trimethoprim
T_{mPAH} — tubular maximum for
 para-aminohippuric acid
TMPD — tetramethyl-p-phenyline-
 diamine
TMS — trimethylsilyl
TMTD — tetramethylthiuram
 disulfide
TMV — tobacco mosaic virus
TN —
 total negatives
 true negative
Tn — normal intraocular tension
TND — term normal delivery
TNF — tumor necrosis factor
TNI — total nodal irradiation
TNM — tumor, nodes and meta-
 stases
TNR — tonic neck reflex
TNT — 2,4,6-trinitrotoluene
TNTC — too numerous to count
TNV — tobacco necrosis virus
TO —
 no evidence of primary tumor
 original tuberculin
 target organ
 telephone order

TO (*continued*)

    tinctura opii [L] tincture of opium

    tubo-ovarian

t.o. − tinctura opii [L] tincture of opium

TOA − tubo-ovarian abscess

TOCP − tri-*o*-cresyl phosphate

T of A − transposition of aorta

tol. − tolerated

tonoc. − tonight

TOP − termination of pregnancy

TOPV − trivalent oral poliovirus vaccine

TORCH − *to*xoplasmosis, *r*ubella, *c*ytomegalovirus and *h*erpes simplex

TORP − total ossicular replacement prosthesis

TOT − "tincture of time"

tot. prot. − total protein

TOWER − testing, orientation, work, evaluation, rehabilitation

TP −

    temperature and pressure

    terminal phalanx

    testosterone propionate

    threshold potential

    thrombocytopenic purpura

    thymic polypeptide

    thymidine phosphorylase

    total positives

    total protein

    transforming principle

    triphosphate

    true positive

    tryptophan

    tube precipitin

    tuberculin precipitation

TPA −

    tannic acid, polyphospho-molybdic acid, amido acid

TPA (*continued*)

    Treponema pallidum agglutination

TPB − tryptone phosphate broth

TPBF − total pulmonary blood flow

TPC −

    thromboplastic plasma component

    Treponema pallidum complement

TPCF − *Treponema pallidum* complement-fixation (test)

TPCP − *Treponema pallidum* cryolysis complement-fixation (test)

TPD − thiamine propyl disulfide

TPEY − telluritepolymixin egg yolk (agar)

TPF − thymus permeability factor

TPG −

    transplacental gradient

    tryptophan peptone glucose (broth)

TPH − transplacental hemorrhage

TPHA − treponemal hemagglutination (test)

TPI −

    treponemal immobilization test (cardiolipin)

    Treponema pallidum immobilization (test)

    triosephosphate isomerase

TPIA − *Treponema pallidum* immobilization (immune) adherence

TPM −

    temporary pacemaker

    triphenylmethane

TPN −

    total parenteral nutrition

    triphosphopyridine nucleotide

TPNH – reduced triphosphopyridine nucleotide
TPO –tryptophan peroxidase
TPP – thiamine pyrophosphate
TPPN – total peripheral parenteral nutrition
TPR –
temperature, pulse and respiration
testosterone production rate
total peripheral resistance
total pulmonary resistance
TPS –
trypsin
tumor polysaccharide substance
TPT –
tetraphenyl tetrazolium
total protein tuberculin
typhoid-paratyphoid (vaccine)
TPTHS – total parathyroid hormone secretion
T-PTX – thyroparathyroidectomy
TPTZ – tripyridyltriazine
TPVR – total pulmonary vascular resistance
Tq. – tourniquet
TR –
tetrazolium reduction
therapeutic radiology
time release
total resistance
total response
tuberculin R (new tuberculin)
tuberculin residue
tubular reabsorption
turbidity-reducing
Tr. –
tincture
trace
TRA – transaldolase
trach. –
tracheostomy

trach. (*continued*)
tracheotomy
tract. – traction
TRAM –
Treatment Rating Assessment Matrix
Treatment Response Assessment Method
TRBF – total renal blood flow
TRC –
tanned red cell
total ridge count
TRCH – tanned-red-cell hemagglutination
TRF –
T-cell–replacing factor
thyrotropin-releasing factor
TRH – thyrotropin-releasing hormone
TRI –
tetrazolium reduction inhibition
total response index
$T_3(RIA)$ – serum triiodothyronine measured by radioassay
$T_4(RIA)$ – serum thyroxine measured by radioimmunoassay
Triac. – triiodothyroacetic acid
TRIC – trachoma-inclusion conjunctivitis
trid. – triduum [L] three days
Trig. – triglycerides
TRIS – tris(hydroxymethyl) aminomethane
TRIT – triiodothyronine
trit. – tritura [L] triturate
TRK – transketolase
TRMC – tetramethylrhodaminoisothiocyanate
tRNA – transfer RNA (ribonucleic acid)
troch. – trochiscus [L] troche

TRP –
   total refractory period
   tubular reabsorption of phosphorus
Trp. – tryptophan
TRPT – theoretical renal phosphorus threshold
TRSV – tobacco ringspot virus
TRU – turbidity-reducing unit
T_3RU – triiodothyronine resin uptake (test)
Try. – tryptophan
TS –
   temperature-sensitive
   test solution
   thoracic surgery
   total solids
   toxic substance
   transsexual
   tricuspid stenosis
   triple strength
   tropical sprue
   tubular sound
   tumor-specific
TSA –
   technical surgical assistance
   trypticase soy agar
   tumor-specific antigen
T_4SA – thyroxine-specific activity
TSB – trypticase soy broth
TSC –
   technetium sulfur colloid
   thiosemicarbazide
TSD –
   target skin distance
   Tay-Sachs disease
   theory of signal detectability
TSE – trisodium edetate
TSF – tissue-coding factor
TSH – thyroid-stimulating hormone
TSH-RF – thyroid-stimulating hormone–releasing factor

TSI –
   thyroid-stimulating immunoglobulins
   triple sugar iron (agar)
TSI agar – triple sugar iron agar
TSN – tryptophan peptone sulfide neomycin (agar)
TSP – total serum protein
tsp. – teaspoonful
TSPAP – total serum prostatic acid phosphatase
T/spine – thoracic spine
TSR –
   testosterone-sterilized rat
   thyroid-to-serum ratio
TSS –
   toxic shock syndrome
   tropical splenomegaly syndrome
TST – tumor skin test
TSTA – tumor-specific transplantation antigen
TSU – triple sugar urea (agar)
TSY – trypticase soy yeast
TT –
   tablet triturate
   tetanus toxoid
   tetrathionate
   tetrazol
   thrombin time
   thymol turbidity
   total thyroxine
   total time
   transit time
   transthoracic
   tuberculin tested
TTC – triphenyltetrazolium chloride
TTD – tissue tolerance dose
TTH –
   thyrotropic hormone
   tritiated thymidine

TTI −
    tension-time index
    time-tension index
TTL − transistor-transistor logic
TTP −
    thrombotic thrombocytopenic
      purpura
    thymidine triphosphate
TTPA − triethylene thiophos-
    phoramide
TTS − temporary threshold shift
TTT − tolbutamide tolerance test
TU −
    thiouracil
    Todd units
    toxic unit
    transmission unit
    tuberculin unit
    turbidity unit
T_3U − triiodothyronine resin up-
    take (test)
tuberc. − tuberculosis
TUD − total urethral discharge
TUG − total urinary gonadotropin
TUR − transurethral resection
TURB − transurethral resection
    of the bladder
TURBT − transurethral resection
    of bladder tumor
TURP − transurethral resection of
    the prostate
tus. − tussis [L] cough
TV −
    tetrazolium violet

TV (continued)
    tidal volume
    total volume
    trial visit
    Trichomonas vaginitis
    tuberculin volutin
TVC −
    timed vital capacity
    total volume capacity
    transvaginal cone
    triple voiding cystogram
TVD − transmissible virus de-
    mentia
TVF − tactile vocal fremitus
TVH − total vaginal hysterectomy
TVL − tenth value layer
TVU − total volume urine
TW −
    tap water
    total (body) water
TWA − time-weighted average
TWE − tap water enema
TWL − transepidermal water loss
TX −
    traction
    transplant
    treatment
T & X − type and crossmatch
ty. −
    type
    typhoid
Tyr − tyrosine
TZ − Tuberculin zymoplastiche

U

U −
    International Unit of enzyme
      activity
    unerupted

U (continued)
    unknown
    upper
    uracil

U (*continued*)
   uranium
   uridine
   urine
   urologist
   urology
^{235}U — isotope of uranium of mass number 235
U. — unit
u — unified atomic mass unit
UA —
   umbilical artery
   unaggregated
   uric acid
   urinalysis
   urine analysis
   uterine aspiration
u.a. — usque ad [L] up to, as far as
UA/C — uric acid-creatinine ratio
UAE — unilateral absence of excretion
UAN — uric acid nitrogen
UB — ultimobranchial body
UBA — undenatured bacterial antigen
UBBC — unsaturated vitamin B_{12}-binding capacity
UBC brace — University of British Columbia brace
UBF — uterine blood flow
UBG — urobilinogen
UBI — ultraviolet blood irradiation
UBP — ureteral back pressure
UC —
   ulcerative colitis
   ultracentrifugal
   unchanged
   unclassifiable
   unit clerk
   urea clearance
   urethral catheterization
   urinary catheter

UC (*continued*)
   uterine contractions
U/C — urine culture
U & C — usual and customary
UCBR — unconjugated bilirubin
UCD — usual childhood diseases
UCG — urinary chorionic gonadotropin
UCHD — usual childhood diseases
UCI — urinary catheter in
UCL — urea clearance (test)
UCO — urethral catheter out
UCP — urinary coproporphyrin
UCR —
   unconditioned response
   usual, customary and reasonable
UCS — unconditioned stimulus
ucs. — unconscious
UD —
   ulnar deviation
   urethral discharge
   uridine diphosphate
   uroporphyrinogen decarboxylase
u.d. — ut dictum [L] as directed
UDC — usual diseases of childhood
UDP — uridine diphosphate
UDPG — uridine diphosphoglucose
UDPGA — uridine diphosphoglucuronic acid
UDP-galactose — uridine diphosphogalactose
UDP-glucose — uridine diphosphoglucose
UDP-glucuronate — uridine diphosphoglucuronate
UDPGT — uridine diphosphoglycyronyl transferase
UDRP — uridine diribose phosphate
UE — upper extremity

UES — upper esophageal sphincter
UFA — unesterified fatty acid
UG — urogenital
UGF — unidentified growth factor
UGI — upper gastrointestinal
UH — upper half
UHF — ultra high frequency
UHL — universal hypertrichosis
  lanuginosa
UI — uroporphyrin isomerase
UIBC — unsaturated iron-binding
  capacity
U.I.C.C. — Union International
  Contra le Cancrum (Interna-
  tional Union against Cancer)
UIF — undegraded insulin factor
UIP — usual interstitial pneumoni-
  tis
UIQ — upper inner quadrant
UJT — unijunction transistor
UK —
  unknown
  urokinase
UL —
  undifferentiated lymphoma
  upper lobe
U & L — upper and lower
ULN — upper limits of normal
ULQ — upper left quadrant
ULT — ultrahigh temperature
ult. — ultimus [L] ultimately, last
ult. praes. — ultimum praescriptus
  [L] last prescribed
UM —
  unmarried
  upper motor
  uracil mustard
Umax. — maximum urinary osmolality
umb. —
  umbilical
  umbilicus

UMNL — upper motor neuron
  lesion
UMP —
  uridine monophosphate (uri-
    dine-5'-phosphate)
  uridylic acid
UN — urea nitrogen
uncomp. — uncompensated
uncond. — unconditioned
uncond. ref. — unconditioned reflex
unct. — unctus [L] smeared
ung. — unguentum [L] ointment
unilat. — unilateral
unk. or unkn. — unknown
uns. —
  unsatisfactory
  unsymmetrical
unsat. — unsaturated
unsym. — unsymmetrical
UO —
  ureteral orifice
  urinary output
UOQ — upper outer quadrant
Uosm. — urinary osmolality
UP —
  upright posture
  ureteropelvic
  uroporphyrin
U/P — urine-plasma ratio
UPG — uroporphyrinogen
UPI — uteroplacental insufficiency
UPJ — ureteropelvic junction
UPOR — usual place of residence
UQ —
  ubiquinone
  upper quadrant
UR —
  unconditioned reflex
  unconditioned response
  upper respiratory

UR (*continued*)
  utilization review
ur. — urine
URD — upper respiratory disease
URF — uterine-relaxing factor
urg. — urgent
URI — upper respiratory infection
URO — uroporphyrin
urol. — urology
URQ — upper right quadrant
URT — upper respiratory tract
URTI — upper respiratory tract
  infection
US —
  ultrasonic
  ultrasound
  unconditioned stimulus
USAN — United States Adopted
  Names
U.S.M.H. — United States Marine
  Hospital
USN — ultrasonic nebulizer
USO — unilateral salpingo-oophor-
  ectomy
U.S.P. — United States Pharma-
  copeia
U.S.P.H.S. — United States Public
  Health Service

USR — unheated serum reagin
  (test)
ust. — ustus [L] burnt
UT — urinary tract
UTBG — unbound thyroxine-
  binding globulin
UTD — up to date
ut dict. — ut dictum [L] as direct-
  ed
utend. — utendus [L] to be used
utend. mor. sol. — utendus more
  solito [L] to be used in the
  usual manner
UTI — urinary tract infection
UTP — uridine triphosphate
UU — urine urobilinogen
UUN — urine urea nitrogen
UUP — urine uroporphyrin
UV —
  ultraviolet
  umbilical vein
  urinary volume
U_v — Uppsala virus
UVA — ultraviolet radiation
UVJ — ureterovesical junction
UVL — ultraviolet light
UVR — ultraviolet radiation
ux. — uxor [L] wife

V

V —
  coefficient of variation
  unipolar chest lead
  vaccinated
  valine
  valve
  vanadium
  variation
  vector
  vein

V (*continued*)
  velocity
  ventilation
  verbal
  vertex
  virulence
  virus
  vision
  visual acuity
  voice

V (*continued*)
  volt
  voltage
  volume
V. – *Vibrio*
v–: – vicinal isomer
v. –
  specific volume
  vena [L] vein
  versus
  very
  vide [L] see
  vitamin
  volt
VA –
  vacuum aspiration
  ventriculoatrial
  vertebral artery
  visual acuity
  volt-ampere
V_A – alveolar ventilation
V.A. – Veterans Administration
Va –
  alveolar ventilation
  visual acuity
  volt-ampere
vac. –
  vaccine
  vacuum
VACTERL – *v*ertebral, *a*nal, *c*ardiac, *t*racheal, *e*sophageal, *r*enal and *l*imb
vag. –
  vagina
  vaginal
VAKT – visual, association, kinaesthetic, tactile
Val – valine
VALE – visual acuity, left eye
VAMP – vincristine, amethopterine, 6-mercaptopurine and prednisone

V_A/Q_C ratio – ventilation-perfusion ratio
var. –
  variant
  variation
  variety
VARE – visual acuity, right eye
VASC – Verbal Auditory Screen for Children
vasc. – vascular
vas. vit. – vas vitreum [L] a glass vessel
VAT – ventricular activation time
VATER – *v*ertebral defects, imperforate *a*nus, *t*racheoesophageal fistula and *r*adial and *r*enal dysplasia
VB –
  viable birth
  vinblastine
VBL – vinblastine
VBOS – veronal-buffered oxalated saline
VBP – vinblastine, bleomycin and Platinol
VBS – veronal-buffered saline
VBS:FBS – veronal-buffered saline – fetal bovine serum
VC –
  acuity of color vision
  vena cava
  ventilatory capacity
  vincristine
  vital capacity
  vocal cord
V/C – ventilation-circulation ratio
V_C – pulmonary capillary blood volume
VCA – viral capsid antigen
VCC – vasoconstrictor center
VCG – vectorcardiogram
VCI – volatile corrosion inhibitor

V-cillin — penicillin V

VCN — vancomycin hydrochloride, colistimethate sodium, nystatin

V_{CO} — carbon monoxide (endogenous production)

V_{CO_2} — carbon dioxide output

VCR — vincristine

VCS — vasoconstrictor substance

VCT — venous clotting time

VCU — voiding cystourethrogram

VCUG — vesicoureterogram

VD —
vapor density
venereal disease
virus diarrhea

Vd — volume dead air space

V_d — apparent volume of distribution (V area)

vd — double vibrations

VDA — visual discriminatory acuity

VDBR — volume of distribution of bilirubin

VDC — vasodilator center

VDEL — Venereal Disease Experimental Laboratory

VDEM — vasodepressor material

VDG — venereal disease—gonorrhea

vdg. — voiding

VDH — valvular disease of the heart

VDL — visual detection level

VDM — vasodepressor material

VDP — vincristine, daunorubicin, prednisone

VDRL — Venereal Disease Research Laboratory

VDRS — Verdun Depression Rating Scale

VDRT — Venereal Disease Reference Test

VDS —
vasodilator substance
venereal disease—syphilis

VDV — ventricular end-diastolic volume

$V_D V_T$ — physiologic dead space in percent of tidal volume

VE —
vaginal examination
vesicular exanthema
visual efficiency
volumic ejection

V & E — Vinethene and ether

V_E —
airflow per unit of time
respiratory minute volume

VEA — ventricular ectopic activity

VEE — Venezuelan equine encephalomyelitis

VEE virus — Venezuelan equine encephalomyelitis virus

vehic. — vehiculum [L] vehicle

vel. or veloc. — velocity

VEM — vasoexcitor material

V_{Emax} — maximum flow per unit of time

vent. —
ventral
ventricular

vent. fib. — ventricular fibrillation

VEP — visual evoked potential

VER — visual evoked response

vert. —
vertebra, vertebral
vertical

ves. —
vesica [L] bladder
vesicular

vesic. — vesicula [L] a blister

vesp. — vesper [L] evening

ves. ur. — vesica urinaria [L] urinary bladder

VET — vestigial testis

Vet. −
   veteran
   veterinary
v. et. − vide etiam [L] see also
VF −
   ventricular fibrillation
   ventricular fluid
   visual field
   vocal fremitus
V.f. − field of vision
V factor − verbal comprehension
   factor
VFDF − very fast death factor
Vfib. − ventricular fibrillation
VFP − ventricular fluid pressure
VG − ventricular gallop
VGH − very good health
VH −
   vaginal hysterectomy
   venous hematocrit
   viral hepatitis
VHD −
   valvular heart disease
   viral hematodepressive disease
VHDL − very high-density lipoprotein
VHF −
   very high frequency
   visual half-field
VI −
   vaginal irrigation
   variable interval
   virgo intacta
   virulence
   volume index
Vi − virginium
VIA − virus-inactivating agent
vib. − vibration
VIBS − vocabulary, information,
   block design, similarities
VIC − vasoinhibitory center
vic. − vices [L] times
vid. − vide [L] see

VIG − vaccinia-immune globulin
vin. − vinum [L] wine
VIP −
   vasoactive intestinal polypep-
      tide
   vasoinhibitory peptide
   very important patient
   voluntary interruption of
      pregnancy
vir. −
   viridis [L] green
   virulent
VIS − vaginal irrigation smear
vis. −
   vision
   visiting
   visitor
visc. −
   visceral
   viscosity
   viscous
vit. −
   vitamin
   vitellus [L] yolk
vitamin
   v. A − vitamin A
   v. A_1 − vitamin A_1 (retinol)
   v. A_2 − vitamin A_2 (dehydro-
      retinol)
   v. B − vitamin B
   v. B complex − vitamin B
      complex
   v. B_1 − vitamin B_1 (thiamine)
   v. B_2 − vitamin B_2 (riboflavin)
   v. B_6 − vitamin B_6
   v. B_{12} − vitamin B_{12} (cyanoco-
      balamin)
   v. B_{12b} − vitamin B_{12b} (hy-
      droxocobalamin)
   v. B_c − vitamin B_c (folic acid)
   v. B_c conjugate − vitamin B_c
      conjugate (folic acid)

vitamin (*continued*)
  v. C – vitamin C (ascorbic acid)
  v. D – vitamin D (calciferol)
  v. D_2 – vitamin D_2 (ergocalciferol)
  v. D_3 – vitamin D_3 (cholecalciferol)
  v. E – vitamin E (alpha-tocopherol)
  v. G – vitamin G (riboflavin)
  v. H – vitamin H (biotin)
  v. K – vitamin K
  v. K_1 – vitamin K_1 (phytonadione)
  v. K_2 – vitamin K_2 (menaquinone)
  v. K_3 – vitamin K_3 (menadione)
  v. L – vitamin L
  v. L_1 – vitamin L_1
  v. L_2 – vitamin L_2
  v. M – vitamin M (folic acid)
vit. cap. – vital capacity
vit. ov. sol. – vitello ovi solutus [L] dissolved in yolk of egg
vitr. –
  vitreous
  vitrum [L] glass
viz. – videlicet [L] namely
VLB – vincaleucoblastine (vinblastine)
VLDL or VLDLP – very low-density lipoprotein
VLSI – very large scale integration
VM –
  vasomotor
  ventricular muscle
  vestibular membrane
  viomycin
  voltmeter

VMA –
  vanillylmandelic acid
  vanilmandelic acid
VMH – ventromedial hypothalamic (neurons)
VMR – vasomotor rhinitis
VN –
  virus-neutralization
  Visiting Nurse
  Vocational Nurse
V.N.A. – Visiting Nurse Association
VO – verbal order
V_{O_2} –
  oxygen consumption
  oxygen uptake
voc. – vocational
VOD – venous occlusive disease
V.O.D. – visio oculus dextra [L] vision, right eye
vol. –
  volar
  volatilis [L] volatile
  volume
  volumetric
  voluntary
  volunteer
vol/vol – volume ratio (volume per volume)
VOM –
  vinyl chloride monomer
  volt-ohm-milliammeter
V.O.S. – visio oculus sinister [L] vision, left eye
v.o.s. – vitello ovi solutus [L] dissolved in yolk of egg
V.O.U. – visio oculus uterque [L] vision, each eye
voxel – volume element
VP –
  vasopressin
  venipuncture

VP (*continued*)
  venous pressure
  Voges-Proskauer (reaction)
  volume-pressure
  vulnerable period
V & P — vagotomy and pyloroplasty
V_P — plasma volume
VPB — ventricular premature
  beat
VPC —
  vapor-phase chromatography
  ventricular premature con-
    traction
  volume packed cells
  volume per cent
VPD — ventricular premature depolarization
VPL — ventroposterolateral
  (nucleus)
VPP — viral porcine pneumonia
VPRC — volume of packed red
  cells
vps — vibrations per second
V/Q — ventilation-perfusion
VR —
  valve replacement
  variable ratio
  vascular resistance
  venous return
  ventilation ratio
  vocal resonance
  vocational rehabilitation
V_r —
  relaxation volume
  ventral root
V.R.A. — Vocational Rehabilitation Administration
VRBC — red blood cell volume
VR & E — vocational rehabilitation and education
VRI — viral respiratory infection
VRL — Virus Reference Library

VRP — very reliable product
  (written on prescription)
VRV — ventricular residual volume
VS —
  vaccination scar
  venisection
  verbal scale (IQ)
  vesicular sound
  vesicular stomatitis
  villonodular synovitis
  vital signs
  volumetric solution
Vs. — venaesectio [L] venesection
vs. —
  single vibration
  versus (against)
  vibration seconds
  voids
v.s. — vide supra [L] see above
VsB. — venaesectio brachii [L]
  bleeding in the arm
VSD — ventricular septal defect
VSOK — vital signs normal
VSS — vital signs stable
VSULA — vaccination scar upper
  left arm
VSV — vesicular stomatitis virus
VSW — ventricular stroke work
VT —
  tetrazolium violet
  vacuum tuberculin
  vasotonin
  ventricular tachycardia
V & T — volume and tension
V_T — tidal volume
VTE — vicarious trial and error
V-test — Voluter test (radiology)
VTG — volume thoracic gas
VTI — volume thickness index
VTM — mechanical tidal volume
VTSRS — Verdun Target Symp-
  tom Rating Scale

VTVM – vacuum tube voltmeter
VV –
  varicose veins
  viper venom
  vulva and vagina
v/v – volume of solute per volume
  of solution
vv. – venae [L] veins

V/VI – grade 5 on a 6-grade basis
VW –
  vessel wall
  von Willebrand's disease
V wave – vertex sharp transient
Vx. – vertex
VZ – varicella-zoster
VZV – varicella-zoster virus

W –
  tryptophan
  water
  watt
  Weber (test)
  week
  weight
  west
  white
  whole
  widow
  widowed
  widower
  width
  wife
  wolframium (tungsten)
  word fluency
  work
W+ – weakly positive
^{185}W – radioactive tungsten
W. – wehnelt (unit of hardness of
  roentgen rays)
w. –
  week
  wife
  with
WA – when awake

WAIS – Wechsler's Adult Intelligence Scale
WAP – wandering atrial pacemaker
WASP – World Association of
  Societies of Pathology
WB –
  washable base
  water bottle
  Wechsler-Bellevue scale
  weight-bearing
  wet-bulb
  whole blood
  whole body
  Willowbrook (virus)
Wb – weber
WBC –
  white blood cell
  white blood count
WBC/hpf – white blood cells per
  high power field
WBE – whole body extract
WBF – whole blood folate
WBH – whole blood hematocrit
WBR – whole body radiation
WBS – whole body scan
WBT – wet bulb temperature

WC −
　water closet
　wheelchair
　white cell
　white cell casts
　whooping cough
　work capacity
WC′ − whole complement
WCC − white cell count
WD −
　wallerian degeneration
　well-developed
　well-differentiated
　wet dressing
　with disease
　wrist disarticulation
w/d − well developed
wd. − ward
WDLL − well-differentiated lymphocytic lymphoma
wds. − wounds
WDWN − well-developed, well-nourished
WE −
　western encephalitis
　western encephalomyelitis
WEE −
　western equine encephalitis
　western equine encephalomyelitis
WEE virus − western equine encephalomyelitis virus
WF −
　Weil-Felix (reaction)
　white female
W/F − white female
W.F.O.T. − World Federation of Occupational Therapists
WFR − Weil-Felix reaction
WG − water gauge
WGA − wheat germ agglutinin
WH − well-healed

W.H.A.P. − Women's Health and Abortion Project
WHO −
　WHO histologic classification of ovarian tumors
　World Health Organization
whp. − whirlpool
whr. − watt hour
W.H.R.C. − World Health Research Center
WHVP − wedged hepatic venous pressure
WIA − wounded in action
wid. −
　widow
　widower
WISC − Wechsler's Intelligence Scale for Children
WK − Wernicke-Korsakoff (syndrome)
wk. −
　weak
　week(s)
WK disease − Wilson-Kimmelstiel disease
WL −
　waiting list
　wavelength
　work load
WL test − waterload test
WM −
　white male
　whole milk
W/M − white male
wm. − whole mount
W.M.A. − World Medical Association
WMF − white middle-aged female
WMM − white middle-aged male
WMR − work metabolic rate
W.M.R. − World Medical Relief
WMX − whirlpool, massage, exercise

WN — well-nourished
WNF — well-nourished female
WNL — within normal limits
WNM — well-nourished male
WO —
    wash out
    written order
W/O — water in oil
w/o — without
WP —
    weakly positive
    wet pack
    whirlpool
    working point
WPB — whirlpool bath
WPRS — Wittenborn Psychiatric Rating Scale
WPW — Wolff-Parkinson-White (syndrome)
WR —
    Wassermann reaction
    weakly reactive
wr. — wrist
WRAT — Wide Range Achievement Test

WRC —
    washed red cells
    water-retention coefficient
WRE — whole ragweed extract
WRVP — wedged renal vein pressure
WS —
    water-soluble
    water swallow
ws. — watts-second
wt. —
    weight
    white
wt/vol — weight per volume
wt/wt — weight ratio (weight per weight)
WV — whispered voice
w/v — weight of solute per volume of solution
WV-MBC — ratio of walking ventilation to maximum breathing capacity
w/w — weight of solute per weight of total solution
WZa — wide zone alpha

X —
    crossed with
    cross or transverse
    extra
    homeopathic symbol for the decimal scale of potencies
    Kienböck's unit of x-ray dosage
    magnification
    multiplied by
    reactance
    removal of
    respirations (anethesia chart)
    start of anesthesia

X (*continued*)
    times
    unknown quantity
$\overline{X}, \overline{x},$ —
    average of all X's
    sample mean
X. — *Xenopsylla*
x — axis
$\overline{x}$ — mean
Ξ, ξ — xi (14th letter of the Greek alphabet)
XA — xanthurenic acid
Xa — chiasma
xanth. — xanthomatosis

XC – excretory cystogram
XDP – xeroderma pigmentosum
Xe – xenon
XES – X-ray energy spectrometer
XL – extra large
XLD – xylose-lysine-deoxycholate (agar)
XM – crossmatch
X_m – magnetic susceptibility
XMP – xanthosine monophosphate (xanthosine-5'-phosphate)
XOR – exclusive operating room
XP – xeroderma pigmentosum
XR – x-ray

XRT – x-ray technician
XS –
   excess
   xiphisternum
XT – exotropia
$X_2 t.$ – chi-square test
Xta – chiasma, chiasmata
XU – excretory urogram
Xu – x-unit
XX – normal female chromosome type
XX/XY – sex karyotypes
XY – normal male chromosome type
Xyl. – xylose

Y –
   tyrosine
   yellow
   young
   yttrium
Y. – *Yersinia*
y – year(s)
Υ, υ – upsilon (20th letter of the Greek alphabet)
YADH – yeast alcohol dehydrogenase
YAG – yttrium aluminum garnet
Yb – ytterbium

YCB – yeast carbon base
yd. – yard(s)
YE – yellow enzyme
YEH_2 – reduced yellow enzyme
YF – yellow fever
YNB – yeast nitrogen base
y.o. – year(s) old
YOB – year of birth
YP – yield pressure
yr. – year(s)
YS – yolk sac
y.s. – yellow spot (of the retina)
yt. – yttrium

Z

Z –
   atomic number
   impedance
   ionic charge number
   standard score

Z (*continued*)
   zero
   zone
Z. – Zuckung [Ger] contraction
z – standardized device

Z, ζ – zeta (sixth letter of the
  Greek alphabet)
Z/D – zero defects
ZE – Zollinger-Ellison (syndrome)
Z/G or ZIG – zoster immune
  globulin
ZI^a – isotope with atomic number
  Z and atomic weight A
Zn – zinc
Zn. fl. – zinc flocculation (test)
$ZnSO_4$ – zinc sulfate

zool. –
  zoological
  zoology
ZPG – zero population growth
Zr – zirconium
^{95}Zr – radioactive zirconium
ZSR – zeta sedimentation ratio
  (method)
Zz. – zingiber [L] ginger
Z.Z.'Z." – increasing degrees of
  contraction

Medical Eponyms

A

Aaron's sign

Aarskog's syndrome — a hereditary syndrome marked by abnormal distances between paired organs and by a broad upper lip, anomalous scrotal fold, relaxed ligaments, and small hands. Called also *faciodigito-genital dysplasia*

Aarskog-Scott syndrome — same as *Aarskog's syndrome*

Abadie's clamp, sign

Abbe's operation(s) — a lateral intestinal anastomosis; division of an esophageal stricture

Abbé's condenser, flap, illuminator, ring, string, method, treatment

Abbé-Estlander operation — the transfer of a full-thickness flap from one lip to fill a defect in the other

Abbé-Zeiss apparatus, counting cell, counting chamber

Abbott's elevator, gouge, method, tube

Abbott-Lucas approach

Abbott-Miller tube

Abbott-Rawson tube

Abderhalden's dialysis, reaction, test

Abderhalden-Fanconi syndrome — osteomalacia, renal glycosuria, aminoaciduria, phosphaturia, and cystine deposition throughout the body

Abderhalden-Fauser reaction

Abegg's rule

Abelin's reaction, test

Abell's uterine suspension

Abelson's cannula

Abercrombie's syndrome — amyloid degeneration

Abercrombie's degeneration, tumor

Abernethy's fascia, sarcoma

abortus Bang ring (ABR) test

Abrahams's cannula, elevator, knife, sign

Abrami's disease — same as *Hayem-Widal syndrome*

Abramov-Fiedler myocarditis

Abrams's heart reflex, needle, punch, reflex, test

Abramson's tube

Abrikosov's (Abrikossoff's) tumor

Abt-Letterer-Siwe syndrome — a proliferation of nonlipid histio-

Abt-Letterer-Siwe syndrome (*continued*)
cytes in the visceral organs, causing red-to-brown, firm nodules to appear, followed by a maculopapular rash or multiple nodules that ulcerate and hemorrhage

Achard's syndrome — arachnodactyly

Achard-Castaigne method, test

Achard-Thiers syndrome — association of diabetes and hirsutism in postmenopausal women; sometimes said to involve an increased incidence of uterine cancer

Achenbach's syndrome — sudden appearance of hematomas of the hand with piercing pain and edema

Achilles bursa, bursitis, jerk, reflex, tendon

Achor-Smith syndrome — nutritional deficiency with pernicious anemia, sprue, and pellagra, due to potassium depletion

Achucárro's stain

Acosta's disease — acute mountain sickness

Acree-Rosenheim reaction, reagent, test

Acrel's ganglion

Adair's forceps, procedure

Adair-Allis forceps

Adair-Dighton syndrome — same as *van der Hoeve's syndrome*

Adamantiades-Behçet syndrome — same as *Behçet's syndrome*

Adami's theory

Adamkiewicz's demilunes, reaction, test

Adams's aspirator, clasp, position, retractor, saw, test

Adams's disease — same as *Adams-Stokes disease*

Adams's operation(s) — subcutaneous intracapsular division of the neck of the femur for ankylosis of the hip; subcutaneous division of the palmar fascia; excision of a wedge-shaped piece from the eyelid

Adams-Stokes disease — heart block with sudden unconsciousness

Adams-Stokes syndrome — same as *Morgagni-Adams-Stokes syndrome*

Adams-Stokes syncope

Adasoy's procedure

Addis's count, method, test

Addison's disease — hypofunction of the adrenal glands with prostration and progressive anemia

Addison's anemia, keloid, melanoderma, planes, point, scleroderma

Addison-Biermer disease — pernicious anemia

Addison-Gull disease — vitiligines of the skin, chronic jaundice, splenomegaly and hepatomegaly

Adelmann's operation — disarticulation of a finger

Adelmann's method

Aden's fever, ulcer

Adie's syndrome — reaction in which one pupil contracts more slowly than the other

Adie's pupil

Adie-Holmes syndrome — same as *Adie's syndrome*

Adler's forceps, punch, test, theory
Adson's syndrome — same as *Naffziger's syndrome*
Adson's maneuver, test
Adson-Brown forceps
Adson-Murphy needle
Aeby's muscle, plane
Afzelius's erythema
Agazotti's mixture
Agnew's keratome, splint
Agnew-Verhoeff incision
Agostini's reaction, test
Ahlfeld's method
Ahlquist-Durham clip
Ahumada–del Castillo syndrome — amenorrhea, low gonadotropin secretion and galactorrhea, not related to pregnancy
Aicardi's syndrome — diffuse central nervous system anomalies in female infants
Åkerlund's deformity, diaphragm
Akin's bunionectomy
Akureyri disease — benign myalgic encephalomyelitis
Alajouanine's syndrome — symmetric lesions of the sixth and seventh cranial nerves with double facial paralysis and external oculomotor paralysis associated with double clubfoot and strabismus
Alanson's amputation
Albarrán's disease — presence of *Escherichia coli* in the urine
Albarrán's gland, test, tubules
Albee's operation(s) — operation for ankylosis of the hip; transplantation of a portion of the tibia
Albee-Delbet operation — for fracture of the neck of the femur

Albers-Schönberg disease/syndrome — osteopetrosis — a hereditary disease characterized by abnormal density of bone
Albers-Schönberg marble bones, method
Albert's disease — inflammation of the bursa
Albert's operation — excision of the knee to secure ankylosis
Albert's syndrome — painful inflammation of the bursa located between the os calcis and the Achilles tendon
Albert's diphtheria stain, position, suture
Albert-Andrews laryngoscope
Albertini's treatment
Albini's nodules
Albinus's muscle
Albl's ring
Albrecht's bone
Albright's syndrome — same as *Albright-McCune-Sternberg syndrome*
Albright's dystrophy, hereditary osteodystrophy, solution
Albright-Butler-Bloomberg syndrome — vitamin D–resistant rickets
Albright-Hadorn syndrome — a disorder of potassium metabolism associated with osteomalacia and sudden hypokalemic muscular paralysis
Albright-McCune-Sternberg syndrome — fibrous dysplasia of bone with endocrine dysfunction
Alcock's canal
Alcock-Hendrickson lithotrite
Alcock-Timberlake obturator

Alden's retractor

Alder's constitutional granulation anomaly

Alder-Reilly anomaly

Aldrich's syndrome — same as *Wiskott-Aldrich syndrome*

Aldrich's mixture

Aldrich-McClure test

Aldridge-Studdefort urethral suspension

Alexander's disease — an infantile form of leukodystrophy

Alexander's operation(s) — shortening of the round ligaments of the uterus; ligation of the vertebral arteries for relief of epilepsy; prostatectomy

Alexander's syndrome — congenital factor VII deficiency resulting in hemophilia-like hemorrhagic diathesis with epistaxes, deep muscular hematomas and internal hemorrhages

Alexander's deafness, gouge, hearing loss, incision, method, punch

Alexander-Adams operation — shortening of the round ligaments of the uterus

Alexander-Farabeuf elevator, periosteotome

Alezzandrini's syndrome — degenerative retinitis

Alfraise's test

Alibert's disease — a progressive lymphoma of the skin

Alibert's keloid, mentagra

Alibert-Bazin syndrome — a rare, usually fatal, disease of the reticuloendothelial system

Allarton's operation — median lithotomy

Allemann's syndrome — familial, hereditary double kidney and clubbed fingers

Allen's fossa, maneuver, paradoxic law, rule, test, treatment

Allen-Barkan knife

Allen-Brown shunt

Allen-Doisy test, unit

Allen-Masters syndrome — pelvic pain resulting from laceration during delivery

Allesandri-Guaceni test

Allingham's operation(s) — inguinal colotomy; excision of the rectum by an incision into the ischiorectal fossae

Allingham's ulcer

Allis's clamp, forceps, inhaler, sign

Allis-Coakley forceps

Allis-Duval forceps

Allis-Ochsner forceps

Allison's atrophy, clamp, retractor

Allport's hook, retractor, searcher

Allport-Babcock retractor, searcher

Almeida's disease — South American blastomycosis

Almén's reagent, test

Alouette's operation — amputation at the hip with a semicircular outer flap to the great trochanter and a large internal flap from within outward

Alouette's amputation

Alper's disease — degeneration of the cerebral gray matter with preservation of the white matter, manifested by progressive mental deterioration, spasticity, myoclonus, generalized convulsions, choreoathetosis, ataxia and early death

Alper's test

Alport's syndrome − progressive sensorineural hearing loss with pyelonephritis or glomerulonephritis

Alsberg's angle, triangle

Alsever's solution

Alström's syndrome − retinal degeneration with nystagmus and loss of central vision

Alström-Hallgren syndrome − a familial syndrome characterized by obesity, diabetes mellitus, deafness, retinitis pigmentosa and mental disorders

Alström-Olsen syndrome − familial inborn visual abnormality due to genetic retinal lesions with no neurological or endocrine changes

Althausen's test

Altmann's fluid, granules, theory

Altmann-Gersh method

Alvarez's prosthesis

Alvarez-Rodriguez catheter

Alvegniat's pump

Alvis's curet

Alyea clamp

Alzheimer's disease/syndrome − presenile dementia

Alzheimer's cells, corpuscles, dementia, sclerosis, stain

Amalric's syndrome − deafness with macular dystrophy and central visual defects

Amann's coefficient, test

Amato's bodies

Ambard's coefficient, constant, equation, formula, law

Amberg's line

Ames test

Amici's disk, line, striae

Ammon's operation(s) − blepharoplasty by a flap from the cheek; dacryocystotomy, resection of a spindle-shaped piece of skin over the bridge of the nose for epicanthus

Ammon's filaments, fissure, horn, quick test, scleral prominence

amniotic infection syndrome of Blane − fetal sepsis following swallowing and aspiration of contaminated amniotic fluid

Amoss's sign

Amplatz's catheter

Amsler's charts, marker

Amsterdam's dwarf, type

Amussat's operation − a long transverse incision for exposure of the colon

Amussat's probe, valve

Anagnostakis's operation(s) − for entropion; for trichiasis

Ancell-Spiegler cylindroma

Andernach's ossicles

Anders's disease − deposit of fatty masses in subcutaneous tissues throughout the body

Anders's syndrome − same as *Dercum's syndrome*

Andersch's ganglion, nerve

Andersen's disease − glycogen-storage disease

Andersen's syndrome − bronchiectasis, pancreatic cystic fibrosis, and vitamin A deficiency

Andersen's triad

Anderson's operation − longitudinal splitting of a tendon to produce lengthening of the tendon

Anderson's medium, phenomenon, procedure, splint, test

Anderson-Adson retractor
Anderson-Goldberger test
Andes disease — chronic mountain sickness
Andogsky's syndrome — bilateral cataracts involving the entire lens
Andrade's syndrome — a form of amyloidosis marked by sensory disorders and progressive paralysis
Andrade's indicator, type of amyloidosis
Andral's decubitus, sign
André's test
André-Thomas sign
Andreasch's test
Andresen's appliance
Andrewes's test
Andrews's disease — eruptions of pustules on palms and soles due to bacterial infection elsewhere in the body
Andrews's bacterid, forceps
Andrews-Hartman forceps, retractor, rongeur
Andrews-Pynchon tube
Anel's operation — dilation of the lacrimal duct followed by an astringent injection
Anel's probe, syringe
Angelchik's prosthesis
Angeli's sulfone
Angell's curet
Angelucci's syndrome — extreme excitability and vasomotor disturbance, associated with vernal conjunctivitis
Anghelescu's sign
Angle's classification, malocclusion, splint
Anglesey's leg
Angström's law, unit

Anichkov's (Anitschkow's) cell, myocyte
Annam ulcer
Annandale's operation(s) — the removal of the condyles of the femur; the fixation of displaced cartilages of the knee joint by stitches
Anrep effect
Ansbacher's unit
Anschütz's chloroform
Anson-McVay herniorrhaphy
Anstie's limit, reagent, rule, test
Anthony's capsule stain, retractor, tube
Anthony-Fisher balloon
Antole-Condale elevator
Anton's syndrome — same as *Anton-Babinski syndrome*
Anton's symptom
Anton-Babinski syndrome — denial or unawareness of blindness in cortical blindness
Antonucci's test
Apert's disease/syndrome — craniostenosis associated with syndactyly
Apert-Crouzon disease — a hereditary disease consisting of hand and foot malformations with craniofacial abnormalities
Apert-Gallais syndrome — same as *Cooke-Apert-Gallais syndrome*
Apgar's scale, score
Apley's grind test, maneuver, sign
Appolito's suture
Apt test
Arakawa's reaction, reagent, test
Arakawa-Higashi syndrome — hypochromic anemia with megaloblastic bone marrow

Aran's law

Aran-Duchenne disease — spinal muscular atrophy

Arantius's bodies, canal, duct, ligament, nodules, ventricle

Arbuckle's probe

Arcelin's method

Archer's forceps

Archetti's test

Arey's rule

Argand's burner

Argonz–Del Castillo syndrome — a combination of galactorrhea with amenorrhea and low urinary follicle-stimulating hormone not associated with pregnancy or acromegaly

Argyle's catheter, tube

Argyle-Salem tube

Argyll Robertson pupil, sign

Arias's syndrome — hyperbilirubinemia with jaundice of the skin, sclera and mucous membranes

Arias-Stella cells, phenomenon, reaction

Aries-Pitanguy mammaplasty

Aristotle's anomaly

Arkin's disease — same as *Bayford-Autenrieth dysphagia*

Arloing-Courmont test

Arlt's disease — a contagious infection by *Chlamydia trachomatis* characterized by keratoconjunctivitis, papillary hypertrophy, follicles and scarring, often leading to blindness

Arlt's operation — any of several operations on the eye and eyelid

Arlt's recess, sinus, trachoma

Arlt-Jaesche operation — transplantation of the ciliary bulbs from the edge of the lid for correction of distichiasis

Armanni-Ebstein cells, change, lesion

Armanni-Ehrlich degeneration

Armstrong's disease — lymphocytic choriomeningitis

Arndt's law

Arndt-Gottron disease/syndrome — scleromyxedema

Arndt-Schulz law

Arneth's syndrome — muffled speech caused by complete hepatization of the lung tissue

Arneth's classification, count, formula, index

Arning's carcinoid

Arnold's nerve reflex cough syndrome — reflex cough from irritation of the area supplied by the auricular branch of the vagus nerve

Arnold's bodies, canal, fold, ganglion, ligament, nerve, neuralgia, sterilizer, substance, test

Arnold-Chiari syndrome — malformation of the cerebellum with hydrocephalus

Arnold-Chiari deformity, malformation

Arnold and Gunning method

Arnott's bed, dilator

Aron's test

Aronson's culture medium, method

Arrhenius's doctrine, equation, formula, theory

Arrhigi's point

Arroyo's sign

Arruga's expressor, forceps, retractor, speculum

Arruga-Gill forceps

Arthus's phenomenon, reaction

Artmann's chisel

Arzberger's pear (pear-shaped vessel)

Asboe-Hansen's disease — a skin disease of newborn girls characterized by bullous, keratogenic, pigmented dermatitis

Asboe-Hansen's incontinentia pigmenti

Asch's operation — correction of deflection of the nasal septum

Asch's forceps, splint

Ascher's syndrome — relaxation of the skin of the eyelid, double lip and nontoxic thyroid gland enlargement

Ascher's glass-rod phenomenon, veins

Ascherson's membrane, vesicles

Aschheim-Zondek hormone, test

Aschner's phenomenon, reflex, sign, test

Aschner-Danini test

Aschoff's bodies, cells, node, nodules

Aschoff-Tawara node

Ascoli's reaction, test, treatment

Aselli's glands, pancreas

Ashby's agar, culture medium

Asherman's syndrome — adhesions within the endometrial cavity, often causing amenorrhea and infertility

Ashford's mamilliplasty

Ashhurst's splint

Ashman's phenomenon

Askenstedt's method

Asperger's psychopathy

Assézat's triangle

Assmann's focus, tuberculous infiltrate

Atkins's knife

Atkins-Cannard tube

Atkins-Tucker laryngoscope

Atkinson's lid block

Atkinson and Kendall test

Atlee's clamp, dilator

Aub-Dubois table

Auberger's blood group

Aubert's phenomenon

Audouin's microsporon

Audry's syndrome — same as *Uehlinger's syndrome*

Auenbrugger's sign

Auer's bodies, phenomenon

Auerbach's ganglion, plexus

Aufranc's gouge, hip prosthesis, retractor

Aufranc-Turner hip prosthesis

Aufrecht's disease — alterations of the parenchyma of the liver and kidney in infectious jaundice

Aufrecht's sign

Aufricht's retractor, speculum

Aufricht-Lipsett rasp

Augustine's nail

Aujeszky's disease — pseudorabies

Aujeszky's itch

Ault's clamp

Auricchio and Chieffi test

Auspitz's disease — same as *Alibert-Bazin syndrome*

Auspitz's dermatosis

Austin's knife

Austin Flint murmur, phenomenon, respiration

Austin Moore arthroplasty, prosthesis

Austin and Van Slyke method

Autenrieth and Funk method

Auvard's cranioclast, speculum
Auvard-Remine speculum
Auvray's incision
Aveline Gutierrez parotidectomy
Aveling's repositor
Avellis's syndrome — unilateral
    paralysis of the larynx and
    soft palate with loss of pain
    and temperature senses
Avellis's paralysis
Avellis-Longhi syndrome — same
    as *Avellis's syndrome*
Avery's culture medium
Avicenna's gland
Avila's approach
Avogadro's constant, law, number
Axenfeld's syndrome — congenital
    ocular maldevelopment
Axenfeld's anomaly, calcareous
    degeneration, conjunctivitis,
    test
Axenfeld-Krukenberg spindle

Axenfeld-Schürenberg syndrome
    — oculomotor paralysis alter-
    nating with spasm
Ayala's equation, index, quotient
Ayer's forceps, test
Ayer-Tobey test
Ayerst's knife
Ayerza's disease — a form of poly-
    cythemia vera marked by cya-
    nosis, dyspnea, bronchitis,
    bronchiectasis and hyperplasia
    of bone marrow and associ-
    ated with sclerosis of the pul-
    monary artery
Ayerza's syndrome — pulmonary
    hypertension with dilatation
    of pulmonary arteries
Ayre's brush, knife
Ayre-Scott knife
Aztec ear, idiocy
Azua's pseudoepithelioma

B

Baaser's dermatostomatitis
Baastrup's disease/syndrome — a
    disorder in which the spinous
    processes of adjacent vertebrae
    are in contact (kissing spine)
Babbitt's metal
Babcock's operation — removal of
    the saphenous vein
Babcock's forceps, herniorrhaphy,
    needle, raspatory, test, trocar
Baber's syndrome — congenital
    cirrhosis of the liver
Babès's treatment, tubercles
Babès-Ernst bodies, corpuscles,
    granules

Babington's disease — same as
    Osler's syndrome
Babinski's syndrome — association
    of cardiac and arterial disorders
    with late syphilis
Babinski's law, phenomenon, re-
    flex, sign, test
Babinski-Fröhlich syndrome —
    adiposogenital dystrophy
Babinski-Nageotte syndrome —
    multiple lesions affecting the
    pyramidal and sensory tracts
Babinski-Vaquez syndrome — same
    as *Babinski's syndrome*
Babinski-Weil test

Babkin's reflex
Baccelli's mixture, sign
Bachman's reaction, test
Bachmann's bundle
Bachmeier's test
Backhaus's clamp, dilator, forceps
Bacon's anoscope, forceps, raspatory, retractor, rongeur
Badal's operation — laceration of the infratrochlear nerve for pain of glaucoma
Badgley's nail, retractor
Baehr-Löhlein lesion
Baehr-Schiffrin disease — same as *Moschowitz's disease*
Baelz's disease/syndrome — congenital and familial papules at the duct openings of the mucous glands of the lips with fissures radiating from the angles of the mouth
Baer's cavity, law, membrane, method, nystagmus, plane, vesicle
Baerensprung's erythrasma
Baermann's test
Baeyer's test
Bäfverstedt's syndrome — benign inflammatory hyperplasia of cutaneous lymphocytes
Bagot's mixture
Bahnson's clamp, retractor
Bailey's cannula, clamp, dilator, forceps, Gigli-saw guide, leukotome, rongeur
Bailey-Cowley clamp
Bailey-Gibbon rib contractor
Bailey-Glover-O'Neil commissurotomy, knife, valvulotome
Bailey-Morse clamp, knife
Bailey-Williamson forceps

Baillarger's syndrome — same as *Frey's syndrome*
Baillarger's bands, layer, lines, sign, striae, striations, stripes
Bailliart's ophthalmodynamometer, tonometer
Bainbridge's clamp, forceps, reflex
Baird's forceps
Bakamjian's pedicle flap
Baker's cyst, forceps, method, tube, velum
Bakes's dilator
Bakwin-Eiger syndrome — multiple fractures in early life with bowing of all extremities
Bakwin-Krida syndrome — same as *Pyle's disease*
Balamuth's culture medium
Balbiani's body, nucleus, rings
Baldwin's operation — formation of an artificial vagina by transplantation of a piece of ileum between the bladder and the rectum
Baldy's operation — retrodisplacement of the uterus
Baldy-Webster operation — same as *Webster's operation*
Baldy-Webster uterine suspension
Balfour's disease — green cancer — a condition marked by development of localized green masses of abnormal cells
Balfour's bodies, gastrectomy, gastroenterostomy, infective granule, retractor, test, treatment
Balint's syndrome — cortical paralysis of visual fixation
Balkan's fracture frame, splint
Ball's method, valves
Ballance's sign

Ballantine's clamp
Ballantine-Drew coagulator
Ballantyne-Runge syndrome —
    prolonged gestation syndrome
Ballen-Alexander retractor
Ballenger's curet, elevator, forceps,
    periosteotome, urethroscope
Ballenger-Forster forceps
Ballenger-Hajek chisel, elevator
Ballenger-Lillie bur
Ballenger-Sluder tonsillectome
Ballentine's forceps
Ballentine-Peterson forceps
Ballet's disease — paralysis of one
    or more of the nerves supply-
    ing the extrinsic eye muscles
Ballet's sign
Ballingall's disease — maduromy-
    cosis
Balme's cough
Baló's disease — inflammation of
    the white substance of the
    brain in which demyelination
    occurs in concentric rings
Balser's fatty necrosis
Bamatter's syndrome — a familial
    syndrome marked by progeria
    with nanism, microcornea,
    corneal opacity, enlarged
    joints, osseous dysplasia, flab-
    by skin and tooth discolora-
    tion
Bamberger's disease(s) — polysero-
    sitis with effusion of fluid into
    the pleural and peritoneal
    cavities; spasm or tic of the
    lower extremities
Bamberger's area, fluid, hemato-
    genic albuminuria, sign
Bamberger-Marie disease — hyper-
    trophic pulmonary osteoarth-
    ropathy

Bamby's clamp
Bamle's disease — epidemic
    pleurodynia
Bancroft's filaria, filariasis
Bancroft-Plenk gastrectomy
Bandeloux's bed
Bandl's ring
Bane's forceps, rongeur
Bang's disease — undulant fever
Bang's bacillus, method, test
Bankart's retractor
Banner's snare
Bannister's disease — angioneu-
    rotic edema
Bannwarth's syndrome — sub-
    acute chronic lymphocytic
    meningitis with facial paraly-
    sis
Bantam's coagulator
Banti's disease/syndrome — con-
    gestive splenomegaly
Banting's cure, diet, treatment
Bar's syndrome — pain in the area
    of the gallbladder, ureters and
    appendix with occasional fever
Bar's incision
Barach's index
Bárány's syndrome — a combina-
    tion of unilateral headache,
    ipsilateral deafness, vertigo,
    tinnitus and inability to point
    a finger
Bárány's apparatus, pointing test,
    sign, symptom
Barbara's pelvimeter
Barber's dermatosis
Barclay's niche
Barcoo's disease — desert sore — a
    form of tropical ulceration of
    the face, hands and lower ex-
    tremities
Barcoo rot, vomit

Barcroft's apparatus
Bard's syndrome — pulmonary metastases in cancer of the stomach
Bard's catheter, dilator, electrode, resectoscope, sign
Bard-Parker blade, dermatome, forceps, scissors
Bardach's test
Bardam's catheter
Bardeen's disk
Bardel's serum
Bardenheuer's extension, incision
Bardet-Biedl syndrome — a recessive, heritable disorder marked by mental retardation, polydactyly and hypogenitalism
Bareggi's reaction, test
Baréty's method
Barfoed's reagent, test
Barfurth's law
Bargen's serum, streptococcus
Barger's method
Barile-Yaguchi-Eveland (BYE) agar
Barkan's operation — goniotomy for congenital glaucoma
Barkan's forceps, goniotomy, knife
Barker's operation(s) — excision of the hip joint; a method of excising the astragalus
Barker's needle, point
Barkman's reflex
Barkow's colliculus, ligament
Barlow's disease — infantile scurvy
Barlow's syndrome — late apical systolic murmur due to protrusion of the posterior mitral-valvular leaflet into the atrial cavity
Barlow's forceps
Barnard's carcinoma
Barnes's bag, compressor, curve, dilator, speculum

Barnes-Dormia stone basket
Barnes-Simpson forceps
Barnhill's curet
Baron's elevator, knife, retractor, tube
Barr's body, bolt, hook, nail, retractor, speculum
Barral's test
Barraquer's disease — any disturbance of fat metabolism marked by progressive diminution of body fat
Barraquer's operation — removal of lens in cataract by suction
Barraquer's brush, erysiphake, forceps, method, scissors, sutures, trephine
Barraquer-Colibri eye speculum
Barraquer-DeWecker scissors
Barraquer-Simons syndrome — same as *Simons's disease*
Barraquer-Zeiss microscope
Barraya's forceps
Barré's signs
Barré-Guillain syndrome — acute febrile polyneuritis
Barré-Liéou syndrome — vertigo of cervical arthrosis
Barré-Masson syndrome — glomus tumor
Barrett's syndrome — chronic peptic ulcer of the lower esophagus
Barrett's epithelium, esophagus, forceps, knife, tenaculum, ulcer
Barrett-Adson retractor
Barrett-Allen forceps
Barrett-Murphy forceps
Barron's ligation
Barsky's operation — repair of a cleft hand

Barsky's cleft lip repair, elevator, pharyngoplasty

Bársony-Polgár syndrome — a diffuse, esophageal spasm caused by disruption of the advance of peristaltic waves by an irregular contraction

Bársony-Teschendorf syndrome — same as *Bársony-Polgár syndrome*

Bart's hemoglobin

Bart-Pumphrey syndrome — a familial, hereditary syndrome consisting of knuckle pads, leukonychia and deafness

Bartelmez's club ending

Barth's hernia

Barthelemy's disease — a symmetric eruption of papules or nodules in children and young adults with tuberculosis

Bartholin's anus, duct, foramen, glands

Bartholomew's rule of fourths

Bartlett's stripper

Barton's operation — for ankylosis, by sawing through the bone and removing a V-shaped section

Barton's bandage, dressing, forceps, fracture

Barton-Cone tongs

Bärtschi-Rochain syndrome — headache, paresthesia, scotoma, stiffness in the neck, pain on pressure of the vertebrae and vertigo

Bartter's syndrome — primary juxtaglomerular cell hyperplasia

Baruch's law, scissors, sign

Barwell's operation — osteotomy for genu valgum

Basedow's disease — a thyroid disorder of unknown etiology, usually called *Graves's disease*

Basedow's goiter, paralysis, triad

Basham's mixture, solution, test

Basile's screw

Bass-Watkins test

Bassen-Kornzweig syndrome — abetalipoproteinemia

Basset's operation — dissection of the inguinal glands for cancer of the vulva

Bassini's operation — for the radical cure of inguinal hernia

Bastedo's rule

Bastian's aphasia, law

Bastian-Bruns law, sign

Bastow's raspatory

Batch-Spittler-McFadden amputation

Bateman's disease — a viral skin disease marked by formation of firm, translucent, depressed papules containing caseous matter

Bateman's prosthesis, purpura

Bates's operation — the division of a urethral stricture from within outward with a special type of urethrotome

Bather's leukemia

Batten's disease — same as *Batten-Mayou disease*

Batten-Mayou disease — a juvenile form of cerebral sphingolipidosis

Battey's disease — a tuberculosis-like lung disease caused by "Battey bacilli"

Battey bacilli

Battle's operation — for appendicitis, with retraction of the rectus muscle

Battle's incision, sign

Battle-Jalaguier-Kammerer incision

Battley's sedative

Baudelocque's operation — an incision through the posterior cul-de-sac of the vagina for removal of the ovum, in extrauterine pregnancy

Baudelocque's diameter, line

Bauer's test, valve

Bauer-Feulgen technique

Bauer-Trusler-Tondra cleft lip repair

Bauhin's gland, valve

Baum's operation — stretching of the facial nerve by an incision below the ear

Baumann's coefficient, test

Baumann-Goldmann test

Baumès's law, symptom

Baumé's scale

Baumgarten's glands

Baumrucker's resectoscope

Baunscheidt's treatment

Bayer's test

Bayford-Autenrieth dysphagia

Bayle's disease — paralytic dementia

Bayle's granulations

Baylor's splint

Baynton's bandage

Bayrac's test

Bazin's disease — a chronic, necrotizing vasculitis of unknown origin, usually occurring on the calves of young women

Béal's conjunctivitis

Beale's ganglion cells

Beall's mitral valve prosthesis

Bean's syndrome — association of erectile, bluish, cavernous hemangiomas of the skin with bleeding hemangiomas of the gastrointestinal tract

Beard's disease/syndrome — neurasthenia

Beard's cystotome, knife, speculum, treatment

Beardsley's dilator, forceps, tube

Bearn-Kunkel syndrome — a condition seen in young women marked by cirrhosis of the liver with hypergammaglobulinemia and increase of plasma cells in the liver

Beatson's operation — ovariotomy in inoperable breast cancer

Beatty-Bright friction sound

Beau's disease/syndrome — cardiac insufficiency

Beau's lines

Beaupre's forceps

Beauvais's disease — rheumatoid arthritis

Beaver's blade, curet, electrode, keratome, retractor

Beaver-DeBakey blade

Beccari's process

Bechtel's prosthesis, screw

Beck's disease — a disease affecting young people in Siberia, marked by swelling of the phalanges, enlargement of joints and retardation of growth

Beck I operation — an operation for supplying collateral circulation to the heart

Beck II operation — a two-stage operation for supplying col-

Beck II operation (*continued*)
lateral circulation to the heart,
performed two to three weeks
apart

Beck's syndrome — occlusion of
the anterior spinal artery resulting in various neurological
complications

Beck's cardiopericardiopexy, forceps, gastrostomy, raspatory,
triad

Beck-Jianu gastrostomy

Beck-Mueller tonsillectome

Beck-Satinsky clamp

Beck-Schenck tonsillectome

Becker's disease — cardiomyopathy leading to fatal congestive heart failure

Becker's muscular dystrophy,
nevus, phenomenon, retractor,
scissors, sign, test, trephine

Becker-Lennhoff index

Beckman-Adson retractor

Beckman-Colver speculum

Beckman-Eaton retractor

Beckman-Weitlaner retractor

Beckmann's apparatus, formula,
thermometer

Beckwith's syndrome — a hereditary disorder marked by extreme cytomegaly of the fetal
adrenal cortex

Beckwith-Wiedemann syndrome —
a recessive, hereditary syndrome marked by exophthalmos, macroglossia and
gigantism

Béclard's amputation, hernia,
nucleus, sign, triangle

Béclère's method

Becquerel's rays

Bednar's aphtha

Bedson's test

Beer's operation — flap operation
for cataract

Beer's collyrium, knife, law

Beevor's sign

Begbie's disease — a thyroid disorder of unknown etiology,
usually called *Graves's disease*

Begg's appliance, technique

Béguez César disease — a lethal,
progressive, autosomal recessive disorder marked by massive leukocytic inclusions,
pancytopenia and hepato-
splenomegaly

Behçet's disease/syndrome — a
complex of disorders including severe uveitis, optic atrophy, lesions of the mouth and
genitalia and other symptoms
suggestive of diffuse vasculitis

Behçet's aphthae

Béhier-Hardy sign, symptom

Behla's bodies

Behnken's unit

Behr's disease — degeneration of
the retinal macula in adult
life

Behr's syndrome — optic atrophy-
ataxia syndrome

Behr's pupil, sign

Behre-Benedict test

Behring's law, tuberculin

Beigel's disease — a fungal disease
of the hair in which hair shafts
bear nodular masses of fungi

Beisman's sign

Békésy's audiometry

Bekhterev's (Bechterew's) disease
— rheumatoid spondylitis

Bekhterev's (Bechterew's) arthritis, layer, nucleus, nystagmus,

Bekhterev's (Bechterew's)
(*continued*)
reaction, reflex, sign, spondy-
litis, symptom, test, tract
Bekhterev-Mendel reflex
Bekhterev-Strumpell-Marie syn-
drome — ankylosing polyar-
thritis
Belfield's operation — vasotomy
Bell's disease — acute delirium
Bell's delirium, law, mania, muscle,
nerve, palsy, paralysis, phe-
nomenon, sign, spasm, suture,
test, treatment
Bell-Dally dislocation
Bell-Magendie law
Bellini's ducts, ligament, tubules
Bellocq's cannula, sound, tube
Bellows's cryoextractor
Bellucci's scissors
Belsey's esophagoplasty, hernior-
rhaphy
Belzer's apparatus
Benaron's forceps
Benassi's method
Bence Jones bodies, cylinders,
globulin, protein, proteinuria,
reaction, urine
Benda's stain
Bender's gestalt test
Bendien's test
Benedict's gastroscope, method,
solution, test
Benedict-Denis method, test
Benedict-Franke method
Benedict-Hitchcock method
Benedict-Hopkins-Cole reagent
Benedict-Leche method
Benedict-Murlin method, test
Benedict-Osterberg method
Benedict-Theis method
Benedikt's syndrome — ipsilateral
oculomotor paralysis, contra-

Benedikt's syndrome (*continued*)
lateral hyperkinesia, paresis of
the arm and leg and ataxia
Beneventi's retractor
Bengolea's forceps
Béniqué's sound
Benjamin's anemia
Bennell's bandage
Bennet's syndrome — erythroblas-
tic anemia, osteoporosis, and
steatorrhea in children
Bennet's corpuscles
Bennett's disease — leukemia
Bennett's operation — for varico-
cele, by partial excision of the
pampiniform plexus
Bennett's angle, forceps, fracture,
movement, retractor
Bensley's neutral gentian orange G
stain
Benson's disease — spherical, cal-
cium-containing opacities in
the vitreous humor
Benson's separator
Bent's operation — shoulder ex-
cision with flap from the del-
toid region
Bentley's filter
Benzhaf's serum
Béraneck's tuberculin
Bérard's aneurysm, ligament
Berardinelli's syndrome — congen-
ital hyperpituitarism of hypo-
thalamic origin
Béraud's valve
Berbecker's pliers
Berbridge's scissors
Berenreuther's test
Berens's dilator, forceps, implant,
keratome, retractor, scissors,
speculum
Berens-Rosa eye implant
Bergeim's method

Bergenhem's operation – surgical implantation of the ureter into the rectum

Berger's disease – glomerulonephritis

Berger's operation – interscapulothoracic amputation

Berger's method, paresthesia, rhythm, sign, symptom

Bergeron's disease – chorea of childhood marked by violent, rhythmic spasms, but running a benign course

Bergeron's chorea

Bergman's sign

Bergmann's syndrome – hiatus hernia in which pressure exerted on the thoracic organs produces dysphagia, tachycardia, hiccups and discomfort and pain in the cardiac region

Bergmann's operation – incision of the tunica vaginalis, performed for hydrocele

Bergmann's cells, cords, fibers, incision, rule

Bergmann-Israel incision

Bergmann-Meyer test

Bergmeister's papilla

Bergonié's method, treatment

Bergonié-Tribondeau law

Bergstrand's disease – osteoid osteoma

Berke's operation – for ptosis of the upper eyelid, with resection of the levator muscle through a skin incision

Berke-Motais operation – for ptosis of the upper eyelid, with suspension of the ptotic lid from the superior rectus muscle

Berkefeld's filter

Berlin's disease – edema of the macular region of the retina

Berlin's syndrome – a familial abnormality marked by short stature

Berlin's edema

Berlind-Auvard speculum

Berman's clamp, locator

Berman-Moorhead locator

Bermenam-Werner probe

Berna's retractor

Bernard's syndrome(s) – acute familial hemolysis; also same as *Bernard-Horner syndrome*

Bernard's canal, duct, layer, puncture

Bernard-Horner syndrome – ptosis, miosis, anhidrosis and endophthalmos due to paralysis of the cervical sympathetic nerves

Bernard-Sergent syndrome – acute adrenocortical insufficiency

Bernard-Soulier syndrome – a coagulation deficiency marked by thrombocytopenia

Bernay's retractor, sponge

Bernberg's intrauterine device

Berndt's hip ruler

Berne's forceps

Bernhardt's disease – same as *Bernhardt-Rot disease*

Bernhardt's formula, paralysis, paresthesia

Bernhardt-Rot disease – tingling, itching and paresthesia in the area of distribution of the external femoral nerve

Bernheim's syndrome – right heart failure without pulmonary congestion

Bernheimer's fibers
Bernouilli's distribution
Bernstein's gastroscope, test
Bernuth's syndrome — sporadic
    hemophilia
Berry's circles, clamp, forceps,
    ligament, raspatory
Berry-Dedrick phenomenon
Bertel's method
Berthelot's test
Bertin's bone, columns, ligament,
    ossicles
Bertolotti's syndrome — sacraliza-
    tion of the fifth lumbar verte-
    bra with scoliosis
Bertoni-Raymondi test
Bertrand's method, reagent, test
Bertrandi's sutures
Berwick's dye
Berzelius's test
Besnier's prurigo, rheumatism
Besnier-Boeck disease — sarcoid-
    osis
Besnier-Boeck-Schaumann disease/
    syndrome — same as *Besnier-
    Boeck disease*
Bespaloff's sign
Besredka's antivirus, reaction
Best's disease — congenital macu-
    lar degeneration
Best's carmine stain, forceps, tele-
    scope
Bethe's method
Bethea's method, sign
Bettendorff's test
Bettmann's test
Betz's cell area, cells
Beuren's syndrome — a congenital
    syndrome combining multiple
    cardiovascular disorders, den-
    tal abnormalities, mental re-
    tardation, peculiar facies and a
    coarse, metallic voice

Bevan's operation — for unde-
    scended testicle
Bevan's incision
Bevan Lewis cells
Beyer's forceps, rongeur
Bezold's abscess, ganglion, mas-
    toiditis, perforation, sign,
    triad
Bial's reagent, test
Bianchi's syndrome — a sensory
    aphasia with loss of ability to
    comprehend writing, seen in
    lesions of the left parietal lobe
Bianchi's nodules, valve
Biber-Haab-Dimmer dystrophy
Bibron's antidote
Bicek's retractor
Bichat's canal, fissure, foramen,
    ligament, membrane, tunic
Bickel's ring
Bickerstaff's encephalitis
Bidder's ganglia, organ
Biederman's sign
Biedert's cream mixture
Biedl's disease — a hereditary dis-
    order characterized by mental
    retardation, obesity, retinitis,
    hypogonadism and polydac-
    tyly
Bieg's entotic sign
Bielschowsky's disease — same as
    Bielschowsky-Jansky disease
Bielschowsky's method, stain,
    technique
Bielschowsky-Jansky disease — the
    late infantile form of cerebral
    sphingolipidosis
Bielschowsky-Lutz-Cogan syn-
    drome — internuclear ophthal-
    moplegia
Biemond's syndrome — a hered-
    itary disorder marked by
    mental deficiency, obesity,

Biemond's syndrome (*continued*)
progressive loss of retinal
response and polydactyly

Biemond's ataxia

Bier's operation — osteoplastic
amputation of the leg with a
bone flap cut out of the tibia
and fibula above the stump

Bier's amputation, anesthesia,
hyperemia, spots, treatment

Biermer's disease — pernicious
anemia

Biermer's anemia, sign

Biermer-Ehrlich anemia

Biernacki's sign

Biesenberger's operation — reduction mammaplasty

Biesiadecki's fossa

Biett's disease — discoid lupus
erythematosus

Biett's collar

Bietti's syndrome — xerosis con-
junctivae with iridopupillary
anomalies

Bietti's dystrophy

Bigelow's operation — crushing of
a calculus in the bladder followed by washing out of the
fragments

Bigelow's ligament, litholapaxy,
lithotrite, septum

Bilderbeck's disease — acrodynia

Bilhaut-Celoquet wedge resection

Bill's traction handle

Billeau's curet

Billroth's disease — meningocele
from fracture of the skull

Billroth's operation(s) — partial
resection of the stomach with
anastomosis; pylorogastrec-
tomy with anterior gastroenterostomy; excision of the

Billroth's operation(s) (*continued*)
tongue by transverse incision
below the symphysis of the
jaw

Billroth's cords, forceps, hypertrophy, strands, tube

Bimler's appliance

Binda's sign

Binelli's styptic

Binet's age, test

Binet-Simon test

Bing's erythroprosopalgia, test

Bing-Neel syndrome — hyperglob-
ulinemia with involvement of
the central nervous system,
marked by fever, anorexia,
emaciation, irritability, personality changes and mental
deterioration

Binkhorst's eye implant

Binswanger's disease — presenile
dementia caused by demyelination of the subcortical white
matter of the brain

Binswanger's dementia, encephalitis

Binz's test

Biot's breathing, respiration, sign

Birch-Hirschfeld lamp, tumor

Bird's disease — susceptibility to
infection as a result of oxalic
poisoning

Bird's formula, respirator, sign,
treatment

Birkett's forceps, hernia

Birkhaug's test

Birnberg's bow

Birtcher's cautery, coagulator,
hyfrecator

Bischoff's test

Bishop's score, sphygmoscope

Bishop-Black tendon tucker

Bishop-Coop enterostomy
Bishop-DeWitt tendon tucker
Bishop-Harmon forceps, irrigator
Bishop-Peter tendon tucker
Bismarck brown
Bissell's operation — excision of a
    portion of the round and
    broad ligaments for uterine
    retroversion
Bitot's patches, spots
Bittner agent, virus
Bittorf's reaction
Bivine's method
Bizzarri-Guiffrida knife, laryngo-
    scope
Bizzozero's cells, corpuscles, plate-
    lets
Bjerrum's scotoma, scotometer,
    screen, sign
Björk's drill
Björk-Shiley mitral valve prosthesis
Björnstad's syndrome — congenital
    cochlear deafness
Björnström's algesimeter
Black's formula, method, reagent,
    test
Black-Wylie dilator
Blackberg-Wanger test
Blackett-Healy method
Blackfan-Diamond anemia
Blackman's reaction
Blainville's ear
Blair's hook, knife, retractor
Blair-Brown graft, procedure,
    retractor
Blake's curet, disks, forceps
Blakemore-Sengstaken tube
Blakesley's forceps, retractor,
    trephine
Blalock's anastomosis, forceps,
    procedure
Blalock-Hanlen operation — the
    creation of a large, atrial

Blalock-Hanlen operation
    (*continued*)
    septal defect as a palliative
    procedure for transposition
    of the great vessels
Blalock-Niedner clamp
Blalock-Taussig operation — anas-
    tomosis of the subclavian
    artery to the pulmonary
    artery to shunt some systemic
    circulation into the pulmonary
    circulation
Blanchard's cryptotome, forceps,
    method, treatment
Bland-White-Garland syndrome —
    anomalies of the coronary
    artery from the pulmonary
    artery associated with enlarge-
    ment of the heart
Blandin's ganglion, glands
Blandin-Nuhn glands
Blandy's urethroplasty
Blane's amniotic infection syn-
    drome — fetal sepsis follow-
    ing swallowing and aspiration
    of contaminated amniotic
    fluid
Blaschko's lines
Blasius's duct
Blaskovics's operation — resec-
    tion of a semilunar piece of
    skin from the canthal fold,
    for blepharoptosis
Blasucci's catheter
Blatin's syndrome — the tremu-
    lous impulse sometimes felt
    upon palpation over a hydatid
    cyst
Blatin's sign
Blaud's pills
Blegvad-Haxthausen syndrome —
    osteogenesis imperfecta and
    blue sclera, with atrophy of

Blegvad-Haxthausen syndrome (*continued*)
the skin and zonular cataract

Blencke's disease — metaepiphyseal osteodystrophy of the calcaneum

Blessig's cysts, groove, lacuna, spaces

Blessig-Iwanoff cyst

Blinks's effects

Bloch's scale

Bloch-Stauffer dyshormonal dermatosis

Bloch-Sulzberger syndrome — a congenital defect in females consisting of lesions of the skin, eyes, nails, teeth, central nerous system and hair

Bloch-Sulzberger incontinentia pigmenti, melanoblastosis

Block-Steiger test

Blocq's disease/syndrome — inability to stand or walk although the legs are normal — often a sign of conversion hysteria

Blondel's serum

Blondlot's rays

Bloodgood's disease — cystic disease of the breast

Bloodgood's inguinal herniorrhaphy

Bloodwell's forceps

Bloom's syndrome — congenital telangiectatic erythema

Bloor's method, test

Bloor, Pelkan, and Allen method

Blot's perforator

Blount's disease — same as *Blount-Barber disease*

Blount's osteotome, osteotomy

Blount-Barber disease — aseptic necrosis of the medial condyle of the tibia

Blount-Barber syndrome — same as *Erlacher-Blount syndrome*

Bloxam's test

Bluemel's treatment

Blum's syndrome — deficiency of sodium chloride, fixation of chlorine in tissues, and excess urea in the urine

Blum's reagent, substance, test

Blumberg's ligament, sign

Blumenau's nucleus, test

Blumenbach's clivus, plane, process

Blumenthal's disease — erythroleukemia

Blumenthal's lesion

Blumer's shelf

Blyth's test

Boari's operation — transplantation of the vas deferens, enabling emptying into the urethra

Boari's button

Boas's algesimeter, point, test

Boas-Oppler bacillus, lactobacillus

Bobroff's operation — osteoplastic operation for spina bifida

Bochdalek's duct, foramen, ganglion, gap, hernia, pseudoganglion, sinus, valve

Bock's ganglion, nerve

Bock-Benedict method

Bockhart's impetigo

Bodal's test

Bodansky's unit

Bodenheimer's anoscope, speculum

body of Luys syndrome — a violent form of motor restless-

body of Luys syndrome (*continued*)
ness, involving only one side of the body, caused by a lesion of the hypothalamic nucleus
Boeck's disease — sarcoidosis
Boeck's itch, lupoid, sarcoid, scabies
Boeck-Drbohlav culture medium
Boedeker's test
Boehm's anoscope, proctoscope, sigmoidoscope
Boerhaave's syndrome — spontaneous rupture of the esophagus
Boerhaave's glands
Boerner-Lukens test
Boettcher's forceps, hemostat, trocar
Bogaert's disease — a rare hereditary disorder characterized by abnormal cholesterol metabolism and bile acid formation causing progressive ataxia, mental deterioration, cataracts and multiple xanthomas
Bogdän-Buday disease — abscesses of the liver and possibly of the lungs, spleen and joints following extrahepatic injuries
Bogg's method, reagent
Bogomolets's serum
Bogorad's syndrome — paroxysmal lacrimation appearing after facial palsy
Bogros's space
Bogue's operation — multiple ligation of the veins in varicocele
Böhler's clamp, fracture frame, splint
Böhler-Braun splint

Bohlman's pin
Böhm's operation — tenotomy of an ocular muscle for strabismus
Bohmansson's test
Bohme's reagent
Bohn's epithelial pearls, nodules
Bohr's atom, effect
Boies's elevator, forceps
Boley's gauge
Bolk's retardation theory
Bollinger's bodies, granules
Bolton's point, triangle
Bolton-nasion plane
Boltz's reaction, test
Bomford-Rhoads anemia
Bonaccolto's forceps, scleral ring
Bonain's solution
Bonanno's test
Bonchardat's reagent
Bond's forceps, splint
Bongiovanni-Eisenmenger syndrome — a chronic liver disease that features hyperadrenalism, marked by elevation of serum gamma globulin and total proteins, high urinary corticosteroid level, and increased glycogen storage activity
Bonhoeffer's symptom
Bonina-Jacobson tube
Bonn's forceps
Bonnaire's method
Bonnano's tube
Bonner's position
Bonnet's syndrome(s) — visual hallucinations in the elderly, not associated with mental disorders; trigeminosympathetic neuralgia
Bonnet's capsule, enucleation of eyeball, sign

Bonnet-Dechaume-Blanc syndrome — tortuosity of the vessels of the retina, with arteriovenous angioma of the optic nerve, thalamus and mesencephalon

Bonnevie-Ullrich syndrome — a complex syndrome characterized by webbing of the neck, lymphangiectatic edema of the hands and feet, dwarfism and other anomalies

Bonney's clamp, forceps, hysterectomy

Bonnier's syndrome — a complex of symptoms caused by a lesion of the lateral vestibular nucleus, involving vertigo, pallor and other aural and ocular disturbances

Bonnot's gland

Bonta's knife

Bonwill's triangle

Bonzel's operation — surgical separation of the external margin of the iris from the ciliary body

Böök's syndrome — a rare familial syndrome marked by premolar aplasia, excessive sweating and premature grayness

Borchardt's test

Borden's test

Bordet's amboceptor, phenomenon, test

Bordet-Gengou agar, bacillus, phenomenon, reaction

Bordier-Fränkel sign

Börjeson-Forssman-Lehmann syndrome — mental deficiency, epilepsy, hypogonadism and hypometabolism

Bornholm's disease — epidemic pleurodynia

Boros's esophagoscope

Borrel's blue, bodies

Borries's syndrome — localized encephalitis with cerebrospinal fluid changes, headache, fever and other symptoms suggesting abscess of the brain

Borsch's bandage

Borsieri's line, sign

Borst-Jadassohn epithelioma

Borthen's operation — iridotasis

Bose's operation — a type of tracheotomy

Bose's hook, tracheotomy

Bosher's knife

Bossi's dilator

Bostock's disease — hay fever

Bostock's catarrh

Boston's exanthem, sign, test

Bosviel's syndrome — hemorrhage from a ruptured uvular hematoma

Bosworth's drill, retractor, speculum

Bosworth-Shawler incision

Botallo's duct, foramen, ligament

Botelho's test

Botkin's disease — infectious hepatitis

Böttcher's cells, crystals

Böttger's test

Bottini's operation — making a channel through the prostate to cure prostate enlargement

Bottu's test

Botvin's forceps

Bouchard's disease — dilatation of the stomach from inefficiency of the gastric muscles

Bouchard's coefficient, index, nodes, nodules, sign

Bouchardat's test, treatment

Boucheron's speculum

Bouchet-Gsell disease — a benign meningitis seen in people who work with swine and pork

Bouchut's respiration, tubes

Boudin's law

Bouillaud's disease — rheumatic endocarditis

Bouillaud's syndrome — the coexistence of pericarditis and endocarditis in acute articular rheumatism

Bouillaud's sign

Bouin's fluid, solution

Bouin-Ancel test

Bourdon's test

Bourgery's ligament

Bourget's test

Bourneville's disease/syndrome — tuberous sclerosis

Bourns's respirator

Bouveret's disease/syndrome — paroxysmal tachycardia

Bouveret's ulcer

Boveri's test

Bovie's cautery, electrosurgical unit, knife

Bovin's fixation

Bowditch's law

Bowen's disease — intraepidermal squamous cell carcinoma

Bowen's epithelioma, osteotome, precancerous dermatosis

Bowen-Grover meniscotome

Bowlby's splint

Bowman's capsule, disks, glands, lamina, layer, membrane, muscle, probe, scissors, space, theory, tubes

Box-DeJager adenotome

Boyce's position, sign

Boyd's amputation, incision

Boyd-Stearns syndrome — rickets beginning during infancy, dwarfism, osteoporosis and malnutrition associated with metabolic disorders

Boyden's sphincter, test meal

Boyer's bursa, cyst

Boyes-Goodfellow hook retractor

Boyksen's test

Boyle's law

Boyle Davis mouth gag

Boynton's needle holder

Boys-Allis forceps

Bozeman's operation — turning the cervix uteri into the bladder and suturing it for the relief of vesicouterovaginal or ureterouterine fistula

Bozeman's catheter, clamp, forceps, position, speculum, sutures

Bozeman-Frisch catheter

Bozeman-Wertheim needle holder

Bozicevich's test

Bozzi's foramen

Bozzolo's sign

Braasch's bulb catheter, cystoscope, forceps

Braastad's retractor

Brace's test

Brachet's mesolateral fold

Brachmann–de Lange syndrome — a congenital syndrome in which severe mental retardation is associated with numerous anomalies, including dwarfism, webbed neck, brachycephaly and others

Bracht's maneuver

Bracht-Wächter bodies, lesions
Bracken's forceps
Brackett's probe
Brackin's incision
Braden's reservoir
Bradford's forceps, frame
Bradley's disease — epidemic
 nausea and vomiting
Bradshaw's albumosuria
Bradshaw-O'Neill clamp
Bragard's sign
Bragg's peak of proton beam
Bragg-Paul pulsator
Braid's effect, strabismus
Brailey's operation — stretching
 the supratrochlear nerve to
 relieve pain in glaucoma
Brailsford-Morquio disease — a
 rare form of mucopoly
 saccharidosis marked by
 severe dwarfism and lumbar
 kyphosis
Brain's reflex
Bram's test
Brand's bath
Brande's test
Brandt's syndrome — a familial
 syndrome of childhood mark-
 ed by diarrhea, steatorrhea,
 alopecia, paronychia with nail
 dystrophy, pustulous dermati-
 tis and blepharitis and con-
 junctivitis
Brandt's method, technique, treatment
Brandt-Andrews maneuver,
 method
Branham's bradycardia, sign
Bransford-Lewis dilator
Brant's splint
Brantley-Turner retractor
Brasil's alcoholic picro-formol

Brauch-Romberg symptom
Brauer's cardiolysis
Braun's anastomosis, canal, cranio-
 clast, culture medium, forceps,
 graft, hook, ring, tenaculum,
 test
Braun-Husler reaction, test
Braun-Jaboulay gastrectomy,
 gastroenterostomy
Braun-Wangensteen graft
Braune's canal
Braunwald's sign
Braunwald-Cutter prosthesis
Bravais-jacksonian epilepsy
Brawley's rasp, retractor
Braxton Hicks's contractions,
 sign, version
Brazelton behavioral scale
Breck's pin
Breda's disease — yaws
Brehmer's method, treatment
Breisky's disease —atrophy of the
 female genitalia, most com-
 monly occurring in older
 women
Breisky's pelvimeter
Breisky-Navratil speculum
Breitman's adenotome
Bremer's test
Brennemann's syndrome — mes-
 enteric and retroperitoneal
 lymphadenitis
Brenner's operation — a modifica-
 tion of *Bassini's operation* in
 which the abdominal muscles
 are sutured to the cremaster
 muscle
Brenner's forceps, formula, test,
 tumor
Brentano's syndrome — a disorder
 of muscle glycogen metabolism
 during pregnancy, with deple-

Brentano's syndrome (*continued*) tion of liver glycogen and creatinuria

Breschet's canals, hiatus, sinus, veins

Brescio-Cimino arteriovenous fistula

Breslau's method

Bret's syndrome — on radiographs one lung presents a clear picture and the other an opaque shadow

Breton's law

Bretonneau's disease — diphtheria

Bretonneau's angina, diphtheria

Breus's mole

Brewer's infarcts, point, speculum

Brewster's retractor

Bricker's operation — creation of an ileal conduit with a flat stoma for the collection of urine

Brickner's position, sign

Brieger's cachexia, reaction, test

Briggs's transilluminator

Brigham's forceps

Bright's disease — a broad term for kidney disease, usually glomerulonephritis

Bright's blindness, eye, granulations

Brighton's balloon

Brill's disease — a recurrence of typhus, sometimes occurring many years after the initial acute episode

Brill-Baehr-Rosenthal disease — same as *Brill-Symmers syndrome*

Brill-Symmers disease/syndrome — giant follicular lymphoma

Brill-Zinsser disease — same as *Brill's disease*

Brinell hardness number

Brinkerhoff's anoscope, speculum

Brinton's disease — diffuse fibrous proliferation of the submucosal connective tissue of the stomach

Brion-Kayser disease — infection caused by *Salmonella* of all groups except *S. typhosa*

Briquet's syndrome — shortness of breath due to hysterical paralysis of the diaphragm

Briquet's ataxia

Brissaud's disease — habitual spasmodic movement or contraction of any part

Brissaud's dwarf, infantilism, reflex, scoliosis

Brissaud-Marie syndrome — unilateral spasm of the tongue and lips, usually due to hysteria

Brissaud-Marie sign

Brissaud-Sicard syndrome — spasmodic hemiplegia caused by lesions of the cerebral commissure

Bristow's procedure

Bristowe's syndrome — a series of symptoms characteristic of tumor of the corpus callosum

Brittain's arthrodesis, chisel

Broadbent's apoplexy, registration point, sign, test

Broadbent-Bolton plane

Broberger-Zetterström syndrome — idiopathic hypoglycemia in children without increase in urinary excretion of adrenalin

Broca's amnesia, angle, aphasia, area, ataxia, band, center, convolution, fissure, formula, gyrus, plane, point, pouch, region

Brock's operation — an incision into the ventricle and dilation of the pulmonary valve

Brock's syndrome — atelectasis of the right middle pulmonary lobe, with pneumonitis

Brock's dilator, incision, infundibulectomy, valvotomy, valvulotome

Brock-Suckow polyposis

Brockenborough's sign

Brockenbrough's needle

Brocq's disease — parasporiasis

Brocq's pseudopelade

Brocq-Pautrier glossitis

Brödel's white line

Broden's methods

Broders's classification, index

Brodie's disease — chronic synovitis

Brodie's abscess, bursa, finger, joint, knee, ligament, pain, pile, probe, reaction, sign, tumor

Brodin's syndrome — duodenal stenosis caused by lymphadenitis associated with appendicitis

Brodmann's areas

Brodney's cannula, clamp

Broesike's fossa

Bronson's magnet

Bronson-Turz retractor

Brooke's disease — trichoepithelioma

Brooke's epithelioma, tumor

Brooks's punch, scissors

Brophy's operation — for cleft palate

Brophy's bistoury, forceps, mouth gag, periosteotome, scissors, tenaculum

Brophy-Deschamps needle

Broviac's catheter

Brown's vertical retraction syndrome — adhesion of the ocular muscles of the fetus

Brown's applicator, clamp, dermatome, periosteotome, reaction, test, tonsillectome

Brown-Adson forceps

Brown-Blair dermatome

Brown-Brenn technique

Brown-Buerger cystoscope, forceps

Brown-Dohlman eye implant

Brown-Pearce carcinoma, epithelioma, tumor

Brown-Pusey trephine

Brown-Séquard disease/syndrome — ipsilateral paralysis due to damage of one side of the spinal cord

Brown-Séquard's epilepsy, hemiplegia, injection, lesion, paralysis, sign, treatment

Brown-Symmers disease — fatal, acute serous encephalitis in children

Browne's hypospadias repair, opacity, tubes, urethral reconstruction

Brownian-Zsigmondy movement

Browning's vein

Broyles's aspirator, bronchoscope, esophagoscope, laryngoscope, nasopharyngoscope

Bruce's bundle, septicemia, tract

Bruce-Muir tract

Bruch's glands, layer, membrane

Bruck's disease — deformity of bones, ankylosis of joints, and atrophy of muscles

Bruck's reaction, test

Brücke's fibers, lens, lines, muscle, protein-free pepsin, reagent, test, tunic

Brudzinski's reflex, sign

Bruening's bronchoscope, otoscope, snare, speculum

Bruening-Citelli rongeur

Brug's filaria, filariasis

Brugsch's syndrome — acropachyderma

Brugsch's index, test

Brunati's sign

Bruner's speculum

Brunetti's chisel

Brunhilde's virus

Brunn's epithelial nests, membrane, method

Brunner's chisel, forceps, glands, incision, raspatory

Brünninghausen's method

Bruns's disease — pneumopaludism — a lung disease of malarial origin

Bruns's syndrome — intermittent headache, vertigo, vomiting and visual disturbance upon sudden movement of the head

Bruns's apraxia of gait, glucose medium, sign

Brunschwig's operation — pancreatoduodenectomy done in two stages

Brunschwig's forceps

Brunsting's syndrome — grouped vesicular lesions about the head and neck, usually occurring in older men

Brunton's otoscope

Bruser's incision

Brushfield's spots

Brushfield-Wyatt syndrome — a congenital condition marked by hemianopia, contralateral

Brushfield-Wyatt syndrome (continued) hemiplegia, cerebral angioma and mental retardation

Bryant's operation — lumbar colotomy

Bryant's line, sign, traction

Bryce's test

Bryce-Teacher ovum

Bryson's sign

Buchner's bodies

Bucholz's prosthesis

Buchwald's atrophy

Buck's operation — a wedge-shaped incision of the patella and the ends of the tibia and fibula

Buck's curet, extension, fascia, osteotome, traction

Bücklers's dystrophy

Bucknall's procedure

Buckstein's insufflator

Bucky's diaphragm, rays

Bucky-Potter diaphragm

Bucy's knife, retractor

Bucy-Frazier suction tube

Bud's bar

Budd's disease — chronic hepatic enlargement

Budd's cirrhosis, jaundice

Budd-Chiari syndrome — symptomatic obstruction of the hepatic veins, usually of unknown origin

Budge's center

Budin's joint, rule

Büdinger-Ludloff-Läwen syndrome — traumatic separation of the cartilage of the patella with fissures

Buerger's disease — thromboangiitis obliterans

Buerger's bougie, symptom

Buerger-Grütz disease — idiopathic hyperlipemia

Buerger-McCarthy forceps, scissors

Buergi's theory

Bufano's test

Bugbee's electrode

Buhl's disease — an acute sepsis affecting newborn infants, marked by hemorrhages into the skin, mucous membranes, navel and intestinal organs

Buhl's desquamative pneumonia

Buhl-Dittrich law

Bühler's baby test

Buie's cannula, electrode, forceps, hemorrhoidectomy position, tube

Buie-Hirschman anoscope, clamp, speculum

Buie-Smith retractor, speculum

Buisson's articulation

Buist's method

Buller's bandage, shield

Bullis fever

Bumke's pupil

Bumper's fracture

Bumpus's forceps, resectoscope

Bunge's amputation, law, spoon

Büngner's bands, cell cordons

Bunim's forceps

Bunnell's drill, splint, sutures

Bunsen burner

Bunsen's coefficient

Bunsen-Roscoe law

Bunts's catheter

Bunyamwera virus

Bunyan's bag

Burch's caliper, evisceration

Burch-Greenwood tendon tucker

Burchardt-Liebermann test

Burckhardt's operation — incision into a retropharyngeal abscess from the outside of the neck

Burckhardt's corpuscles, dermatitis

Burdach's columns, fasciculus, fibers, fissure, nucleus, tract

Burdick's cautery, electrosurgical unit

Burdizzo's vasectomy

Bureau-Barrière disease — a nonfamilial form of Hicks's syndrome marked by pseudosyringomyelic ulcerative lesions of the foot, found chiefly in middle-aged males who have had frequent injuries

Burford's retractor, spreader

Burford-Finochietto retractor, spreader

Burger's scalene triangle, sign, test

Bürger-Grütz syndrome — hyperlipoproteinemia

Burghart's sign, symptom

Burke's syndrome — progressive pulmonary dystrophy

Burkitt's lymphoma, tumor

Burnam's test

Burnett's syndrome — hypercalcemia and severe renal insufficiency attributed to ingestion of milk over long periods of time

Burnett's disinfecting fluid, solution

Burnham's forceps, scissors

Burnier's syndrome — dwarfing, optic atrophy and adiposogenital dystrophy from decreased functioning of the anterior pituitary

Burns's amaurosis, chisel, ligament, space, telescope

Burow's operation — plastic operation for the removal of tumors

Burow's blepharoplasty, solution, vein
Burton's line, sign
Buruli ulcer
Burwell's bur
Bury's disease — a chronic eruption of flattened nodules occurring on the buttocks, wrists, elbows and knees with final scarring
Busacca's floccule, nodule
Buscaino's reaction, test
Busch's scissors
Buschke's disease — cryptococcosis
Buschke's scleredema
Buschke-Löwenstein tumor
Buschke-Ollendorff syndrome — dermatofibrosis
Busquet's disease — exostoses on the dorsum of the foot
Busse's saccharomyces

Busse-Buschke disease — same as *Buschke's disease*
Butcher's saw
Bütschli's emulsion, granules, nuclear spindle
Butter's cancer
Butterfield's cystoscope
Buxton's clamp
Buzzi's operation — creation of an artificial pupil by a needle passed through the cornea
Bwamba fever virus
Bychowski's test
Byford's retractor
Byler's disease — familial cholestasis with hepatosplenomegaly and dwarfism
Bywaters's syndrome — edema, oliguria and other manifestations of renal failure following a crushing injury

C

Cabot's ring bodies, splint
Cacchi-Ricci disease — a hereditary disorder marked by multiple cystic dilations of the renal collecting tubes — sponge kidney
Cache Valley virus
Caffey's disease/syndrome — infantile cortical hyperostosis
Caffey-Silverman disease/syndrome — same as *Caffey's disease*
Cagot ear
Cahoon's method
Caillan's test

Cain's complex
Cairns's operation — to relieve glaucoma
Cairns's forceps, retractor
Cajal's cells, interstitial nucleus, stain
Caldani's ligament
Caldwell's method, position
Caldwell-Luc operation — an opening into the maxillary antrum through the supradental fossa above the maxillary premolar teeth
Caldwell-Moloy classification
Calhoun-Merz needle

Calibri's forceps
Call-Exner bodies
Callahan's flange, forceps, method
Callander's amputation
Callaway's test
Calleja's islands, islets
Callison's fluid
Calmette's ophthalmoreaction, reaction, serum, test, tuberculin, vaccine
Calmette-Guerin bacillus
Calori's bursa
Calot's operation — forcible reduction of kyphosis
Calot's node, treatment, triangle
Caltagirone's chisel, knife
Calvé's syndrome — vertebral osteochondritis
Calvé's cannula
Calvé-Legg-Perthes syndrome — osteochondrosis of capitular epiphysis of femur
Calvé-Perthes disease — same as *Calvé-Legg-Perthes syndrome*
Calvert's test
Calvin's cycle
Camera's syndrome — vertebral and paravertebral lumbosciatic osteopathy caused by inflammatory lesions of the lower lumbar spine and sacrum
Camerer's law
Cameron's appliance, gastroscope
Cameron-Haight elevator
Cameron-Lorenz cautery
Cameroon fever
Cammann's stethoscope
Cammidge's reaction, test
Camp-Coventry method
Campani's test
Campbell's catheter, forceps, ligament, osteotome, sound, test, trocar

Camper's angle, fascia, ligament, line
Camurati-Engelmann disease — diaphyseal dysplasia
Canada-Cronkhite syndrome — familial gastrointestinal polyposis
Canavan's disease — spongy degeneration of the central nervous system
Canavan's sclerosis
Canfield's knife
Cannizzaro's reaction
Cannon's syndrome — increased adrenal epinephrine secretion during emotional stress
Cannon's nevus, point, reflex, ring
Cannon-Rochester elevator
Cantani's test, treatment
Cantelli's sign
Cantlie's foot tetter
Cantor tube
Caparosa's bur, crimper
Capdepont's syndrome — hereditary disease transmitted as an autosomal dominant trait in which tooth development is marked by dark discoloration, poorly formed dentin and abnormally low mineral content
Capgras's syndrome — the schizophrenic illusion that impostors have replaced friends or relatives
Capgras's symptom
Caplan's syndrome — the presence of intrapulmonary nodules
Cappagnoli's test
Capps's sign
Capranica's test
Capuron's points
Carabelli's cusp, sign, tubercle
Carassini's spool

Carcassonne's ligament

Cardarelli's aphthae, sign, symptom

Carden's amputation

Cardillo's retractor

Carey-Coombs murmur

Cargile's membrane, sutures

Carini's syndrome — congenital ichthyosis at birth marked by smooth, deep red skin with cracks at the flexures, followed by peeling of the scales

Carlens's catheter, forceps, mediastinoscope, tube

Carleton's spots

Carmack's curet

Carmalt's clamp, forceps, hemostat

Carman's sign

Carmel's clamp

Carmichael's crown

Carmody-Batson operation — reduction of fractures of the zygoma and zygomatic arch

Carmody's aspirator, drill, forceps

Carmody-Brophy forceps

Carnett's sign

Carnochan's operation — removal of Meckel's ganglion and part of the fifth nerve for neuralgia

Carnot's test

Carnoy's solution

Caroli's disease — folding of the neck of the gallbladder, causing biliary dyskinesia and hypertonia

Carpenter's syndrome — a congenital syndrome marked by premature closing of cranial sutures and webbing of fingers

Carpenter's dissector, knife

Carpentier's anuloplasty, valve

Carpentier-Edwards valve

Carpue's operation — Indian method of rhinoplasty

Carr's tourniquet

Carr-Price test

Carr-Walker method

Carrel's method, treatment, tube

Carrel-Dakin fluid, treatment

Carrell's patch

Carrez's test

Carrión's disease — South American infectious disease caused by *Bartonella bacilliformis*

Carrion's prosthesis

Carroll's elevator, osteotome

Carroll-Legg osteotome

Carroll-Smith-Petersen osteotome

Carson's catheter

Carter's operation(s) — formation of an artificial pupil by a small opening into the cornea and perfoming an iridotomy; reconstruction of the bridge of the nose by transplanting bone from the rib

Carter's clamp, retractor, splenectomy, splint

Cartwright's blood group, prosthesis

Carus's circle, curve

Cary-Blair transport medium

Casal's collar, necklace

Casalá-Mosto disease — eczematid-like purpura marked by small red maculae of the lower extremities, extending to the entire body

Casamajor's test

Casilli's test

Casman's broth

Casoni's reaction, test

Caspar's ring opacity

Caspersson's type B cells

Cassel's operation — excision of exostoses of the ear through the external auditory meatus

Casselberry's cannula, position

Casser's (Casserio's, Casserius's) fontanelle, ligament, muscle

Cassidy's syndrome — intestinal carcinoma associated with a sharp rise of blood serotonin, arterial hypertension, cyanotic spots, dyspnea, colic and diarrhea

Cassidy-Brophy forceps

Cassirer's syndrome — cyanosis of the extremities with discoloration of the skin of the fingers, wrists and ankles

Castallo's retractor, speculum

Castaneda's method, stain

Castellani's disease — an infectious disease of the bronchi caused by *Spirochaeta bronchialis*

Castellani's syndrome — febrile hepatosplenomegaly with arthritis, marked by malaise, fever and arthritic pain

Castellani's bronchitis, mixture, paint, test, treatment

Castellani-Low symptom

Castelli-Paparella tube

Castellino's sign

Castle's factor

Castleman's lymphoma, tumor

Castroviejo's dermatome, dilator, forceps, keratome, punch, speculum, trephine

Castroviejo-Arruga forceps

Castroviejo-Kalt needle holder

Cathelin's method, segregator

Cattani's serum

Cattell's Infant Intelligence Scale, T-tube

Catu virus

Caulk's punch

Causse-Shea prosthesis

Cavanaugh's bur

Cavare's disease — familial periodic paralysis

Cave's incision, retractor, spatula

Cavin's osteotome, shunt

Caylor's scissors

Cazenave's disease(s) — erythematous scaly patches of the face, ears and scalp with atrophy and scars; a chronic form of pemphigus in adults with flaccid bullae and later generalized exfoliation

Cazenave's vitiligo

Cecil's operation — a three-stage operation for urethral stricture

Cecil-Culp urethroplasty

Cederschiöld's massage

Ceelen-Gellerstedt syndrome — essential pulmonary hemosiderosis

Cegka's sign

Celebes vibrio

Celestin's prosthesis, tube

Celsius scale, thermometer

Celsus's kerion, lithotomy

Cerenkov's radiation

Cesaris Demel bodies

Céstan's syndrome — same as *Céstan-Chenais syndrome*

Céstan-Chenais syndrome — lesions of the brain stem, causing hemiplegia, hemisynergia, endophthalmia, miosis and ptosis

Céstan-Raymond syndrome — obstruction of the basilar artery, marked by quadriplegia and nystagmus

Chabaud's mixture

Chaddock's reflex,sign

Chaffin's catheter, tube

Chaffin-Pratt tube

Chagas's disease — same as *Chagas-Cruz disease*

Chagas-Cruz disease — a form of trypanosomiasis caused by *Trypanosoma cruzi*

Chagres fever, virus

Chamberlain's forceps, incision, mediastinotomy, method

Chamberland's filter

Chamberlen's forceps

Chambers's pessary

Champetier de Ribes's bag

Championière's disease — fibrinous bronchitis

Chandelier's sign

Chandler's disease — primary idiopathic nontraumatic necrosis of the femoral head, seen most often in early middle age

Chandler's felt collar splint, forceps, fusion, method, retractor

Chantemesse's reaction

Chaoul's therapy, tube

Chapman's mixture, pill, test

Chapman-Stone agar

Chapple's syndrome — unilateral facial weakness or paralysis in the neonate, with weakness or paralysis of the vocal cord and muscles of deglutition

Chapple's sign

Chaput's method

Charcot's disease — neuropathic arthropathy

Charcot's syndrome(s) — amyotrophic lateral sclerosis; intermittent claudication; intermittent fever due to cholangitis

Charcot's arthritis, arthropathy, arthrosis, bath, cirrhosis, edema, fever, foot, gait, joint, pains, sclerosis, sign, triad, vertigo, zone

Charcot-Böttcher crystalloids

Charcot-Leyden crystals

Charcot-Marie atrophy, type

Charcot-Marie-Tooth disease — progressive neuropathic muscular atrophy

Charcot-Marie-Tooth atrophy, type

Charcot-Marie-Tooth-Hoffmann syndrome — neuropathic muscular atrophy

Charcot-Neumann crystals

Charcot-Vigouroux sign

Charcot-Weiss-Barker syndrome — stimulation of a hyperactive carotid sinus causing a marked fall in blood pressure

Chardack's pacemaker

Chardack-Greatbatch pacemaker

Charles's law, needle

Charlin's syndrome — neuritis of the nasal ciliary nerve

Charlouis's disease — yaws

Charlton's needle, trocar

Charmot's syndrome — macroglobulinemia with splenomegaly, seen in adults of the Congo region

Charnley's arthrodesis, arthroplasty, forceps, prosthesis, retractor

Charnley-Mueller arthroplasty, prosthesis

Charrière's scale

Charrin's disease — infection with *Pseudomonas aeruginosa*

Chase-Sulzberger phenomenon

Chaslin's gliosis

Chassaignac's axillary muscle, paralysis, tubercle

Chassard-Lapiné maneuver, method, position

Chatfield-Girdleston splint

Chauffard's syndrome — polyarthritis, enlargement of lymph nodes and fever, usually caused by some form of non-human tuberculosis

Chauffard's point

Chauffard-Still syndrome — same as *Chauffard's syndrome*

Chauffeur's fracture

Chaussé's method, procedure

Chaussier's areola, line, tube

Chautard's test

Chauveau's bacillus, bacterium

Chauvenet's method

Chavany-Brunhes syndrome — a genetic syndrome characterized by persistent headache and psychoneurotic disorders associated with calcification of the falx cerebri

Cheadle's disease — infantile scurvy

Cheatle's disease — benign cystic disease of the breast

Cheatle's forceps

Cheatle-Henry incision

Chédiak's anomaly, reaction, test

Chédiak-Higashi syndrome — abnormalities of the nuclear structure of leukocytes with cytoplasmic inclusions, and often with hepatosplenomegaly, lymphadenopathy, anemia and thrombocytopenia. Called also *Béguez César disease*

Chédiak-Higashi anomaly

Chédiak-Steinbrinck anomaly

Chédiak-Steinbrinck-Higashi syndrome — same as *Chédiak-Higashi syndrome*

Chédiak-Steinbrinck-Higashi anomaly

Cheever's operation — complete tonsillectomy through the neck

Chelsea-Eaton speculum

Cheney's syndrome — osteoporosis, with changes in the skull and mandible

Chenuda virus

Cherchevski's (Cherchewski's) disease — ileus of nervous origin

Cherney's incision

Chernez's incision

Cheron's forceps, serum

Cherry's extractor, osteotome, probe, scissors

Cherry-Adson forceps

Cherry-Austin drill

Cherry-Kerrison forceps

Chervin's method, treatment

Chester's disease — xanthomatosis of the long bones with spontaneous fractures

Chevalier Jackson bronchoscope, esophagoscope, gastroscope, laryngoscope, speculum, tube

Chevallier's glossitis

Chevassu's tumor

Cheyne's disease — hypochondria

Cheyne's dissector, elevator, nystagmus

Cheyne-Stokes asthma, nystagmus, psychosis, respiration, sign

Chiari's disease — same as *Budd-Chiari syndrome*

Chiari's syndrome — same as *Chiari-Budd syndrome*

Chiari II syndrome — elongation of the medulla and cerebellar vermis through the foramen magnum into the upper spinal canal

Chiari's network, reticulum

Chiari-Arnold syndrome — same as *Arnold-Chiari syndrome*

Chiari-Budd syndrome — thrombosis of the hepatic vein

Chiari-Frommel syndrome — abnormal prolongation of postpregnancy lactation

Chicago disease — North American blastomycosis

Chick-Martin method, test

Chiene's operation(s) — removal of a wedge from the inner condyle of the femur for cure of knock knee; exposure of the retropharyngeal space by lateral cervical incision

Chiene's incision, lines, test

Chievitz's layer, organ

Chilaiditi's syndrome — interposition of the colon between the liver and diaphragm

Chilcott's cannula

Child's forceps, pancreatectomy

Child-Phillips forceps, needle

Chimani-Moos test

Chlumsky's button

Choix fever

Chopart's operation(s) — amputation of the foot with the calcaneus, talus and other parts of the tarus being retained; plastic operation of the lip

Chopart's amputation, articulation, joint

Chopra's antimony test

Chorine's test

Chotzen's syndrome — a congenital disorder marked by premature closure of the cranial sutures and webbing of the fingers

Choyce's eye implant

Christ-Siemens syndrome — a congenital ectodermal defect

Christ-Siemens-Touraine syndrome — same as *Christ-Siemens syndrome*

Christchurch chromosome

Christensen's phenomenon

Christensen-Krabbe disease — progressive cerebral poliodystrophy with blindness, seizures and deafness, usually beginning in the first year of life

Christian's disease — a chronic idiopathic form of histiocytosis marked by bone defects, exophthalmos and diabetes insipidus

Christian-Weber disease — a nodular, nonsuppurative form of lupus erythematosus

Christison's formula

Christmas disease — deficiency of plasma thromboplastin

Christmas factor

Christopher's spots

Chrobak's test

Church's scissors

Churchill's iodine caustic

Churg-Strauss syndrome — allergic granulomatous angiitis

Chvostek's anemia, sign, symptom, test, tremor

Chvostek-Weiss sign

Ciaccio's glands, method, stain

Ciamician-Magnanini's test

Ciarrocchi's disease — erosion between the interdigital webs of the fingers, caused by *Candida albicans*

Cicherelli's forceps, rongeur

Cinelli's chisel

Cinelli-McIndoe chisel

Cipollina's test

Citelli's syndrome — mental backwardness and drowsiness arising from adenoidal or sinus infection

Citelli-Meltzer punch

Civatte's disease — hyperpigmentation and telangiectasia of the skin

Civatte's poikiloderma

Civiale's operation — crushing of a vesical calculus within the bladder with a lithotrite

Civinini's canal, ligament, process, spine

Clado's anastomosis, band, fossa, ligament, point

Clagett's cannula, needle

Clairborne's clamp

Clapton's line

Clara's cells

Clark's operation — a plastic operation for urethral fistula

Clark's restiform body, rule, scale, test

Clark-Collip method

Clark-Guyton forceps

Clark-Lubs culture medium

Clark-Verhoeff forceps

Clarke's cells, column of spinal cord, nucleus, ulcer

Clarke-Hadfield syndrome — cystic fibrosis of the pancreas

Classon's scissors

Clauberg's agar, culture medium, test, unit

Claude's syndrome — paralysis of the third oculomotor nerve on one side and asynergia on the other

Claude's hyperkinesis sign

Claude Bernard–Horner syndrome — same as *Bernard-Horner syndrome*

Claudius's cells

Clausen's method

Clawicz's chisel

Clayton's osteotome, splint

Cleaves's method

Cleeman's sign

Cleopatra projection

Clérambault-Kandinsky syndrome — a mental disturbance in which one believes his mind is under the control of some outside influence or person

Clérambault-Kandinsky complex

Clerf's aspirator, dilator, forceps, laryngoscope

Clerf-Arrowsmith safety pin closer

Clive's test

Cloquet's canal, fascia, ganglion, gland, hernia, ligament, needle sign, node, pseudoganglion, septum

Cloudman's melanoma

Clough-Richter's syndrome — anemia in which erythrocytes undergo severe autoagglutination

Clouston's syndrome — hidrotic ectodermal dysplasia

Cloward's blade, drill, hammer, osteotome, punch, rongeur

Cloward-Hoen retractor

Clute's incision

Clutton's joint

Coakley's operation — for frontal sinus disease

Coakley's cannula, forceps, hemostat, sutures

Coats's disease — chronic, progressive exudative retinopathy

Coats's retinitis, ring

Coban's dressing, wrap

Cobb's syndrome — a disorder of the spinal cord similar to *Sturge-Weber syndrome*

Cobb's elevator, osteotome

Cobbett's knife

Cobelli's glands

Cock's operation — urethrotomy

Cockayne's syndrome — a heritable disorder marked by dwarfism, pigmentary degeneration of the retina, optic atrophy, deafness and mental retardation

Codivilla's operation — for pseudarthrosis

Codivilla's extension

Codman's clamp, incision, sign triangle, tumor

Cody's tack

Coe virus

Coffey's incision, technique, uterine suspension

Coffey-Humber treatment

Coffin-Lowry syndrome — mental retardation with distorted facies and digital anomalies

Coffin-Siris syndrome — same as *Coffin-Lowry syndrome*

Cogan's syndrome(s) — nonsyphilitic interstitial keratitis, followed by deafness and associated with infectious disease; congenital oculomotor apraxia

Cogan's dystrophy

Cohen's elevator, forceps, test

Cohen-Eder cannula, tongs

Cohn's solution, test

Cohnheim's areas, artery, fields, theory

Colcher-Sussman method

Cole's frame, retractor, sign, test

Coleman's syndrome — injury of the cervical spine associated with head and shoulder injury

Coleman's Schiff reagent

Coleman-Shaffer diet

Coley's fluid, toxin

Colibri's forceps, speculum

Coller's forceps

Colles's fascia, fracture, law, ligament, mother, space

Colles-Baumès law

Collet's syndrome — same as *Collet-Sicard syndrome*

Collet-Sicard syndrome — glossolaryngoscapulopharyngeal hemiplegia

Collier's fold

Collin's dissector, forceps, law, osteoclast, pelvimeter, speculum, tube

Collin-Duvall forceps

Collings's electrode, knife

Collip's unit

Collis's mouth gag, technique

Collison's drill, screw

Colliver's symptom

Collyer's pelvimeter

Colonna's operation(s) — a reconstruction operation for intracapsular fracture of the femoral neck; capsular arthroplasty of the hip

Colt's cannula

Colver's dissector, forceps, needle, retractor

Colver-Coakley forceps

Comel's acrorhigosis
Comessatti's test
Comly's syndrome — methemo-
globinemia caused by drinking
water with high concentrations
of nitrates
Commando's operation — for
management of oral cancer
Comolli's sign
Compere's chisel, gouge, osteo-
tome
Compton's effect
Concato's disease — progressive
malignant polyserositis
Condorelli's disease — acro-osteo-
dystrophy, amenorrhea and
parathyroid disorders
Condy's fluid
Cone's caliper, cannula, forceps,
retractor, tube
Cone-Bucy cannula
Congo red test
Conn's syndrome — primary
aldosteronism
Conn's tourniquet
Connell's incision, sutures
Conolly's system
Conor and Bruch disease — epi-
demic in the Mediterranean
region and South Africa,
caused by infection from
Rickettsia conorii
Conrad-Crosby needle
Conradi's disease — a rare, hered-
itary syndrome marked by
multiple opacities in the
epiphyses, dwarfism, cataract,
general debility and dulled
mentation
Conradi's line
Conradi-Hünermann syndrome —
a rare bone disease in infants,

Conradi-Hünermann syndrome
(*continued*)
marked by manifestations of
discrete calcific densities in
the hyaline cartilage
Constantine's catheter
Contejean's test
Contino's epithelioma, glaucoma
Converse's chisel, curet, knife,
method, osteotome, saw,
scissors, speculum
Converse-MacKenty elevator
Conway's technique
Conzett's goniometer
Cook's retractor, speculum
Cooke's count, criterion, formula,
index, test
Cooke-Apert-Gallais syndrome —
congenital adrenal hyperplasia
in females resulting in defective synthesis of adrenocortical steroids
Cooley's disease — diminished
synthesis of beta chains of
hemoglobin, marked by micro-
cytic anemia, hepatosplenomegaly, skeletal deformities
and cardiac enlargement
Cooley's anemia, clamp, dilator,
forceps, graft, trait, tube
Cooley-Bloodwell-Cutter prosthesis
Cooley-Pontius blade, shears
Coolidge's tube
Coombs's test
Cooper's disease — chronic cystic
disease of the breast
Cooper's bougie, cannula, fascia,
gouge, hernia, irritable breast,
irritable testis, ligament, neuralgia
Coopernail's sign
Coors's filter

Cope's clamp, law, needle, sign, test

Cope-DeMartel clamp

Copeland's retinoscope

Copeman-Ackermann syndrome — painful lumbar sclerolipoma marked by hard, subcutaneous nodules

Coppridge's forceps

Corbett's forceps

Corbus's disease(s) — a rapidly destructive infection producing erosion of the glans penis and often destruction of the entire external genitalia; infection thought to be due to a spirochete

Cordes's forceps, punch

Cordes-New forceps, punch

Cords's angiopathy

Corey's forceps, tenaculum

Cori's disease — glycogenosis of the liver, with muscle and heart involvement from glucosidase deficiency

Cori's cycle, ester

Corley-Denis method

Cornelia de Lange's syndrome — same as *Brachmann–de Lange syndrome*

Corner's plug, tampon

Corner-Allen test, unit

Cornet's forceps

Corning's anesthesia, method, puncture

Corper's culture medium

Correra's line

Corri's method

Corrigan's disease — aortic insufficiency

Corrigan's cautery, cirrhosis, line, pneumonia, pulse, respiration, sign

Corti's arches, canal, cells, fibers, ganglion, membrane, organ, rods, tunnel

Corvisart's disease — chronic hypertrophic myocarditis

Corvisart's complex, facies

Corwin's forceps, hemostat

Coryllos's elevator, raspatory, retractor, thoracoscope

Coryllos-Bethune rib shears

Coryllos-Doyen elevator

Coryllos-Moure rib shears

Coryllos-Shoemaker rib shears

Coschwitz's duct

Cossio's syndrome — interauricular septal defect associated with plastic pericarditis

Costa's test

Costello-Dent syndrome — hypo-hyperparathyroidism

Costen's syndrome — a complex of symptoms resulting from trauma to or arthritis of the temporomandibular joint — pain, malocclusion, muscle tremor and ankylosis

Cotard's syndrome — a form of depressive insanity with delusions and suicidal impulses

Cotte's operation — removal of the presacral nerve

Cotting's operation — for ingrown toenail

Cottle's caliper, clamp, elevator, forceps, incision, osteotome, speculum, tenaculum, tube

Cottle-Arruga forceps

Cottle-Jansen forceps

Cottle-Joseph hook

Cottle-Kazanjian forceps

Cottle-MacKenty elevator

Cottle-Neivert retractor
Cottle-Walsham forceps
Cotton's fracture, procedure
Cotugno's disease — sciatica
Cotunnius's aqueduct, canal,
    nerve, space
Coulomb's law
Coulter's counter
Councill's catheter, dilator,
    stone basket
Councilman's bodies, lesions
Councilman-Mallory blood serum
Coupland's elevator, tube
Cournand's catheter, needle
Cournand-Grino needle
Courvoisier's gallbladder, incision,
    law, sign
Courvoisier-Terrier syndrome —
    dilatation of the gallbladder
    with retention jaundice due to
    obstruction
Coutard's law, method
Couto's disease — fatty degenera-
    tion of the visceral organs
Couvelaire's syndrome — prema-
    ture separation of a normally
    implanted placenta in associa-
    tion with albuminuria, azo-
    temia and shock
Couvelaire's uterus
Cova's point
Cowden's syndrome — a familial
    syndrome involving abnormal-
    ities of the central nervous
    system and defects of many
    body structures, including
    hypertrophy of the breasts
    with fibrocystic disease and
    early malignant degeneration
Cowen's sign
Cowie's guaiac test
Cowling's rule

Cowper's gland, ligament
Cox's treatment, vaccine
Coxsackie virus
Cozzolino's zone
Crabtree's dissector, effect
Crafoord's clamp, forceps, scissors
Crafoord-Cooley tunneler
Crafts's test
Craig's culture medium, forceps,
    pin, scissors, test
Craig-Sheehan retractor
Cramer's 2.5 reagent, splint, test
Crampton's muscle, test
Crandall's syndrome — hearing
    defects associated with
    hypogonadism
Crane's chisel, mallet, osteotome
Crapeau's snare
Credé's antiseptic, maneuver,
    method, ointment
Creevy's dilator, stone dislodger
Crenshaw's forceps
Creutzfeldt-Jakob disease — a rare,
    usually fatal, viral encephalop-
    athy accompainied by degen-
    eration of the pyramidal and
    extrapyramidal systems and
    by progressive dementia
Creyx-Lévy syndrome — a reverse
    form of *Sjögren's syndrome*
Crichton-Browne's sign
Crigler's evacuator
Crigler-Najjar syndrome — a con-
    genital familial form of non-
    hemolytic jaundice
Crile's blade, clamp, forceps,
    hemostat, spatula
Crile-Crutchfield clamp
Crile-Matas operation — produc-
    tion of regional anesthesia by
    intraneural infiltration
Crimean hemorrhagic fever virus

Cripps's obturator

Crismer's test

Crisp's aneurysm

Critchett's operation — excision of the anterior part of the eyeball

Crocker's disease — chronic inflammation of the skin of the extremities

Crocq's disease — acrocyanosis

Crohn's disease — a chronic, granulomatous, inflammatory disease of unknown etiology invading any part of the gastrointestinal system, frequently leading to intestinal obstruction

Crombie's ulcer

Cronin's implant, method

Cronin-Lowe reaction, test

Cronkhite's syndrome — same as *Cronkhite-Canada syndrome*

Cronkhite-Canada syndrome — a sporadic condition of gastrointestinal polyposis

Crooke's cells, changes, hyaline degeneration

Crooke-Russell basophils, changes

Crookes's lens, space, tube

Crosby's syndrome — hereditary nonspherocytic hemolytic anemia

Crosby's capsule, knife

Crosby-Cooney operation — for drainage of fluid from the peritoneal cavity in ascites

Cross-Bevan reagent

Crotti's retractor

Crouzon's disease — craniofacial dysostosis

Crowel-Beard procedure

Crozat's appliance

Cruickshank's clamp

Crutchfield's clamp, drill, tongs

Crutchfield-Raney tongs

Cruveilhier's disease — spinal muscular atrophy

Cruveilhier's artery, atrophy, fascia, joint, ligaments, navicular fossa, nodules, paralysis, plexus, sign, tumor, ulcer

Cruveilhier-Baumgarten syndrome — cirrhosis of the liver with patent umbilical veins

Cruveilhier-Baumgarten cirrhosis, murmur

Cruz's trypanosomiasis

Cruz-Chagas disease — same as *Chagas's disease*

Cryer's elevator

Csapo's abortion

Csillag's disease — a chronic atrophic skin disease characterized by indurated papules and keratotic plugs

Cubbins's screw

Cuignet's method, test

Cullen's sign

Culley's splint

Cullom-Mueller adenotome

Culp's ureteropelvioplasty

Cummings's catheter

Cummings-Pezzer catheter

Cunisset's test

Cunningham's clamp

Curdy's knife, sclerotome

Curie's law, therapy

Curling's factor, ulcer

Curry's nail, needle, splint

Curschmann's disease — the peritoneal covering of the liver is converted into a white, undifferentiated mass

Curschmann's mask, spiral

Curschmann-Batten-Steinert syndrome — atrophic myotonia, especially in the lingual and thenar muscles

Curtis's forceps

Curtius's syndrome(s) — hypertrophy of one side of the entire body; ovarian insufficiency marked by menstrual disturbances and leukorrhea, constipation and vasomotor disorders

Cushing's disease — Cushing's syndrome, in which the hyperadrenocorticism is due to excessive pituitary secretion of adrenocorticotropic hormone

Cushing's operation(s) — exposure of the gasserian ganglion and three divisions of the fifth nerve; a type of ureterorrhaphy without support

Cushing's syndrome(s) — a condition occurring chiefly in women and marked by facial adiposity, osteoporosis of the spine, hypertension, amenorrhea and diabetes mellitus, resulting from hyperadrenocorticism due to neoplasm of the adrenal cortex; tumors of the cerebello-pontine angle

Cushing's syndrome(s) (*continued*) and acoustic tumors marked by impairment of hearing, cerebellar ataxia, and eventual impairment of the sixth and seventh nerve function with elevated intracranial pressure

Cushing's basophilism, law, medulloblastoma, phenomenon, suture, tumor, ulcer

Cushing-Hopkins elevator

Cushing-Rokitansky ulcer

Cushman's drain

Custer's cells

Cutler's eye implant

Cutler-Beard technique

Cutler-Power-Wilder test

Cutola's test

Cutting's test

Cuvier's canal, ducts, sinuses

Cyon's experiment, nerve

Cyriax's syndrome — pain similar to that of angina pectoris but caused by slipped rib cartilage pressing on the interchondral joint nerves

Czapek-Dox agar, solution

Czermak's keratome, lines, spaces

Czerny's disease — periodic hydrarthrosis of the knee

Czerny's anemia, diathesis, incision, sutures

Czerny-Lembert sutures

Daae's disease — same as *Daae-Finsen disease*

Daae-Finsen disease — epidemic pleurodynia

Dabney's grippe

Daclin test

Da Costa's disease(s) — misplaced gout; neurocirculatory asthenia

Da Costa's syndrome(s) — a hereditary skin disorder marked by hyperkeratotic plaques and erythrodermic areas of varying size and shape; neurocirculatory asthenia

D'Acosta's syndrome — anoxia from diminished oxygen intake at high altitudes, with difficulty in breathing and giddiness

Daems's clamp

Daguet's ulceration

Dakin's antiseptic, fluid, solution

Dakin-Carrel method

Dale's phenomenon, reaction

Dale-Laidlaw capillary clotting time method

Dalen-Fuchs nodules, spots

Dalrymple's disease — inflammation of the ciliary body and cornea

Dalrymple's sign

Dalton's law

Dalton-Henry law

D'Amato's reaction, sign, test

Dameshek's syndrome — same as *Cooley's anemia*

Damocrates's confection

Damoiseau's curve, sign

Damshek's needle, trephine

Dana's operation — posterior rhizotomy

Dana's syndrome — degenerative changes in the white matter of the spinal cord, associated with pernicious anemia

Danberg's forceps

Danbolt-Closs syndrome — same as *Brandt's syndrome*

Dancel's treatment

Dandy's forceps, hemostat, rhizotomy, ventriculostomy

Dandy-Walker syndrome — congenital hydrocephalus caused by obstruction of the foramina of Magendie and Luschka

Dandy-Walker deformity

Daniel's operation — exploration for nonpalpable lymph nodes on the scalene muscles, to determine the absence or presence of lymphoma, metastatic tumors and sarcoidosis

Daniels's clamp, tonsillectome

Danielssen's disease — same as *Danielssen-Boeck disease*

Danielssen-Boeck disease — leprosy, marked by hyperesthesia and followed by anesthesia, paralysis, ulcers, gangrene and mutilation

Danielus-Miller modification of Lorenz's method

Danlos's disease/syndrome — same as *Ehlers-Danlos syndrome*

Danysz's effect, phenomenon

Dar es Salaam bacterium

Dare's method

Darier's disease/syndrome — a skin disease usually beginning in childhood, marked by keratotic papules that become crust-covered and produce vegetating tumor-like growths of the head, neck, back, chest and groin

Darier's sign

Darier-Ferrand dermatofibroma, dermatofibrosarcoma

Darier-Roussy sarcoid

Darkshevich's fibers, ganglion, nucleus

Darling's disease — histoplasmosis

Darling's capsulotome

Darrach's ulnar resection

d'Arsonval current
Darwin's ear
Daubenton's angle, line, plane
Davat's operation — compressing the veins by acufilopressure for cure of varicocele
Davenport's diagram, stain
David's disease(s) — tuberculosis of the spine; an unexplained form of hemorrhagic disease in women
David's speculum
Davidoff's (Davidov's) cells, knife, retractor
Davidsohn's sign, test
Davidson's anemia, forceps, syringe, trocar
Daviel's operation — extraction of cataract through a corneal incision without cutting the iris
Daviel's spoon
Davies's disease — endomyocardial fibrosis
Davies-Colley's operation — removal of a wedge of bone from the outer side of the tarsus for correction of talipes
Davies-Colley's syndrome — same as *Cyriax's syndrome*
Davis's bronchoscope, crown, forceps, graft, hemostat, sign, splint, stone dislodger, uterine suspension
Davis-Crowe mouth gag
Davis-Geck incision
Davy's test
Dawbarn's sign
Dawson's encephalitis
Day's factor, hook, knife, test
De Alvarez's forceps
De Azua's pseudoepithelioma

de Clérambault's syndrome — same as *Clérambault-Kandinsky syndrome*
de Gimard's syndrome — gangrenous purpura
de Grandmont's operation — for ptosis of the eyelid
de la Camp's sign
de Lange's syndrome — same as *Brachmann-de Lange syndrome*
De Martini-Balestera syndrome — same as *Burke's syndrome*
de Musset's sign
de Mussy's point, sign
de Pezzer's catheter
de Quervain's disease — painful tenosynovitis from narrowness of tendon sheath
de Quervain's fracture, thyroiditis
De Salle's line
De Sanctis–Cacchione syndrome — a hereditary condition marked by atrophic lesions of the skin, with mental retardation, retarded growth, gonadal hypoplasia and sometimes neurologic complications
de Signeux's dilator
De Tomasi–Coleman method
De Toni–Caffey syndrome — same as *Caffey-Silverman syndrome*
De Toni–Fanconi syndrome — cystinosis
De Vries's syndrome — a familial congenital condition of both sexes marked by factor V deficiency with bleeding and syndactyly
De Vries's theory
De Watteville current

de Wecker's cannula, scissors, sclerotomy

de Wecker-Pritikin scissors

Dean's applicator, hemostat, periosteotome

Dean-MacDonald clamp

Dean-Webb titration

Deaver's incision, retractor, scissors, tube

DeBakey's blade, forceps, graft, implant, prosthesis, stripper, tube

DeBakey-Bahnson clamp, forceps

DeBakey-Bainbridge forceps

DeBakey-Balfour retractor

DeBakey-Cooley dilator, forceps, retractor

DeBakey-Metzenbaum scissors

Debler's syndrome — familial hemolytic anemia

Débove's disease — splenomegaly

Débove's membrane, treatment, tube

Debré's syndrome(s) — cat-scratch disease; a disease caused by an inborn error of metabolism, resulting in disturbances of carbohydrate and lipid metabolism

Debré's phenomenon

Debré-Fibiger syndrome — pseudospasm of the pylorus marked by vomiting, dehydration and early death

Debré-Marie syndrome(s) — fever followed by edema and polyneuritis, involving all four extremities; dwarfism, genital infantilism and a disorder of water metabolism, marked by hydrophilia, oligodypsia, oliguria, retarded water elim-

Debré-Marie syndrome(s) (continued)
ination and high density of urine

Debré-Mollaret syndrome — same as Debré's syndrome

Debré-Paraf antigen reaction

Debré-Sémélaigne syndrome — muscular hypertrophy, weakness, cretinism and occasionally mental retardation in children

Decker's culdoscope, retractor

Declat's liquid

DeCourcy's clamp

Dedichen's test

Dedo-Pilling laryngoscope

Deehan's typhoid reaction

Deelman's effect

Deen's test

Dees's needle

Deetjen's bodies

Defer's method

Defourmental's forceps

Degener's test

Degnon's sutures

Degos's disease/syndrome — malignant papulosis

Degos's malignant papillomavirus

Degos-Delort-Tricot syndrome — malignant papulosis with atrophy

Dehio's test

Dehn-Clark method

Deiters's nucleus syndrome — same as Bonnier's syndrome

Deiters's cells, frame, nucleus, phalanges, process, tract

DeJager's elevator

Dejean's syndrome — orbital floor lesions associated with exoph-

Dejean's syndrome (*continued*)
thalmos, diplopia, maxillary
pain and numbness along the
trigeminal nerve branches

Déjérine's disease — progressive
hypertrophic interstitial neuropathy

Déjérine's syndrome(s) — polyneuritis secondary to an infection
with *Corynebacterium diph-
theriae;* hemorrhage or thrombosis of the anterior spinal
artery, causing paralysis of the
tongue, arm and leg

Déjérine's sign, type

Déjérine-Klumpke syndrome —
same as *Klumpke's paralysis*

Déjérine-Klumpke paralysis

Déjérine-Landouzy dystrophy,
type

Déjérine-Lichtheim phenomenon

Déjérine-Roussy syndrome —
thrombosis of the thalamo-
geniculate artery that produces
pain, sensory disorders, hemi-
ataxia, hemiplegia and choreo-
athetoid movements

Déjérine-Sottas disease — same as
Déjérine's disease

Déjérine-Sottas syndrome — progressive, hypertrophic interstitial neuropathy

Déjérine-Thomas syndrome — cortical cerebellar degeneration

Déjérine-Thomas atrophy

Dejust's test

del Castillo's syndrome — bilateral
small testes, sterility with azo-
ospermia, small seminiferous
tubules and absence of ger-
minal epithelium

Del Toro's operation — destruction of the apex of a conical
cornea

Delaborde's dilator

Delafield's fluid, hematoxylin

Delaney's retractor

Delaye's paralysis

Delbet's sign

DeLee's catheter, forceps, maneuver, pelvimeter, speculum,
tenaculum

DeLee-Breisky pelvimeter

DeLee-Hillis obstetric stethoscope

DeLee-Perce perforator

DeLee-Simpson forceps

DeLee-Zweifel cranioclast

Delff's test

Delgado's electrode

Delmege's sign

Delore's method

Delorme's operation — pericardi-
ectomy

Delpech's abscess

Delphian node

Demarest's forceps

Demarquay's sign

Demarquay-Richet syndrome — a
congenital orofacial abnormality marked by cleft lip, cleft
palate, fistula of the lower lip
and progeria facies

DeMartel's clamp, forceps, scissors

DeMartel-Wolfson clamp, forceps

Demel's forceps

Demianoff's sign

Deming's nephropexy

Demme's method

Demoivre's formula

Demons-Meigs syndrome — same
as *Meigs's syndrome*

DeMorgan's spots

Demours's membrane

Deneke's spirillium
Denhardt-Dingman mouth gag
Denigès's reagent, test
Denis's method
Denis Browne forceps, needle, procedure, splint
Denis-Leche method
Denker's trocar, tube
Denman's method, spontaneous evolution, version
Dennie's sign
Dennie-Marfan syndrome — spastic paralysis and mental retardation associated with congenital syphilis
Dennis's anastomosis, clamp, forceps
Dennis-Silverman test
Denny-Brown syndrome — primary degeneration of the dorsal root ganglion cells, with degeneration of the muscles associated with bronchogenic carcinoma
Denonvilliers's operation — plastic correction of a defective ala nasi by transferring a triangular flap from the adjacent side of the nose
Denonvilliers's aponeurosis, fascia
Denucé's ligament
Denver's classification
Denys's tuberculin
Denys-Leclef phenomenon
Depage's position
Depage-Janeway gastrostomy
DePalma's hip prosthesis
Depaul's tube
Depuy's arthroplasty, awl, extractor, frame, prosthesis, retractor, rongeur, splint

DePuy-Pott splint
DePuy-Weiss needle
Derbyshire's neck
Dercum's disease/syndrome — pain and tenderness with paresthesia in menopausal women from subcutaneous deposits of fat and pressure on cutaneous nerves
Derf's needle holder
Derlacki's chisel, gouge, knife, punch
Derlacki-Shambaugh chisel, microscope
Derra's clamp, knife, valvulotome
D'Errico's bur, drill, forceps, elevator, trephine
D'Errico-Adson retractor
Derrien's test
Desault's apparatus, bandage, ligation, sign
Descartes's law
Descemet's membrane
Deschamps's carrier, compressor, needle
Deschamps-Navratil needle
Deseret's angiocatheter, drain
Desilet's catheter
Desjardin's forceps, point, probe, scoop
Desmarres's clamp, elevator, forceps, law, scarifier
d'Espine's sign
Detakats-McKenzie forceps
Determann's syndrome — intermittent myasthenia of muscles as a result of arteriosclerosis
Detre's reaction
Deutschländer's disease — tumor of the metatarsal bones
Deutschman's knife

DeVega's anuloplasty

Deventer's diameter

Devergie's disease — a chronic inflammatory disease of the skin marked by scaling macules and follicular papules

Devergie's attitude

Devic's disease/syndrome — encephalomyelopathy with demyelination of the optic nerves and spinal cord causing progressive blindness in both eyes

Devic-Gault syndrome — same as *Devic's syndrome*

Devine's tube

Devonshire's catheter, colic, knife

Dew's sign

Dewar's procedure

Dewey's forceps

Deyerle's drill, pin, punch

d'Herelle's phenomenon

Di Guglielmo disease — a malignant blood dyscrasia marked by progressive anemia, myeloid dysplasia, hepatosplenomegaly, and hemorrhagic tendency
test, tube

Diamond-Blackfan syndrome — a rare hypoplastic anemia of young infants with deficiency of nucleated erythrocytes in the bone marrow

Diana complex

Dick's dilator, reaction, serum, test, toxin

Dicken's test

Dickinson's syndrome — same as *Alport's syndrome*

Dickinson's method

Dide-Botcazo syndrome — bilateral calcarine lesions causing visual disorders, spatial agnosia and amnesia

Dieffenbach's operation(s) — amputation at the hip; plastic closure of triangular defects by displacing a quadrangular flap toward one side of the triangle

Dieffenbach's amputation, forceps

Diertz's shears

Dieter's forceps

Diethrich's clamp

Dietl's crisis

Dietlen's syndrome — cardiac flutter and diaphragmatic tension on inspiration in patients with cardiopericardial and cardiodiaphragmatic adhesions and adhesions at the apex of the heart

Dietrich's syndrome — aseptic epiphyseal necrosis of the metacarpal bone

Dietrich's apparatus

Dieudonné's culture medium

Dieulafoy's aspirator, erosion, theory, triad, ulcer

DiGeorge's syndrome — congenital absence of the thymus and parathyroid glands, with delayed development and marked susceptibility to infection

Dighton-Adair syndrome — same as *van der Hoeve's syndrome*

Dimitri's disease — a congenital syndrome marked by angiomas, glaucoma, intracranial calcification, hemiplegia and epilepsy

Dimitry's erysiphake, trephine
Dimitry-Bell erysiphake
Dimitry-Thomas erysiphake
Dimmer's keratitis
Dingman's abrader, forceps, mouth
gag, osteotome
Dingman-Denhardt mouth gag
Dingman-Senn retractor
Dioscorides's granule
Dirck's fibrils
Disse's spaces
Dittel's operation — enucleation
of the lateral lobes of an en-
larged prostate
Dittel's sound
Dittrich's plugs
Dix's gouge, needle, spud
Dixon's blade, tuberculin
Dixon-Mann's sign
Dixon-Thomas-Smith clamp
Dobbie-Trout clamp
Dobell's solution
Dobie's globule, layer, line
Dochez's serum
Dochez-Avery reaction
Docktor's forceps, needle
Döderlein's bacillus
Dogiel's corpuscle
Dogliotti's valvulotome
Dogliotti-Guglielmini clamp
Doherty's eye implant
Döhle's disease — syphilitic aortitis
Döhle's bodies
Döhle-Amato bodies
Döhle-Heller aortitis
Dohlman's hook
Dold's reaction, test
Doleris's operation — for retro-
deviation of the uterus
Döllinger's ring
Dollinger-Bielschowsky syndrome
— early juvenile ganglioside
lipidosis

Dollo's law
Dolman's test
Domagk's method
Dombrock's blood group
Donald's clamp
Donaldson's test, tube
Donath's phenomenon, test
Donath-Landsteiner syndrome —
hemoglobinuria due to
hemolysis, caused by an auto-
hemolysin in the blood unit-
ing the erythrocytes at low
temperatures
Donath-Landsteiner test
Donders's glaucoma, law, pressure,
test
Donnan's equilibrium
Donné's bodies, corpuscles, test
Donogany's test
Donohue's syndrome — a rare and
lethal familial condition mark-
ed by slow physical and mental
growth, elfin facies, and severe
endocrine disorders
Donovan's bodies
Dooley's nail
Doppler's operation — injection of
phenol into tissues around the
sympathetic nerve leading to
the gonads to increase hor-
mone production and sexual
rejuvenation
Doppler's apparatus, effect, moni-
tor, phenomenon, principle,
shift, ultrasonography
Doppler-Cavin monitor
Dopter's serum
Dorello's canal
Dorendorf's sign
Dorn-Sugarman test
Dorno's rays
Dorothy Reed cells
Dorset's egg culture medium

Dorset-Niles serum
Dorsey's cannula, forceps, leukotome, spatula
Dos Santos's needle
Dott's mouth gag, retractor
Doubilet's sphincterotome
Dougherty's irrigator
Douglas's abscess, bag, cry, cul-de-sac, fold, forceps, graft, ligament, line, mechanism, method, pouch, space, septum, speculum, trocar
Dourmashkin's bougie
Dover's powder
Dowell's hernia repair
Down's syndrome — retarded growth, mongoloid features, and moderate-to-severe mental retardation, associated with chromosomal abnormality
Downes's cautery
Downey's cells
Downing's clamp, knife, retractor
Downs's analysis
Doyen's operation — eversion of the sac for relief of hydrocele
Doyen's clamp, forceps, raspatory, retractor, scissors, speculum
Doyen-Jansen mouth gag
Doyère's eminence, hillock
Doyle's vein stripper
Doyne's familial colloid degeneration, familial honeycomb choroiditis, honeycomb degeneration, iritis
Dragendorff's test
Draper's law
Drapier's needle
Drechsel's test
Dresbach's syndrome — the presence of elliptical erythrocytes in normal persons and in

Dresbach's syndrome (*continued*) patients with some types of anemia
Dresbach's anemia
Dreser's formula
Dressler's disease — intermittent hemoglobinuria
Dressler's syndrome(s) — a condition occurring after myocardial infarction, marked by leukocytosis, chest pain, fever, pleurisy and pneumonitis; intermittent hemoglobinuria
Drew-Smythe catheter
Dreyer's test
Dreyfus's syndrome — congenital flattening of the vertebrae followed by development of hyphoscoliosis, ankylosis of the spine, short neck, dwarfism and muscular weakness and atonia
Drinker's respirator
Drosin's postures
Drummond's artery, sign
Drysdale's corpuscles
Du Noüy's phenomenon
Duane's syndrome — a hereditary syndrome in which ocular muscle function is severely impaired
Duane's test
Dubin-Johnson syndrome — chronic or intermittent jaundice, marked by hyperbilirubinemia and amorphous, granular, brown pigment in the liver
Dubin-Sprinz disease/syndrome — same as *Dubin-Johnson syndrome*
Dubini's disease — a violent and fatal form of chorea caused by

Dubini's disease (*continued*)
   acute infectious disease of the
   central nervous system
Dubini's chorea
Dubois's disease — multiple abscesses of the thymus gland in
   congenital syphilis
Dubois's abscess, formula, method,
   sign, treatment
DuBois-Reymond's law
Dubos's crude crystals, culture
   medium, enzyme, lysin
Duboscq's colorimeter
Dubovitz's syndrome — intrauterine dwarfism
Dubreuil-Chambardel's syndrome
   — dental caries of the incisors,
   usually appearing in early
   adolescence
Dubreuilh's melanosis
Duchenne's disease(s) — spinal
   muscular atrophy; bulbar
   paralysis; tabes dorsalis
Duchenne's syndrome — the col-
   lective signs of bulbar paralysis
Duchenne's muscular dystrophy,
   paralysis, sign, trocar, type
Duchenne-Aran disease — spinal
   muscular atrophy
Duchenne-Erb syndrome — paralysis of the upper roots of the
   brachial plexus caused by
   destruction of the fifth and
   sixth cervical roots
Duchenne-Griesinger disease —
   pseudohypertrophic muscular
   dystrophy
Duchenne-Landouzy dystrophy,
   type
Duckworth's phenomenon, sign
Ducrey's disease — infection of
   the genitalia with *Haemophilus*

Ducrey's disease (*continued*)
   ducreyi, marked by soft
   pustules that rupture and
   form ulcers on the genital
   organs
Ducrey's bacillus
Duddell's membrane
Dudley's hook
Dudley-Klingenstein syndrome —
   tumors of the small intestine,
   with melena and ulcer-like
   symptoms
Dudley-Smith speculum
Duffield's scissors
Duffy's blood group
Dufourmental's rongeur
Dugas's sign, test
Duhamel's operation — for Hirschsprung's disease, by modification of the pull-through
   procedure and establishment
   of a longitudinal anastomosis
   between the proximal gangli-
   onated segment of the colon
   and the rectum
Duhot's line
Duhring's disease — chronic dermatitis marked by erythematous,
   papular, vesicular, eczematous
   or bullous lesions occurring in
   successive combinations
Duhring's pruritus
Dührssen's operation — vaginofix-
   ation of the uterus
Dührssen's incisions
Dujarier's clasp
Dukes's disease — a febrile disease
   of childhood, probably a mild
   form of scarlet fever
Dukes's cannula, method, test,
   tube
Dukes-Filatov disease — same as
   Dukes's disease

Dulong-Petit law
Dumdum fever
Dumont's retractor, scissors
Dumontpallier's test
Dunbar's serum
Duncan's folds, mechanism,
    method, placenta, position,
    ventricle
Duncan-Bird sign
Duncan-Hoen method
Dunfermline's scale
Dungern's test
Dunham's cones, fans, triangles
Dunhill's forceps, hemostat
Dunlap, Swanson and Penner
    method
Dunlop's stripper, traction
Dunn's tongue depressor
Dunning's elevator
Dunphy's sign
Duplay's disease — subacromial
    or subdeltoid bursitis
Duplay's operation — plastic
    procedures for a congenitally
    deformed penis
Duplay's bursitis, fibroma, hook,
    method, procedure, speculum,
    tenaculum
Duplay-Lynch speculum
Dupont's test
Dupré's disease/syndrome —
    symptoms of meningeal irrita-
    tion associated with acute
    febrile illness but without in-
    fection of the meninges
Dupuis's cannula
Dupuy's syndrome — same as
    Frey's syndrome
Dupuy-Dutemps operation —
    blepharoplasty of the lower
    lid with tissue from the oppo-
    site lid

Dupuytren's disease — plantar
    fibromatosis
Dupuytren's operation — amputa-
    tion of the arm at the shoulder
    joint
Dupuytren's abscess, amputation,
    contraction, contracture, en-
    terotome, fracture, hydrocele,
    phlegmon, sign, splint, suture,
    tourniquet
Duran-Reynals's permeability fac-
    tor
Durand's disease — a viral disease
    marked by upper respiratory,
    meningeal and gastrointestinal
    symptoms
Durand-Nicolas-Favre disease —
    venereal lymphogranuloma
Durand-Zunin syndrome — an
    association of the agenesis of
    the septum pellucidum with
    various structural abnormal-
    ities
Durant's disease — an inherited
    condition, transmitted as an
    autosomal dominant trait, in
    which bones are abnormally
    brittle and susceptible to
    fracture
Dürck's granuloma, nodes
Duret's lesion
Durham's decision, culture medi-
    um, rule, trocar, tube
Duroziez's disease — congenital
    mitral stenosis
Duroziez's murmur, sign
Dutton's disease —trypanosomia-
    sis
Dutton's relapsing fever, spirochete
Duval's nucleus
Duval-Allis forceps
Duval-Coryllos rib shears

Duval-Crile forceps
Duvergier's sutures
Duverney's foramen, fracture, gland
DuVries's hammer toe repair
Dwyer's instrumentation
Dyggve-Melchior-Clausen syndrome — osteochondrodysplasia with mental retardation, short stature and deformities of long bones

Dyke-Davidoff syndrome — a condition, possibly due to neonatal injury, affecting one side of the brain and marked by mental retardation, hemiplegia and neurological impairment
Dyke-Young syndrome — macrocytic hemolytic anemia
Dzierzynsky's syndrome — a form of craniomandibulofacial dysostosis

Eadie-Hofstee plot
Eagle syndrome — facial pain from an elongated styloid process
Eagle's test
Eales's disease/syndrome — recurrent hemorrhage into the retina and vitreous
Earle's clamp, probe
Earle L fibrosarcoma, sarcoma
Eastman's clamp, forceps, retractor
Eaton agent pneumonia, pneumonia
Eaton's speculum
Eaton-Lambert syndrome — myasthenia associated with small-cell carcinoma of the bronchus
Ebbinghaus's test
Eber's forceps
Eberth's disease — typhoid fever
Eberth's lines, perithelium
Ebner's fibrils, glands, lines, reticulum
Ebola virus

Ebstein's disease(s) — hyaline degeneration and necrosis of the epithelial cells of the renal tubules; a malformation of the tricuspid valve
Ebstein's angle, anomaly, lesion, treatment
Eck's fistula
Ecker's fissure, fluid, plug
Ecklin's syndrome — a usually fatal form of normoblastic myelocytic anemia of newborn infants, marked by splenomegaly, hepatomegaly, low hemoglobin level, reticulocytosis, erythroblastosis, moderate leukocytosis and jaundice
Ecklin's anemia
Economo's disease — lethargic encephalitis
Economo's encephalitis
Eddowes's syndrome — blue sclera associated with abnormal brittleness and fragility of bone

Edebohls's operation — decapsulation of the kidneys for Bright's disease

Edebohls's incision, position

Edelmann's syndrome(s) — a form of chronic infectious anemia; chronic pancreatitis with secondary involvement of the nervous system and skin

Edelmann's anemia, cell

Edelmann-Galton whistle

Eder's forceps, gastroscope, laparoscope

Eder-Chamberlin gastroscope

Eder-Hufford esophagoscope, gastroscope

Eder-Palmer gastroscope

Edinburgh's retractor, sutures

Edinger's fibers, law, nucleus

Edinger-Westphal nucleus

Edlefsen's reagent, test

Edsall's disease — a form of heat exhaustion accompanied by pain, muscular spasm and weak pulse

Edwards's syndrome — a condition caused by an extra chromosome 18, marked by mental retardation, cranial deformities, micrognathia, corneal opacities, ventricular septal defects and other abnormalities

Edwards's generator, implant, patch, prosthesis

Edwards-Carpentier aortic valve brush

Effler's tack

Eggers's plate, screw, splint

Eggleston's method

Eglis's glands

Ehlers-Danlos disease/syndrome — a congenital syndrome marked by hyperelasticity of the skin, fragility of blood vessels, excessive susceptibility of the skin to trauma, hematomas, loose joints, and pigmented, granulomatous pseudotumors

Ehrenfried's disease — hereditary deforming chondrodysplasia

Ehrenritter's ganglion

Ehret's syndrome — paralysis developing after a painful injury

Ehrhardt's forceps

Ehrlich's acid hematoxylin, biochemical theory, diazo reaction, granules, hemoglobinemic bodies, line, postulate, reagent, side-chain theory, stains, test, tumor

Ehrlich-Hata preparation, remedy, treatment

Ehrlich-Heinz granules

Ehrlich-Türk line

Ehrlich-Weigert formula

Ehrmann's test

Eicher's chisel, hip prosthesis

Eichhorst's disease — neuritis affecting the nerve sheath and interstitial muscle tissue

Eichhorst's atrophy, corpuscles, neuritis, type

Eichstedt's disease — a chronic superficial dermatomycosis caused by *Malassezia furfur,* marked by desquamating macules on the chest and shoulders

Eicken's method

Eijkman's lactose broth, test

Einarson's gallocyanin-chrome method

Einhorn's dilator, saccharimeter, string test, tube

Einstein-Starck law

Einthoven's formula, galvanometer, law, triangle

Eiselt's test

Eisenberg's milk-rice culture medium

Eisenlohr's syndrome — numbness and weakness of the extremities with paralysis of the lips, tongue and palate

Eisenmenger's syndrome — ventricular septal defect with pulmonary hypertension and cyanosis

Eisenmenger's complex, tetralogy

Eitelberg's test

Ekbom's syndrome — a sense of uneasiness or restlessness on going to bed that leads to involuntary twitching of the legs

Ekman-Lobstein syndrome — same as *Lobstein's disease*

El Tor's vibrio

Eldridge-Green lamp

Electra complex

Ellermann-Erlandsen method, test

Ellik's evacuator, meatotome, sound, stone basket

Ellinger's method

Elliot's operation — trephining the sclerocornea for relief of increased tension in glaucoma

Elliot's forceps, position, sign trephine

Elliott's law

Ellis's curve, line, needle holder, sign, spud

Ellis-Garland curve, line

Ellis–van Creveld syndrome — polydactyly, chondrodysplasia with acromelic dwarfism, hidrotic ectodermal dysplasia and congenital heart defects

Ellsner's gastroscope

Eloesser's flap

Elsberg's cannula, incision, test

Elschnig's syndrome — extension of the palpebral fissure laterally, displacement of the lateral canthus and ectropion of the lower eyelid and lateral canthus

Elschnig's bodies, conjunctivitis, forceps, pearls, retractor, scoop, spatula, spots

Elschnig-O'Brien forceps

Elschnig-O'Connor forceps

Elsner's asthma

Ely's operation — skin grafting on granulating surfaces in chronic suppurative otitis media

Ely's sign, test

Elzholz's bodies, mixture

Emanuel-Cutting test

Embden's ester

Embden-Meyerhof cycle, pathway

Emden-Meyerhof-Parnas pathway

Emerson's agar, bronchoscope, effect, stripper, suction tube

Emmert-Gellhorn pessary

Emmet's operation(s) — repair of a lacerated perineum; trachelorrhaphy; surgical creation of a vesicovaginal fistula

Emmet's forceps, retractor, scissors, sutures, tenaculum, trocar

Engel's syndrome — anaphylactic edema of the lungs, with eosinophilia and cough

Engel's alkalimetry, saw
Engel-Lysholm maneuver
Engel-May nail
Engel-Recklinghausen disease — osteitis with fibrous degeneration and formation of cysts
Engel–von Recklinghausen syndrome — same as *Recklinghausen's disease*
Engelmann's disease — same as *Camurati-Engelmann disease*
Engelmann's disk, splint
English disease — rickets
English forceps, position, rhinoplasty
Engman's disease — dermatitis marked by erythematous, crusted, scaling lesions and oozing spots
Engman's syndrome — same as *Zinsser-Engman-Cole syndrome*
Engström's respirator
Ennis's forceps
Enroth's sign
Enslin's triad
Epstein's syndrome(s) — a kidney disorder marked by edema, albuminuria, hypoalbuminemia, hyperlipemia and great susceptibility to infection; pseudodiphtheria
Epstein's blade, method, needle, nephrosis, osteotome, pearls, rasp, symptom
Epstein-Barr virus (EBV)
Equen's magnet
Equen-Neuffer knife
Eraso's method
Erb's disease — same as *Erb-Charcot syndrome*

Erb's syndrome — the aggregate of signs of myasthenia gravis
Erb's atrophy, dystrophy, palsy, paralysis, phenomenon, point, sclerosis, sign, spastic paraplegia, syphilitic spastic paraplegia, waves
Erb-Charcot disease/syndrome — spastic spinal paralysis
Erb-Duchenne paralysis
Erb-Goldflam disease/syndrome — myasthenia gravis
Erb-Landouzy disease — muscular dystrophy
Erb-Oppenheim-Goldflam syndrome — same as *Erb-Goldflam syndrome*
Erb-Zimmerlin type
Erben's phenomenon, reflex, sign
Erdheim's disease — cystic medial necrosis
Erdheim's syndrome — acromegaly with bone and cartilage hypertrophy of the clavicle, vertebral bodies and intervertebral disks
Erdheim's cystic medial necrosis
Erdmann's reagent, test
Erhard's test
Erhardt's clamp, forceps, speculum
Erich's arch bar, forceps, splint
Erichsen's disease — traumatic neurosis following spinal injury
Erichsen's ligature, sign, spine, test
Erlacher-Blount syndrome — bowleg in children, not caused by rickets
Erlanger's sphygmomanometer
Erlenmeyer's flask
Erni's sign
Ernst's radium application

Esbach's method, reagent, test

Escamilla-Lisser syndrome — hypothyroidism in adults, associated with ascites; cardiac, intestinal and bladder atony; anemia; menorrhagia; and carotinemia

Escat's phlegmon

Escherich's bacillus, reflex, sign, test

Escudero's test

Esmarch's bandage, probe, scissors, tourniquet, tubes

Espíldora-Luque's syndrome — blindness in one eye, with contralateral hemiplegia

Esser's operation — a method of securing epithelialization of an unhealed deep wound

Esser's graft

Essex-Lopresti maneuver, method, technique

Essig's splint

Essrig's forceps, scissors

Estes's operation — implantation of an ovary into a uterine cornu, performed when the tubes are absent

Estlander's operation — resection of one or more ribs in empyema

Estlander's cheiloplasty, flap

Estren-Dameshek syndrome — a familial type of hypoplastic anemia marked by pancyto-

Estren-Dameshek syndrome (*continued*)
penia, pallor, weakness and a tendency to bleed

Eternod's sinus

Ethridge's forceps

Eulenburg's disease — a congenital hereditary disease marked by tonic spasm and muscular rigidity

Eustace-Smith's murmur, sign

Evans's disease — familial cardiomegaly

Evans's syndrome — autoimmune hemolytic anemia, leukopenia, thrombocytopenia and purpura

Evans blue, forceps

Evans–Lloyd-Thomas syndrome — suspended heart

Eve's method

Everett's forceps

Everitt's salt

Eversbusch's operation — for correction of ptosis

Eves's snare

Ewald's evacuator, forceps, law, node, test, tube

Ewart's phenomenon, sign

Ewing's angioendothelioma, endothelial sarcoma, sign, tumor

Exner's plexus

Exton's reagent, test

Exton-Rose glucose tolerance test

F. R. Thompson hip prosthesis, rasp
Faber's syndrome – hypochromic anemia
Faber's anemia
Fabre's test
Fabricius's bursa
Fabry's disease – a hereditary sphingolipidosis in which glycolipids are deposited in tissues, especially the kidneys, causing edema, enlargement of the heart and hypertension
Faget's law, sign
Fahey's pin
Fahr's disease – progressive calcific deposition in the walls of cerebral blood vessels
Fahr-Volhard disease – malignant nephrosclerosis
Fahraeus's method, phenomenon, reaction, test
Fahraeus-Lindqvist effect
Fahrenheit's scale, thermometer
Fairbank's disease – idiopathic familial osteophytosis
Fajans's law
Fajersztajn's crossed sciatic sign
Falconer-Weddell syndrome – intermittent compression of the subclavian artery and vein between the clavicle and first thoracic rib, with vascular disorders in the upper limbs
Falk's clamp, forceps, retractor
Falk-Tedesco's test
Fallopio's foramen
Fallopius's aqueduct, ligament

Fallot's disease/syndrome – tetralogy of Fallot
Fallot's pentalogy, tetrad, tetralogy, trilogy
Falope's ring
Falret's disease – manic-depressive psychosis
Falta's syndrome – polyglandular insufficiency, usually combining hypofunction of the anterior gland and myxedema
Falta's coefficient, triad
Fañana's glia
Fanconi's syndrome – a rare hereditary disorder with poor prognosis, marked by pancytopenia and hypoplasia of bone marrow with accompanying musculoskeletal and genitourinary anomalies
Fanconi's anemia, pancytopenia
Fanconi-Albertini-Zellweger syndrome – a congenital disease of bone characterized by a heart defect and other abnormalities
Fanconi-Hegglin syndrome – pulmonary infiltrations with positive Wassermann reactions in nonsyphilitic patients
Fanconi-Petrassi syndrome – hereditary hemolytic anemia with macrocytosis and hyperchromia
Fanconi-Schlesinger syndrome – dwarfism, mental retardation, convergent strabismus, hypercalcemia, azotemia, hypertension and other anomalies

Fanconi-Türler syndrome — a congenital, probably familial, syndrome characterized by cerebellar ataxia associated with uncoordinated eye movement, nystagmus and mental retardation

Fansler's anoscope, proctoscope, speculum

Fantus's antidote, test

Farabeuf's amputation, forceps, raspatory, retractor, saw, triangle

Farabeuf-Lambotte clamp, forceps

Faraday's constant, dark space, law

Farber's disease — a rare, hereditary disorder of ceramide metabolism marked by loss of voice, desquamating dermatitis, foam cell infiltration of bones and joints, granulomatous reaction in heart, lung and kidneys and psychomotor retardation

Farber's syndrome — same as *Farber-Uzman syndrome*

Farber's lipogranulomatosis, test

Farber-Uzman syndrome — a progressive form of hereditary lipidosis marked by nodular erythematous swellings and cardiopulmonary and central nervous system involvement, usually leading to death within the first two years of life

Farlow's tongue depressor

Farlow-Boettcher snare

Farnham's forceps

Farr's law, retractor, test

Farrant's solution

Farre's tubercles, white line

Farrington's forceps

Farrior's forceps, speculum

Farris's forceps

Fauchard's disease — periodontitis

Faught's sphygmomanometer

Faulkner's chisel, curet, trocar

Faulkner-Browne chisel

Fauser's reaction

Faust's method

Fauvel's forceps, granules

Favoloro's retractor

Favre's disease — night blindness and microcystic edema of the macula retinae, associated with development of macular retinoschisis

Favre's bodies

Favre-Durand-Nicholas disease — lymphogranuloma venereum

Favre-Racouchot syndrome — nodular elastoidosis

Fazio-Londe atrophy, type

Fearon's test

Fechner's law

Fede's disease — granuloma of the frenum of the tongue, occurring in children

Federici's sign

Federoff's splenectomy

Federov's eye implant

Feer's disease — acrodynia

Fehland's clamp

Fehleisen's streptococcus

Fehling's solution, test

Feilchenfeld's forceps

Fein's needle, trocar

Feingold's diet

Feiss's line
Feitis's flecked spleen
Feldman's retractor
Feleky's instrument
Felix Vi serum
Felix-Weil reaction
Fell-O'Dwyer apparatus
Felton's paralysis, serum, unit
Felty's syndrome — a combination of rheumatoid arthritis, splenomegaly, leukopenia, anemia, and thrombocytopenia
Fenger's forceps
Fenton's bolt
Fenwick's disease — idiopathic atrophic gastritis
Fenwick's ulcer
Fenwick-Hunner ulcer
Féré-Langmead lipomatosis
Féréol's nodes
Féréol-Graux paralysis
Ferguson's angiotribe, forceps, method, retractor, scissors, stone basket
Ferguson-Metzenbaum scissors
Ferguson-Moon retractor
Fergusson's operation — an incision for surgical removal of the upper jaw
Fergusson's incision, speculum
Fergusson and Critchley's ataxia
Fernandez's reaction
Ferrata's cell
Ferrein's canal, cords, foramen, ligament, pyramid, tubes, tubules
Ferrier's method, treatment
Ferris's dilator, forceps
Ferris-Robb knife
Ferris Smith forceps, knife, retractor, rongeur
Ferris Smith–Gruenwald rongeur

Ferris Smith–Halle bur
Ferris Smith–Kerrison forceps, rongeur
Ferris Smith–Sewal retractor
Ferris Smith–Takahashi rongeur
Ferry-Porter law
Feulgen's reaction, stain, test
Feulgen-Schiff reaction
Févre-Languepin syndrome — a familial syndrome marked by popliteal webbing associated with cleft lip, cleft palate, fistula of the lower lip, syndactyly, onychodysplasia and deformity of the foot
Feyrter's disease — pulmonary plasmocytosis in premature infants
Fichera's method, treatment
Fick's bacillus, first law of diffusion, formula, halo, method, phenomenon, principle, veil
Ficker's diagnosticum
Fiedler's disease — leptospiral jaundice
Fiedler's myocarditis
Fielding's membrane
Fiessinger's syndrome — a severe form of erythema multiforme
Fiessinger-Leroy-Reiter syndrome — nongonococcal urethritis, followed by conjunctivitis and arthritis
Fieux's test
Figueira's syndrome — weakness of the neck muscles, with spasticity of the muscles of the lower extremities
Filatov's disease — infectious mononucleosis
Filatov-Dukes disease — same as *Dukes's disease*
Fildes's culture medium, law

Filhos's caustic
Filipovitch's (Filipowicz's) sign
Fillauer's splint
Finckh's test
Finikoff's method, treatment
Fink's curet, forceps, laryngo-
scope, retractor, tendon tucker
Fink-Jameson forceps
Finkelstein's albumin milk, feeding
Finkler-Prior spirillium
Finney's operation — enlargement
of the pyloric canal and estab-
lishment of an anastomosis
between the stomach and
duodenum
Finney's pyloroplasty
Finnoff's transilluminator
Finochietto's forceps, retractor,
scissors, stirrup
Finsen's apparatus, bath, lamp,
light, rays, treatment
Finsen-Reya lamp
Finsterer's sutures
Fisch-Renwick syndrome — con-
genital deafness, hyperterlor-
ism, ocular heterochromia and
white forelock
Fischer's syndrome — a familial
congenital syndrome, with
keratosis of the palms and feet,
clubbing of the distal phalanges
of the toes and fingers and
various other anomalies
Fischer's needle, sign, test
Fischler's method
Fish's forceps
Fishberg's concentration test,
method
Fishberg-Friedfeld test
Fisher's syndrome — paralysis of
one or more of the ocular
motor nerves

Fisher's cannula, forceps, knife,
retractor
Fisher-Arlt forceps
Fisher-Nugent retractor
Fisher-Race theory
Fishman-Doubilet test
Fisk's method
Fiske's method
Fiske-Subbarow method
Fitz's syndrome — a series of
symptoms indicative of acute
pancreatitis, epigastric pain
and vomiting, followed by
collapse
Fitz's law
Fitz Gerald method, treatment
Fitz-Hugh's syndrome — gonococ-
cic peritonitis of the upper
abdomen
Fitzgerald's forceps
Fitzpatrick's suction tube
Fitzwater's forceps
Flack's node, test
Flagg's laryngoscope
Flajani's disease — exophthalmic
goiter
Flajani's operation — separation
of the external margin of the
iris from the ciliary body
Flanagan's gouge
Flannery's speculum
Flatau's law
Flatau-Schilder disease — a subacute or chronic form of leukoencephalopathy of children
and adolescents. Symptoms
include blindness, deafness
and progressive mental deterioration
Flechsig's areas, column, cuticu-
lum, fasciculus, field, law,
primordial zones, tract

Fleck's phenomenon
Fleig's test
Fleischer's dystrophy, line, kerato-
    conus ring, vortex
Fleischer-Strümpell ring
Fleischl's test
Fleischmann's bursa, follicle, hy-
    groma
Fleischner's disease — osteochon-
    dritis affecting the middle
    phalanges of the hand
Fleischner's syndrome — horizon-
    tal linear atelectasis
Fleischner's method
Fleitmann's test
Fleming's conization of cervix
Flemming's body, center, fixing
    fluid, mass, solution, substance
Fletcher's afterloading tandem,
    medium
Fletcher–Van Doren forceps
Flexner's bacillus, dysentery,
    serum
Flexner-Jobling carcinoma, car-
    cinosarcoma, tumor
Flieringa's scleral ring
Fliess's therapy, treatment
Flint's arcade, law, murmur
Floegel's layer
Flood's ligament
Florence's crystals, reaction, test
Florey's unit
Florschütz's formula
Flouren's doctrine, law, theory
Flower's index
Floyd's needle
Fluhmann's test
Flynn-Aird syndrome — a familial
    syndrome marked by muscle
    wasting, ataxia, dementia,
    epidermal atrophy and ocular
    anomalies

Flynt's needle
Fochier's abscess
Focker's test
Foerster's syndrome — generalized
    amyotonia
Fogarty's catheter, clamp, probe
Foix's syndrome — paralysis of
    the oculomotor nerves, paresis
    of the sympathetic nerves and
    neuroparalytic keratitis
Foix-Alajouanine syndrome —
    subacute necrotizing myelitis
Foley's bag, catheter, forceps,
    pyeloplasty, Y-type uretero-
    pelvioplasty
Foley-Alcock catheter
Folin's method, reagent, test
Folin-Bell's method
Folin-Benedict-Myers method
Folin-Berglund method
Folin-Cannon-Denis method
Folin-Denis method, test
Folin-Farmers method
Folin-Flander method
Folin-Hart method
Folin-Macallum method
Folin-McEllroy test
Folin-McEllroy-Peck method
Folin-Peck method
Folin-Pettibone method
Folin-Shaffer method
Folin-Wright method
Folin-Wu method, test
Folin-Youngburg method
Folius's muscle, process
Fölling's disease — phenylketo-
    nuria
Follmann's balanitis
Foltz's valve
Fomon's knife, periosteotome,
    retractor, scissors
Fonio's solution

Fontana's markings, spaces, stain

Forbes's disease — glycogen storage disease

Forbe's amputation

Forbes-Albirght syndrome — a condition in which a pituitary tumor secretes excessive amounts of prolactin and produces persistent lactation

Fordyce's disease — a developmental anomaly marked by ectopic sebaceous glands that appear as papules on the oral mucosa

Fordyce's angiokeratoma, granules, lesion, spots

Foregger's bronchoscope, laryngoscope

Forel's commissure, decussation, field

Forestier-Certonciny syndrome — senile rheumatic gout

Forestier and Rotés-Querol syndrome — ankylosing vertebral hyperostosis

Forget-Fredette agar

Formad's kidney

Fornet's reaction, ring test

Forney's syndrome — familial mitral insufficiency

Forrester's clamp, splint

Forrester-Brown head halter

Forschheimer's spots

Forsius-Eriksson syndrome — a familial syndrome transmitted as a recessive X-linked trait and marked by albinism, hypoplasia, nystagmus, astigmatism and myopia

Forssell's syndrome — polycythemia associated with kidney diseases

Forssell's sinus

Forssman's antibody, antigen, lipoid

Förster's disease — central choroiditis in which the spots are at first black and then become enlarged and white

Förster's operation(s) — intradurally cutting the seventh, eighth, and ninth dorsal nerve roots on both sides in locomotor ataxia; an operation to produce rapid artificial ripening of a cataract

Förster's choroiditis, forceps, photometer, snare, uveitis

Förster-Penfield operation — excision of scar tissue in the epileptogenic cortical area in traumatic epilepsy

Foshay's reaction, serum, test

Fosler's splint

Foss's clamp, forceps, retractor

Foster's frame

Foster-Ballenger speculum

Foster-Kennedy syndrome — retrobulbar optic neuritis, with atrophy on one side of the lesion and papilledema on the other, occurring in frontal lobe tumor of the brain

Fothergill's disease — scarlet fever associated with painful pharyngitis or peritonsillar abscess

Fothergill's operation — for uterine prolapse

Fothergill's neuralgia, pill, sore throat

Fouchet's test

Foulis's cells

Fourmentin's thoracic index

Fournier's disease — fulminating gangrene of the scrotum

Fournier's gangrene, sign, teeth, test, tibia, treatment

Foville's syndrome — a form of hemiplegia affecting alternate sides

Foville's fasciculus

Fowler's incision, maneuver, position, solution, sound

Fowler-Murphy treatment

Fowler-Weir incision

Fox's disease — a rare skin disease marked by bullous and vesicular eruptions brought on by trauma

Fox's blepharoplasty, eye implant, eye shield, impetigo, speculum, splint

Fox-Fordyce disease — a persistent, itching papular eruption from inflammation of the apocrine sweat glands

F.R. Thompson hip prosthesis, rasp

Frackelton's needle

Fraenkel's nodules, symptom

Frahur's clamp, scissors

Fraley's syndrome — dilation of the renal calices caused by stenosis of the upper infundibulum

Franceschetti's disease — retinal dystrophy marked by multiple yellow-white lesions of the retina

Franceschetti's syndrome — mandibulofacial dysostosis

Franceschetti's dystrophy

Franceschetti-Jadassohn syndrome — a heriditary condition of reticular skin pigmentation with keratosis of the palms

Franceschetti-Jadassohn syndrome (*continued*) and soles. Called also *Naegeli's syndrome*

Francis's disease — tularemia

Francis's forceps, test

Franck's plethysmograph

Francke's needle

Franco's operation — suprapubic cystotomy

François's syndrome — a complex syndrome characterized chiefly by brachycephaly, mandibular hypoglossia, hypotrichosis and bilateral congenital cataracts

François's dysencephaly, dystrophy

François-Haustrate syndrome — otomandibular dysostosis

Frangenheim's forceps

Frank's operation — a method of performing a gastrostomy

Frank-Starling mechanism

Franke's operation — removal of the intercostal nerves for the visceral crises of tabes

Franke's triad

Frankel's disease — indurative pneumonia

Fränkel's appliance, sign, speculum, test, treatment

Fränkel-Voges asparagin culture medium

Franken's test

Frankenhäuser's ganglion

Frankfeldt's forceps, sigmoidoscope

Frankfort's horizontal plane

Frankl-Hochwart's disease — the symptom complex of cochlear, vestibular, facial and tri-

Frankl-Hochwart's disease (*continued*)
geminal nerve irritation occurring in early syphilis

Franklin's disease — plasma proteinemia, characterized by abnormal globulins and associated with malignant disorders of plasmacytic and lymphoid cells

Franklin's glasses, retractor

Franklin-Silverman curet, needle

Franz's syndrome — cessation of vibration after ligation of the vein proximal to an arteriovenous fistula

Franz's retractor

Fraser's syndrome — congenital absence of eyelids with multiple anomalies, including ear malformation, digital deformities and renal maldevelopment

Fraser's forceps

Frater's retractor

Fraunhofer's lines

Frazier's osteotome, retractor, scissors, tube

Frazier-Adson clamp

Frazier-Paparella suction tube

Frazier-Sachs clamp

Frazier-Spiller operation — a subtemporal trigeminal rhizotomy

Frederick's syndrome — auricular fibrillation associated with complete atrioventricular block

Frederick's needle

Fredet-Ramstedt operation — pyloromyotomy

Freeman's clamp, leukotome

Freeman-Sheldon syndrome — craniocarpotarsal dystrophy

Freeman-Swanson prosthesis

Freer's elevator, knife, periosteotome, retractor

Freer-Gruenwald forceps

Frei's disease — lymphogranuloma venereum

Frei's antigen, bubo, test

Freiberg's disease — osteochondrosis of the head of the second metatarsal

Freiberg's infarction, infraction, knife, retractor, traction

Freiburg's method

Freimuth's curet

Frejka's pillow splint

French flap, scale

Frenkel's syndrome — ocular contusion syndrome

Frenkel's movements, treatment

Frerichs's theory

Freud's cathartic method

Freund's operation — chondrotomy for congenital funnel breast

Freund's adjuvant, anomaly, dermatitis, reaction

Freund-Kaminer reaction

Frey's syndrome — localized flushing and sweating of the ear and cheek in response to eating

Frey's eye implant, hairs

Frey-Freer bur

Frey-Gigon method

Freyer's operation — suprapubic enucleation of the hypertrophied prostate

Freyer's drain

Fricke's bandage, dressing

Friderichsen's test

Friderichsen-Waterhouse syndrome — same as *Waterhouse-Friderichsen syndrome*

Fridericia's method
Fried's rule
Friedenwald's syndrome — lifting of a ptosed eyelid on turning the eyes to the right, opening the mouth wide, and sticking out the tongue
Friedenwald's ophthalmoscope
Friedländer's disease — inflammation of the innermost coat of an artery, by which smaller vessels become constricted or obliterated
Friedländer's bacillus, pneumobacillus, pneumonia
Friedman's retractor, test, vein stripper
Friedman-Lapham test
Friedman-Otis bougie
Friedman-Roy syndrome — the association of mental deficiency, strabismus, extensor plantar reflexes, speech defects and clubfoot
Friedmann's disease — recurrent spastic paralysis in children, resulting from congenital syphilis
Friedmann's syndrome(s) — a cycle of symptoms caused by progressive, subacute encephalitis, including headache, vertigo, insomnia, debility and defective memory; a form of petit mal epilepsy in children
Friedreich's disease(s) — a disorder marked by rapid muscle contractions occurring simultaneously or consecutively in various unrelated muscles; facial hemihypertrophy
Friedreich's ataxia, foot, phenomenon, sign, tabes

Friedrich's syndrome — a rare, aseptic form of epiphyseal necrosis of the sternal ends of the clavicles
Friedrich's clamp, raspatory
Friedrich-Petz clamp
Friend's catheter, leukemia
Friesner's knife
Friess-Pierrou syndrome — filariasis with eosinophilia, adenopathies and pneumopathies
Fritsch's catheter, retractor
Fritsch-Asherman syndrome — amenorrhea or hypomenorrhea, dysmenorrhea, habitual abortion and sterility following puerperal or postabortal infection or curettage
Fritz's aspirator
Fröhde's reagent, test
Fröhlich's disease/syndrome — adiposogenital dystrophy caused by adenohypophyseal tumor
Frohn's reagent, test
Froin's syndrome — lumbar spinal fluid with presence of large amounts of protein, rapid coagulation and progressive absence of cells
Froment's paper sign
Frommann's lines
Frommel's disease — same as *Chiari-Frommel syndrome*
Frommel's operation — shortening of the uterosacral ligaments for retrodeviation of the uterus
Frommel-Chiari syndrome — same as *Chiari-Frommel syndrome*
Frommer's dilator, test
Froriep's ganglion, induration, law
Fröschel's symptom
Frost's sutures

Frost-Lang operation — insertion of a gold ball to replace an enucleated eyeball

Fruehjahr's catarrh

Frugoni's disease — infectious eosinophilia

Frugoni's syndrome — thrombophlebitic splenomegaly

Fuchs's syndrome — a progressive ocular disease of unknown cause, marked by heterochromia of the iris, iridocyclitis and cataracts

Fuchs's atrophy, coloboma, crypts, dellen, dimple, dystrophy, forceps, heterochromia, keratitis, lamella, method, position, spot, test

Fuchs-Rosenthal hemocytometer

Fukala's operation — removal of the lens of the eye for treatment of myopia

Fulci's spherules

Fuld's test

Fuld-Goss test

Fülleborn's method

Fuller's operation — incision of the seminal vesicles

Fuller's cell, dressing, tube

Fulton's retractor, rongeur, scissors

Funkenstein's test

Fürbringer's sign, test

Furniss's anastomosis, catheter, clamp, forceps, incision

Furniss-Clute clamp, pin

Furniss-McClure-Hinton clamp

Furst-Ostrum syndrome — platybasia associated with congenital synostosis of the neck and Sprengel's deformity

Fürstner's disease — pseudospastic paralysis with tremor

Furth's tumor

G

Gaboon ulcer

Gabriel's proctoscope

Gabriel Tucker bougie, forceps

Gad's hypothesis

Gaenslen's sign, test

Gaffky's scale, table

Gaillard-Arlt suture

Gailliard's syndrome — location of the heart in the right hemithorax

Gairdner's disease — cardiac distress without apprehension

Gairdner's coin test

Gaisböck's disease/syndrome — stress polycythemia

Galassi's pupillary phenomenon

Galbiati's ischiopubiotomy

Gale's formula

Galeati's glands

Galeazzi's fracture, sign

Galen's anastomosis, bandage, foramen, pore, veins, ventricle

Galezowski's dilator

Gall's craniology

Galli Mainini test
Gallie's herniorrhaphy, needle, transplant
Gallois's test
Galt's trephine
Galton's delta, law, whistle
Gambee's sutures
Gamgee's tissue
Gamna's disease — a form of splenomegaly with thickening of the splenic capsule
Gamna's nodules
Gamna-Gandy nodules
Gamstorp's disease/syndrome — a hereditary, familial syndrome marked by attacks of periodic paralysis, with hyperkalemia and normal urinary potassium during the attacks
Ganassini's test
Gandhi's knife
Gandy's clamp
Gandy-Gamna nodules, spleen
Gandy-Nanta disease — siderotic splenomegaly
Gangi's reaction
Gangolphe's sign
Gannetta's dissector
Gannther's test
Ganser's syndrome — amnesia, disturbances of consciousness, hallucinations, and sensory changes, usually of hysterical origin
Ganser's diverticulum, ganglion, symptom
Gänsslen's disease — familial form of constitutional leukopenia, transmitted as a dominant trait

Gant's operation — division of the femoral shaft for hip joint ankylosis
Gant's clamp, line
Garceau's catheter
Garcin's syndrome — unilateral global involvement of cranial nerves
Gardiner-Brown test
Gardner's syndrome — familial polyposis of the large bowel, with supernumerary teeth, fibrous dysplasia of the skull, osteomas and fibromas
Gardner's headrest, needle
Gardner-Diamond syndrome — a reaction syndrome occurring principally in young women, in which spontaneous, painful ecchymoses occur without trauma—possibly of emotional origin
Gardner-Wells tongs
Garel's sign
Garfield-Holinger laryngoscope
Gariel's pessary
Garland's clamp, curve, forceps,
Garland's clamp, curve, triangle
Garré's disease — sclerosing, non-suppurative osteomyelitis
Garré's osteitis, osteomyelitis
Garretson's bandage
Garrett's dilator
Garriga's test
Garrigue's forceps, speculum
Garrison's forceps, rongeur
Garrod's pads, test
Gärtner's bacillus, phenomenon, tonometer
Gartner's canal, cyst, duct
Garven-Gairns method
Gaskell's bridge, clamp

Gasser's syndrome — a rare syndrome of unknown cause occurring in young children, consisting of renal failure, hemolytic anemia and severe thrombocytopenia

Gasser's ganglion

Gasser-Karrer syndrome — fatal hemolytic anemia

Gastaut's syndrome — unilateral convulsions associated with hemiplegia and epilepsy in young children

Gatch's bed

Gatellier's incision

Gaucher's disease — familial splenic anemia

Gaucher's cell, splenomegaly

Gaul's pits

Gaule's spots

Gault's cochleopalpebral reflex, test

Gauran's test

gaussian curve

Gaustad's syndrome — reversible attacks of confusion, stupor and coma with personality changes and motor disturbances, associated with cirrhosis of the liver

Gauvain's brace, fluid

Gavard's muscle

Gavin-Miller clamp, forceps

Gawalowski's test

Gay's glands

Gay-Force test

Gay-Lussac's law

Gayer's test

Gaylor's forceps, punch

Gaynor-Hart method

Gaza's operation — cutting the appropriate rami communi-

Gaza's operation (*continued*) cantes of the sympathetic nervous system

Gee's disease — same as *Gee-Herter-Heubner disease*

Gee-Herter disease — same as *Gee-Herter-Heubner disease*

Gee-Herter-Heubner disease — childhood celiac disease

Gee-Herter-Heubner syndrome — the infantile form of nontropical sprue

Gee-Thaysen disease — adult celiac disease

Gegenbaur's cell, sulcus

Gehrung pessary

Geigel's reflex

Geiger counter

Geiger-Downes cautery

Geiger-Müller counter

Geissler's test, tube

Geissler-Pluecker tube

Gélineau's syndrome — narcolepsy

Gellé's test

Gellhorn's forceps, pessary, punch

Gelpi's forceps, retractor

Gelpi-Lowrie forceps

Gély's suture

Gemini's clamp, forceps

Gendre's fixative

Genga's bandage

Gengou's phenomenon

Gennari's band, layer, line, stria, stripe

Gensoul's disease — diffuse, purulent inflammation of the floor of the mouth, spreading to the soft tissues of the upper neck, sometimes causing airway obstruction

Gentele's test

Georgi's test

Geraghty's test
Gerald's forceps
Gérard-Marchand fracture
Gerbasi's anemia
Gerbode's dilator
Gerdy's fibers, fontanelle, hyoid fossa, interauricular loop, ligament, tubercle
Gerhardt's disease — a condition chiefly affecting the extremities, marked by paroxysmal vasodilation with burning pain and rise in skin temperatures
Gerhardt's syndrome — bilateral abductor paralysis of the vocal cords
Gerhardt's dullness, phenomenon, reaction, sign, test, triangle
Gerhardt-Semon law
Gerlach's network, tonsil, valve
Gerlier's disease — a disease of the nerves and nerve centers characterized by pain, paresis, vertigo, ptosis and muscular contractions, usually found among farm laborers and stablemen
Germistan virus
Gerota's capsule, fascia, fasciitis, method
Gerrard's test
Gerson-Herrmannsdorfer diet
Gerstmann's syndrome — a combination of right-left disorientation, inability to express thoughts in writing and inability to do simple calculations
Gerzog's knife, speculum
Gerzog-Ralks knife
Gesvelst's network
Getsowa's adenoma
Ghilarducci's reaction

Ghon's complex, focus, primary lesion, tubercle
Ghon-Sachs bacillus
Giacomini's band
Gianelli's sign
Giannuzzi's bodies, cells, crescents, demilunes
Gianotti-Crosti syndrome — eruptive papulous dermatitis of the extremities
Gibbon's hernia, hydrocele
Gibbon-Landis test
Gibbs's theorem
Gibbs-Donnan equilibrium
Gibert's disease — pityriasis rosea
Gibert's pityriasis
Gibney's disease — painful inflammation of the spinal muscles
Gibney's bandage, boot, perispondylitis, strapping
Gibson's disease — a rare disease that may be familial, marked by a decrease in the rate of methemoglobin reduction in the presence of glucose or lactate
Gibson's bandage, glioma, incision, murmur, rule, splint, sutures, vestibule
Gibson-Balfour retractor
Giemsa's stain
Gierke's disease — glycogen storage disease
Gierke's cells, corpuscles
Giertz-Shoemaker rib shears
Gies's biuret reagent, biuret test
Gifford's operation(s) — delimiting keratotomy; destruction of the lacrimal sac by trichloracetic acid
Gifford's curet, forceps, keratotomy, maneuver, reflex, retractor, sign

Gifford-Galassi reflex

Gigli's operation — lateral section of the os pubis with Gigli's wire saw, performed in difficult labor

Gigli's pubiotomy, wire saw

Gilbert's disease — a familial, benign elevation of bilirubin levels without liver damage

Gilbert's syndrome — an association of malignant testicular tumors, with gynecomastia, high titers of chorionic gonadotropic hormones and the presence of folliculin

Gilbert's catheter, cholemia, forceps, sign

Gilbert-Dreyfus syndrome — a familial form of pseudohermaphroditism, marked by male phenotype, hypospadias, gynecomastia, scanty axillary hair, absent beard and nearly normal testes

Gilbert-Graves speculum

Gilbert-Lereboullet syndrome — hereditary nonhemolytic jaundice

Gilchrist's disease — North American blastomycosis

Gilchrist's mycosis

Giliberty's prosthesis

Gill's operation — insertion of a wedge of bone for dropfoot or pes equinus

Gill's blade, forceps, knife, scissors

Gill-Fuchs forceps

Gill-Hess forceps

Gill-Manning decompression laminectomy

Gill-Safar forceps

Gilles de la Tourette's syndrome — motor incoordination, with involuntary repetition of another's words and involuntary utterance of obscenities

Gillespie's operation — excision of the wrist by a lengthwise dorsal incision

Gilliam's operation — retroversion of the uterus

Gillie's operation — a method of reducing fractures of the zygoma and the zygomatic arch

Gillies's operation — for correction of ectropion utilizing a split-skin graft

Gillies's elevator, flap, forceps, graft, incision, scissors

Gillies-Dingman hook

Gillmore's needle

Gilman-Abrams tube

Gilmer's intermaxillary fixation, method, splint, wiring

Gilmore's probe

Gilson's solution

Gilvernet's retractor

de Gimard's syndrome — gangrenous purpura

Gimbernat's ligament, reflex ligament

Gimmick's elevator

Ginsberg's forceps

Giordano's sphincter

Giordano-Giovannetti diet

Giovannini's disease — a fungus infection that produces a nodular disease of the hair

Giraldés's organ

Girard's forceps, method, probe, treatment

Giraud-Teulon law

Girdner's probe

Giuffrida-Ruggieri stigma

Givens's method

Gjessing's syndrome — periodic catatonic stupor and excitement, coinciding with nitrogen retention and responding to thyroid therapy

Glanzmann's disease — a platelet abnormality characterized by defective clot formation and prolonged bleeding

Glanzmann's syndrome — congenital hemorrhagic thrombocytic dystrophy

Glanzmann's thrombasthenia

Glanzmann-Riniker syndrome — X-linked hypogammaglobulinemia, with susceptibility to pyogenic infection

Glanzmann-Saland syndrome — severe polyneuritic paralysis following diphtheria

Glaser's retractor

Glasgow's sign

Glassman-Allis clamp, forceps

Glassman's basket, clamp, forceps

Glatzel's mirror

Glauber's salt

Glénard's disease/syndrome — prolapse or downward displacement of the viscera that may be associated with neurasthenic manifestations

Glenn's operation — for pulmonary atresia

Glenn's anastomosis, procedure

Glenner's forceps, retractor

Gley's cells, glands

Glisson's disease — rickets

Glisson's capsule, cirrhosis, sling

Glover's clamp, forceps, organism, rongeur

Gluck's shears

Gluge's corpuscles

Gluzinski's test

Gmelin's reaction, test

Godélier's law

Godfried-Prick-Carol-Prakken syndrome — a familial syndrome consisting of multiple neurofibromatoses, with atrophoderma vermiculatum, mongoloid facies, mental retardation and heart abnormalities, including congenital heart block

Godtfredsen's syndrome — cavernous sinus–nasopharyngeal tumor syndrome

Goeckerman's treatment

Goelet's retractor

Goethe's suture

Goetsch's skin reaction, test

Goffe's colporrhaphy

Goggia's sign

Gohrbrand's dilator, valvulotome

Golaski's graft

Goldbacher's anoscope, proctoscope, speculum

Goldberg-Maxwell syndrome — male pseudohermaphroditism characterized, when complete, by female external genitalia

Goldblatt's clamp, hypertension, kidney, phenomenon

Golden-Kantor syndrome — steatorrhea associated with the roentgenological picture of "moulage sign," dilation and segmentation of the small intestine

Goldenhar's syndrome — mandibulofacial dysostosis with epibulbar dermoids

Goldflam's disease — same as *Goldflam-Erb disease*

Goldflam-Erb disease — myasthenia gravis

Goldman's curet, knife, punch

Goldman-Fox knife

Goldman-Kazanjian forceps

Goldmann's applanation tonometer

Goldmann-McNeill blepharostat

Golds's forceps

Goldscheider's disease — the epidermis is loosely attached to the corium, giving rise to blisters that usually heal without scarring

Goldscheider's percussion, test

Goldstein's disease — hereditary hemorrhagic telangiectasia

Goldstein's syndrome — a disease of the cerebellum marked by disorders of equilibrium and associated with distorted perception of space, time and weight

Goldstein's cannula, curet, hematemesis, hemoptysis, heredofamilial angiomatosis, irrigator, rays, sign, speculum

Goldthwait's fracture frame, sign, symptom

Golgi's apparatus, body, cells, complex, corpuscles, cycle, fibril, law, organ, stain, theory, types I and II neurons, zone

Golgi-Mazzoni corpuscles

Golgi-Rezzonico apparatus, spiral, threads

Goll's column, fasciculus, fibers, nucleus, tract

Golonbov's sign

Goltz's syndrome — same as *Goltz-Gorlin syndrome*

Goltz's experiment, theory

Goltz-Gorlin syndrome — a hereditary, congenital syndrome of extensive ectodermal and mesodermal dysplasia

Gombault's degeneration, neuritis

Gombault-Philippe triangle

Gomori's method, stains

Gomori-Takamatsu procedure, stains

Gomori-Wheatley stain

Gompertz's law

Gonin's operation — treatment of retinal detachment by thermocautery of the retinal fissure

Gonin-Amsler marker

Gooch's filter, splint

Good's forceps, rasp, scissors

Goodell's dilator, law, sign

Goodenough draw-a-man test, draw-a-person test

Goodenough-Harris drawing test

Goodfellow's cannula

Goodhill's forceps, retractor

Goodpasture's syndrome — glomerulonephritis, usually progressing to death from renal failure

Goodpasture's stain

Goodwin's clamp

Goormaghtigh's apparatus, cells

Gopalan's syndrome — severe burning and aching of the feet associated with hyperesthesia, raised skin temperature and vasomotor changes

Gordon's disease — protein-losing gastroenteropathy

Gordon agent

Gordon's elementary body, forceps, reflex, sign, splint, stethoscope, test

Gordon-Overstreet syndrome — ovarian agenesis, mild virilization, primary amenorrhea, lack of development of the breast, growth retardation and increased excretion of gonadotropins

Gordon-Sweet silver impregnation method

Gordon-Taylor amputation

Gorham's disease — extensive decalcification of a single bone without known cause

Gorham's syndrome — massive osteolysis

Gorlin's syndrome — multiple nevoid basal-cell epitheliomas, jaw cysts and bifid ribs

Gorlin-Chaudhry-Moss syndrome — craniofacial dysostosis, dental and eye abnormalities and patent ductus arteriosus

Gorlin-Goltz syndrome — a hereditary disorder consisting of multiple basal cell carcinomas, multiple anomalies of bone and other defects. Also called *basal cell nevus syndrome*

Gorlin-Psaume syndrome — a condition occurring only in females, marked by mental retardation and anomalies of the mouth, tongue, face and fingers

Gosselin's fracture

Gosset's retractor

Göthlin's index, test

Gott's prosthesis, valve

Gott-Daggett valve

Gottinger's line

Gottlieb's epithelial attachment

Gottron's syndrome — a familial form of progeria affecting the hands and feet

Gottron's sign

Gottschalk's aspirator, saw

Gottstein's basal process, fibers

Gougerot's syndrome — erythematous papular lesions, purpuric macules and dermal or dermohypodermal macules

Gougerot-Blum syndrome — pigmented, purpuric, lichenoid dermatitis

Gougerot-Carteaud syndrome — confluent and reticulated papillomatosis

Gougerot-Nulock-Houwer syndrome — a symptom complex of unknown etiology occurring in women, marked by keratoconjunctivitis and enlargement of the parotid glands. Called also *Sjögren's syndrome*

Gougerot-Ruiter syndrome — allergic vasculitis

Gougerot-Sjögren disease — same as *Sjögren's syndrome*

Goulard's extract, lotion, water

Gould's sutures

Gouley's catheter, sound

Goutz's catheter

Govons's curet

Gowers's syndrome(s) — a paroxysmal condition marked by slow pulse, fall in blood pressure and sometimes convulsions; hereditary distal myopathy; irregularity of the pupillary light reflex seen in tabes dorsalis

Gowers's column, contraction, dystrophy, fasciculus, hemoglobin, maneuver, sign, solution, tract

Goyrand's hernia, injury

graafian follicle

Graber-Duvernay operation — boring minute channels to the center of the head of the femur for modifying circulation within the bone in chronic arthritis

Gracey's curet

Gradenigo's syndrome — paralysis of the sixth cranial nerve, with or without involvement of the ophthalmic branch of the fifth nerve, associated with lesions of the apex of the petrous bone and mastoiditis

Gradle's electrode, forceps, trephine

Graefe's disease/syndrome — gradual paralysis of the eye muscles, affecting first one muscle and then another

Graefe's operation — removal of a cataractous lens by a scleral cut, with laceration of the capsule and iridectomy

Graefe's cystotome, forceps, incision, knife, needle, sign, speculum, spots, test

Graefe-Sjögren syndrome — a hereditary, familial syndrome consisting of retinitis pigmentosa, congenital deafness and spinocerebellar ataxia

Gräfenberg's ring

Graffi's leukemia, mouse chloroleukemia

Graham's elevator, hook, law, scissors, test

Graham-Kerrison punch

Graham Little syndrome — lichen planus associated with acuminate follicular papules

Graham Steell's murmur

Gram's syndrome — juxta-articular adiposis dolorosa

Gram's method, solution, stain

Gram-Weigert stain

Grancher's disease — pneumonia with splenization of the lung

Grancher's sign, system, triad

Grandeau's test

Grandry's corpuscles

Grandry-Merkel corpuscles

Grandy's method

Granger's line, sign

Grant's operation — excision of tumors of the lip

Grant's retractor, separator

Grantham's electrode, needle

Graser's diverticulum

Grashey's aphasia, method

Grasset's law, phenomenon, sign

Grasset-Bychowski sign

Grasset-Gaussel phenomenon

Grasset-Gaussel-Hoover sign

Gratiolet's optic radiation, radiating fibers

Graves's disease — a thyroid disorder of unknown cause, occurring principally in women and marked by exophthalmos, enlarged thyroid gland, nervous tremor, psychic disturbances and emaciation

Graves's scapula, speculum

Grawitz's tumor

Gray's clamp, forceps, resectoscope

Grayton's forceps

Green's caliper, mouth gag, resectoscope, scoop, trephine

Green-Armytage forceps

Green-Sewall mouth gag

Greene' sign

Greenfield's disease — a form of leukoencephalopathy marked by sphingolipid accumulations in neural tissue and by loss of myelin in the central nervous system

Greenhow's disease — excoriation and discoloration of the skin in pediculosis, caused by scratching

Greenhow's incision

Greenhow-Rodman incision

Greenough's microscope

Greenwald's method

Greenwald-Lewman method

Greenwood's forceps, trephine

Gregerson-Boas test

Gregg's syndrome — congenital abnormalities, including cataract, microphthalmia, heart defects and deafness, caused by maternal rubella in pregnancy

Gregory's mixture

Greig's syndrome — extreme width between the eyes due to enlargement of the sphenoid bone, often associated with mental retardation

Greiling's tube

Greither's syndrome — a familial disorder marked by nonscaling hyperkeratosis

Grenet's cell

Greville's bath

Grey Turner's sign

Gridley's stain

Grieshaber's extractor, forceps, keratome, trephine

Griesinger's disease — hookworm infestation

Griesinger's sign, symptom

Griess's test

Griffith's method, sign

Grigg's test

Grignard's compound, reaction, reagent

Grindon's disease — inflammation of the hair follicles

Gringolo's syndrome — ankylopoietic spondylarthritis, hypopyon, iritis, uveitis, polymorphic exudative erythema and ankylosis

Grisel's disease — nasopharyngeal torticollis

Grisolle's sign

Gritti's operation — amputation of the leg through the knee, using the patella as an osteoplastic flap over the end of the femur

Gritti's amputation

Gritti-Stokes amputation

Grob's syndrome — partial alopecia, epicanthus, cleft lip and cleft palate, multiple ridges in the mucous membrane of the jaws, fissures of the tongue, brachydactyly, clinodactyly of the small fingers and mental deficiency

Grocco's sign, test, triangle, triangular dullness

Grocott's adaptation of Gomori's methenamine-silver stain

Groenholm's retractor

Groenouw's type I, type II dystrophy

Groffith's degeneration

Grönblad-Strandberg syndrome — angioid streaks of the retina

Grondahl-Finney operation — esophagogastroplasty, allowing enlargement of the orifice between the esophagus and the stomach

Gross's disease — encysted rectum with dilatation of the anal wall

Gross's clamp, forceps, leukemia, method, retractor, spatula, spud, test, virus

Gross-Pomeranz-Watkins retractor

Grossich's method

Grossman's principle, sign

Grossmann's operation — treatment of retinal detachment by aspiration of subretinal fluid and injection of warm salt solution into the vitreous

Grotthus's law

Grove's cell

Grover's disease — transient acantholytic dermatosis

Gruber's syndrome — a malformation syndrome, lethal in the perinatal period, characterized by intrauterine growth retardation, ocular anomalies, cleft palate, polydactyly, polycystic kidney and other malformations. Called also *Meckel's syndrome*

Gruber's bougies, fossa, hernia, reaction, speculum, suture, test

Gruber-Landzert fossa

Gruber-Widal reaction, test

Gruby's disease — tinea capitis in children caused by fungus infection

Grudziński's osteochondropathy

Gruenwald's forceps, punch, retractor, rongeur

Gruenwald-Bryant forceps

Grünbaum-Widal test

Grünfelder's reflex

Grüning's magnet

Gruskin's test

Grynfelt's hernia, triangle

Grynfelt-Lesgaft triangle

Gsell-Erdheim syndrome — necrotic disintegration of the medial layer of the aorta without inflammatory changes

Guama virus

Guarnieri's bodies, corpuscles, inclusions

Guaroa virus

Guatamahri's nodules

Gubler's syndrome — a form of alternating hemiplegia with ipsilateral facial paralysis

Gubler's hemiplegia, line, paralysis, reaction, sign, tumor

Gubler-Robin typhus

Gudden's atrophy, commissure, law

Gudebrod's sutures

Guedel's airway, blade, laryngoscope

Guelpa's treatment

Guéneau de Mussy's point

Guepar's prosthesis

Guérin's epithelioma, fold, fracture, glands, sinus, tumor, valve

Guérin-Stern syndrome — congenital contractures of extremities

Guggenheim's forceps, scissors

Di Guglielmo's disease — an acute form of erythremic myelosis

Guibor's chart

Guidi's canal

Guild-Pratt speculum

Guilford's syndrome — congenital absence of teeth, inability to

Guilford's syndrome (*continued*)
smell or taste, hypotrichosis
and anhidrosis

Guilford's stapedectomy

Guilford-Schuknecht scissors

Guillain-Barré syndrome — a
disease affecting the peripheral
nervous system and cranial
nerves, marked by demyelination, inflammation, edema
and nerve root decompression.
Called also *Landry's paralysis*

Guillain-Barré polyneuritis

Guilland's sign

Guinard's method, treatment

Guinon's disease — same as *Gilles
de la Tourette's syndrome*

Guisez's tube

Guist's forceps, eye implant, scissors, speculum

Guist-Black speculum

Guldberg and Waage's law

Gull's disease — myxedema

Gull's renal epistaxis

Gull-Sutton disease — arteriolar
nephrosclerosis

Gull-Toynbee law

Gullstrand's law, ophthalmoscope,
slit lamp

Gumprecht's shadow

Gundelach's punch

Gunn's syndrome — unilateral
ptosis of the eyelid

Gunn's dots, law, phenomenon,
sign

Gunning's mixture, reaction,
splint, test

Gunson's method

Günther's disease — congenital
erythropoietic porphyria

Gunther's syndrome — an obscure
form of myositis associated
with myoglobinuria

Günz's ligament

Günzberg's test

Gusberg's curet, punch

Gussenbauer's operation — cutting
an esophageal stricture through
an opening above the stricture

Gussenbauer's suture

Gutglass's forceps

Guthrie's formula, muscle,
test

Gutierrez's syndrome — abdominal
pain in the epigastric or umbilical region, with a history of
chronic constipation associated or unassociated with
urinary disorders and early
signs of chronic nephritis

Guttmann's retractor, sign, speculum

Gutzeit's test

Guy's gouge, knife, pill

Guye's sign

Guyon's operation — amputation
above the malleoli

Guyon's amputation, bougie,
clamp, dilator, sign, sound

Guyon-Benique sound

Guyon-Péan clamp

Guyton's scissors

Guyton-Friedenwald sutures

Guyton-Lundsgaard sclerotome

Guyton-Maumenee speculum

Guyton-Noyes forceps

Guyton-Park speculum

Gwathmey's hook, oil-ether
anesthesia, suction tube

Gynefold's pessary

Haab's degeneration, magnet, reflex

Haagensen's test

Haas's method

Haase's rule

Haber's syndrome — an autosomal dominant, inherited trait marked by permanent flushing and telangiectasia of the face, accompanied by keratotic lesions of the trunk

Habermann's disease — sudden onset of a polymorphous skin eruption composed of macules, papules and vesicles

Hackenbruch's experience

Hacker's operation — for balanitic hypospadias

Haden's syndrome — hereditary hemolytic jaundice without spherocytosis

Hadfield-Clarke syndrome — same as *Clarke-Hadfield syndrome*

Haeckel's law

Haenel's syndrome — absence of pain on pressure to the eye in late stages of neurosyphilis

Haenel's symptom

Haferkamp's syndrome — a variant of *Gorham's syndrome,* marked by generalized malignant hemangiomatosis and osteolysis

Hagedorn's needle

Hagedorn-Jensen method

Hageman's factor

Hager's reagent, test

Hagie's pin

Haglund's disease — bursitis in the region of the Achilles tendon, caused by a disturbance of gait

Haglund's syndrome — fracture of the bony nucleus of the calcaneus at its junction with the Achilles tendon

Hagner's disease — a complex bone disease resembling acromegaly

Hagner's operation — drainage of gonorrheal epididymitis through an incision into the epididymis

Hagner's bag, catheter

Hague's lamp

Hahn's operation — gastrotomy with distal dilatation of the pylorus

Hahn's cannula, gastrotomy, method, oxine, reagent, sign

Haidinger's brushes

Haig Ferguson forceps

Haight's elevator, retractor

Haik's eye implant

Hailey-Hailey disease — benign familial pemphigus

Haines's coefficient, formula, reagent, test

Hajek's forceps, mallet, retractor, rongeur

Hajek-Ballenger dissector, elevator

Hajek-Koffler forceps, punch

Hajek-Skillern punch

Hajna's gram-negative broth medium

Hakim's syndrome — dilatation of the cerebral ventricles, asso-

Hakim's syndrome (*continued*)
    ciated with inadequacy of the
    subarachnoid spaces but with-
    out abnormal cerebrospinal
    fluid pressure

Hakin-Cordis pump

Hakion's catheter

Halban's disease — benign ovarian
    tumors in young women with
    persistence of the corpus lute-
    um, with amenorrhea and
    symptoms resembling preg-
    nancy but no true pregnancy

Halberstaedter-Prowazek bodies

Halbrecht's syndrome — jaundice
    of newborn infants related to
    maternal-fetal **ABO** incompat-
    ibility

Haldane's apparatus, chamber

Hale's forceps, iron stain

Hales's piesimeter

Hall's disease — spurious hydro-
    cephalus in children

Hall's antidote, band, dermatome,
    facies, intrauterine device,
    method, neurotome, sign

Hall-Stone ring

Hallauer's glasses

Hallberg's effect

Hallé's chisel, curet, needle, point,
    speculum

Hallé-Tieck speculum

Haller's ansa, arches, circle, cones,
    crypts, duct, frenum, glands,
    habenula, isthmus, layer, line,
    membrane, plexus, rete, tripod

Hallermann-Streiff syndrome —
    bony abnormalities of the face
    and jaw, with multiple eye de-
    fects, including cataract

Hallermann-Streiff-François syn-
    drome — same as *Hallermann-
    Streiff syndrome*

Hallervorden's syndrome — com-
    plete demyelinization of cer-
    tain nerve fibers

Hallervorden-Spatz syndrome —
    same as *Hallervorden's syn-
    drome*

Hallgren's syndrome — vestibulo-
    cerebellar ataxia, retinal dys-
    trophy, congenital deafness
    and cataract

Halliday's hyperostosis

Hallion's test

Hallopeau's disease — an inherited
    disorder in which blisters are
    present at birth, scarring is
    severe, mucous membranes are
    involved and death from infec-
    tion often occurs in youth

Hallopeau's acrodermatitis, pem-
    phigus

Hallopeau-Siemens syndrome —
    same as *Hallopeau's disease*

Hallpike's maneuver

Hallwach's effect

Halpin's operation — removal of
    the lacrimal gland through the
    middle of the eyebrow

Halsey's needle

Halsted's operation(s) — for the
    radial cure of inguinal hernia;
    radical mastectomy

Halsted's clamp, forceps, incision,
    inguinal herniorrhaphy, man-
    euver, radical mastectomy,
    sutures

Halsted-Meyer incision

Halsted-Willy Meyer incision

Ham's test

Hamberger's schema

Hamburger's interchange, phe-
    nomenon, test

Hamby's forceps, retractor

Hamby-Hibbs retractor

Hamdi's solution

Hamel's test

Hamilton's bandage, forceps, method, test

Hamilton-Stewart formula

Hamm's electrode

Hamman's disease — interstitial emphysema of the lungs from spontaneous rupture of the alveoli

Hamman's murmur, sign

Hamman-Rich syndrome — interstitial fibrosis of the lung, giving rise to right-sided heart failure

Hammar's myoid cells

Hammarsten's test

Hammer's test

Hammerschlag's method, phenomenon, test

Hammersmith's prosthesis

Hammond's disease — continuous sinuous, writhing movements, especially severe in the hands

Hammond's splint

Hampson's unit

Hampton's line

Hamrick's elevator

Hamstorn's syndrome — familial intermittent adynamia

Hanafee's catheter

Hanart's disease — familial spastic paraplegia, associated with congenital mental deficiency, transmitted as a recessive trait

Hanau's laws of articulation

Hancock's operation — amputation of the foot at the ankle, with a part of the astragalus being retained in the flap, the lower surface sawed off and the cut surface of the calcaneus brought into contact with it

Hancock's amputation, valve replacement

Hand's disease — same as *Hand-Schüller-Christian disease*

Hand-Schüller-Christian disease — a chronic form of histiocytosis with accumulation of cholesterol, characterized by defects in the membranous bones, exophthalmos and diabetes insipidus

Handley's incision, lymphangioplasty, method

Hanganatziu-Deicher reaction, test

Hanger's test

Hanhart's syndrome — a congenital syndrome marked primarily by severe micrognathia, high nose root, small eyelid fissures, low-set ears, and variable absence of digits or limbs

Hanhart's nanism

Hanke-Koessler test

Hanks's dilator

Hanks-Bradley dilator

Hann's disease — an association of posterior pituitary lesions with diabetes insipidus

Hanna's splint

Hannon's curet

Hannover's canal, intermediate membrane

Hanot's disease/syndrome — biliary cirrhosis

Hanot-Chauffard syndrome — hypertrophic cirrhosis with diabetes mellitus

Hanot-Kiener syndrome — diffuse mesenchymal hepatitis with nodular lymphomatosis

Hanot-MacMahon-Thannhauser syndrome — pericholangiolitic biliary cirrhosis

Hanot-Rössle syndrome — nonobstructive extrahepatic cholangitis with obstructive intrahepatic cholangitis

Hansen's disease — leprosy

Hansen's bacillus

Hansen-Street nail, pin

Hanson's unit

Hapsburg's disease — hemophilia

Hapsburg's jaw, lip

Harada's syndrome — bilateral edema of the fundus, uveitis, choroiditis and retinal detachment

Harbitz-Müller disease — familial hypercholesterinemia

Harden-Young equation, ester

Harder's glands

Harding-Passey melanoma

Harding-Ruttan test

Hardy's speculum

Hardy-Weinberg equilibrium, law, rule

Hare's syndrome — tumor near the apex of the lung, with neuritic pain and atrophy of the muscles of the upper extremity. Called also *Pancoast's syndrome*

Hargin's trocar

Hargraves's cell

Harkavy's syndrome — the occurrence in periarteritis nodosa of asthma, recurrent pulmonary infiltrations, eosinophilic polyserositis, pleurisy, pericarditis and neurological symptoms

Harken's forceps, prosthesis, valve, valvulotome

Harley's disease — intermittent hemoglobinuria

Harmon's incision

Harnasch's disease — acro-osteolysis of the phalangeal diaphyses of the hand and foot with involvement of the jaws, acromion and clavicle

Harrington's clamp, erysiphake, forceps, solution, tonometer

Harrington-Carmalt clamp

Harrington-Mayo forceps

Harrington-Mixter clamp, forceps

Harrington-Pemberton retractor

Harris's syndrome — hyperinsulinism due to functional disorder of the pancreas

Harris's band, dissector, forceps, hematoxylin, hip prosthesis, lines, migrainous neuralgia, segregator, separator, staining method, sutures, tube

Harris-Ray test

Harrison's curve, groove, knife, prosthesis, scissors, speculum, spot test, sulcus

Harrison-Shea curet

Harrower's hypothesis

Hart's syndrome — an autosomal recessive disorder of amino acid transport, marked by a skin rash on exposure to sunlight, temporary cerebellar ataxia and renal aminoaciduria without evident dysfunction

Hart's method, splint, test

Hartel's method, technique, treatment

Hartigan's foramen

Harting's bodies

Hartley's implant

Hartley-Krause operation — excision of the gasserian ganglion

Hartley-Krause operation (*continued*)
and its roots for relief of facial neuralgia

Hartmann's operation — resection of a diseased part of the colon, with the proximal end of the colon brought out as a colostomy and the distal stump being closed by suture

Hartmann's apraxia, catheter, colostomy, curet, forceps, fossa, point, pouch, procedure, punch, rongeur, speculum

Hartmann-Citelli forceps, punch

Hartmann-Dewaxer speculum

Hartmann-Gruenwald forceps

Hartmann-Herzfeld rongeur

Hartnup's disease — a hereditary, pellagra-like skin rash with cerebellar ataxia, renal aminoaciduria and other bizarre biochemical abnormalities

Hartridge's reversion spectroscope

Hartstein's retractor

Haseltine's clamp

Häser's coefficient, formula

Hashimoto's disease — a progressive disease of the thyroid gland, with degeneration of its epithelial elements and replacement by lymphoid and fibrous tissue

Hashimoto's struma, thyroiditis

Haslinger's bronchoscope, electroscope, esophagoscope, laryngoscope, tracheoscope

Hasner's fold, valve

Hass's disease — disseminated neonatal herpes

Hassall's bodies, corpuscles

Hassall-Henle bodies, warts

Hassin's syndrome — protrusion of the ear on the side of the lesion, combined with *Horner's syndrome*

Hata's phenomenon, preparation

Hatch's catheter

Hatchcock's sign

Hatcher's pin

Haudek's niche, sign

Haultaim's operation — modification of Huntington's operation for replacement of inverted uterus

Hauschka-Klein ascites tumor

Haverfield's cannula, retractor

Haverfield-Scoville retractor

Haverhill's clamp, fever

Hawk's test

Hawkins's forceps, fracture, keloid

Hawks-Dennen forceps

Hawley's chart, retainer

Haxthausen's syndrome — hyperkeratosis

Hay's test

Hayden's curet, elevator

Hayem's corpuscles, encephalitis, icterus, jaundice, solution

Haymen-Widal syndrome — acquired hemolytic anemia marked by a low erythrocyte count, icterus, spherocytosis and splenomegaly

Hayes's clamp, retractor

Hayes-Olivecrona forceps

Haygarth's nodes, nodosities

Haynes's operation — draining the cisterna magna for acute meningitis

Haynes's cannula, pin

Haynes-Griffin splint

Hayton-Williams forceps

Hazen's theorem
Head's zones
Heaf's test
Healy's forceps
Heaney's clamp, curet, forceps, hysterectomy, sutures
Heaney-Ballentine forceps
Heaney-Kantor forceps
Heaney-Rezek forceps
Heaney-Simon retractor
Hearson's capsule
Heath's operation — division of the ascending rami of the lower jaw for ankylosis—performed within the mouth
Heath's curet, dissector, forceps, scissors
Heaton's operation — for inguinal hernia
Heberden's disease(s) — rheumatism of the smaller joints accompanied by nodules around the distal interphalangeal joints; angina pectoris
Heberden's asthma, nodes, rheumatism, sign
Hebra's disease — familial non-hemolytic jaundice
Hebra's syndrome — a chronic skin disorder, usually beginning in infancy, marked by pruritic papules that eventually become covered with blood-colored crust
Hebra's pityriasis, prurigo
Hecht's phenomenon, pneumonia, test
Hecht-Weinberg test
Hecht-Weinberg-Gradwohl reaction, test
Heck's disease — focal epithelial hyperplasia

Hector's tendon
Hedblom's syndrome — acute primary diaphragmitis
Hedblom's elevator, raspatory, retractor
Heerfordt's disease — sarcoidosis marked by chronic inflammation of the parotid gland and the uvea
Heerman's chisel, incision
Heffernan's speculum
Hefke-Turner sign
Hegar's dilator, perineorrhaphy, sign
Hegar-Goodell dilator
Hegenbarth's forceps
Hegglin's syndrome — cardiac insufficiency during diabetic coma
Hegglin's anomaly
Hehner's number, value
Heiberg-Esmarch maneuver
Heidenhaim's syndrome — a progressive, degenerative disease marked by cortical blindness, presenile dementia, ataxia and generalized rigidity of muscle
Heidenhain's cells, demilunes, iron hematoxylin stain, law, pouch, rods
Heifitz's retractor
Heilbronner's sign, thigh
Heilmeyer-Schöner erythroblastosis
Heim-Kreysig sign
Heimlich's maneuver, tube
Heine's operation — cyclodialysis in glaucoma
Heine-Medin disease — poliomyelitis, with involvement of the central nervous system and paralysis

Heineke's operation — resection of the colon to remove tumors, done in multiple stages

Heineke-Mikulicz operation — enlargement of a pyloric stricture

Heineke-Mikulicz's gastroenterostomy, herniorrhaphy, pyloroplasty

Heintz's method

Heinz's bodies, granules

Heinz-body anemias

Heinz-Ehrlich bodies

Heise's forceps

Heisrath's operation — excision of the tarsal folds for trachoma

Heister's diverticulum, fold, valve

Heitz-Boyer clamp

Hektoen's medium, phenomenon

Hektoen, Kretschmer and Welker protein

HeLa cells

Helanca's prosthesis

Helbing's sign

Held's end-feet, limiting membrane

Helfrick's retractor

Heliodorus's bandage

Hellat's sign

Hellendall's sign

Heller's disease — dystrophic, median, canaliform depressions of the fingernails without apparent organic cause

Heller's operation — cardiomyotomy

Heller's syndrome — progressive infantile dementia

Heller's dementia, plexus, procedure, test

Heller-Döhle disease — syphilitic aortitis

Heller-Döhle mesoaortitis

Heller-Nelson syndrome — a variant of *Klinefelter's syndrome,* marked by atrophic testes, hyalinization of the seminiferous tubules and elevation of urinary gonadotropins

Hellerström's disease — erythema characterized by edematous pinkish-red rings, associated with meningitis following a tick bite

Hellin's law

Hellin-Zeleny law

Helly's formol-Zenker fixative, fluid

Helmholtz's ligament, line, theory

Helmholz-Harrington syndrome — congenital clouding of the cornea associated with various abnormalities

Helweg's bundle, tract

Helweg-Larssen syndrome — a familial disease with neurolabyrinthitis developing in the fourth or fifth decade

Helwig's disease — inverted follicular keratosis

Hench-Aldrich index, test

Hench-Rosenberg syndrome — rheumatism with repeated episodes of arthritis, without fever and without irreversible damage to joints

Henderson's chisel, retractor

Henderson-Hasselbalch equation

Henderson-Jones disease — osteochondromatosis

Hendren's clamp, forceps

Hendrickson's drain, lithotrite

Henke's forceps, space, triangle, trigone

Henle's ampulla, ansa, band, canal, cell, fibers, fibrin, fissures, glands, incisure, layer, ligament, loop, membrane, reaction, restiform process, sheath, sinus, sphincter, spine, trapezoid bone, tubercle, tuberosity, tubule

Henle-Coenen sign, test

Hennebert's syndrome — nystagmus and vertigo on air compression of the auditory meatus, seen in congenital syphilis

Hennebert's sign, test

Henner's elevator, retractor

Henning's sign

Henny's rongeur

Henoch's disease — chronic progressive chorea of children

Henoch's chorea, purpura

Henoch-Schönlein syndrome — an eruption of purpuric lesions, associated with joint pains, vomiting of blood, passage of bloody stools and sometimes glomerulonephritis

Henoch-Schönlein purpura

Henriques-Sörensen's method

Henrotin's forceps, speculum

Henry's femoral herniorrhaphy, incision, law, melanin reaction, melanin test, splenectomy

Henschen's method

Hensen's body, canal, cells, disk, duct, knot, line, node, plane, stripe

Henshaw's test

Hensing's fold, ligament

Henton's hook, needle

Hepp's osmometer

Herbert's operation — displacement of a wedge-shaped flap of sclera for formation of a filtering cicatrix in glaucoma

Herbert's pits, prosthesis

Herbert Adams clamp

Herbst's corpuscles

d'Herelle's phenomenon

Herff's clamp

Hering's canals, law, nerve, phenomenon, test, theory

Hering-Breuer reflex

Hering-Hellebrand deviation

Herlitz's syndrome — a familial, congenital and fatal variant of *Fox's disease,* marked by blisters on the skin and mucous membranes, epidermal defects, nail dystrophy and, sometimes, skeletal atrophy

Herman's syndrome — pyramidal and extrapyramidal disorders with disturbances of speech and mentation, occurring after closed head injuries

Herman-Taylor gastroscope

Hermann-Perutz reaction, test

Hermansky-Pudlak syndrome — albinism, pseudohemophilia and pigmented macrophages in the bone marrow

Herrenschwand's syndrome — a difference in color of the irides, caused by sympathetic lesions

Herrick's syndrome — sickle-cell anemia

Herrick's anemia, clamp

Herring's bodies, test

Herring-Binet test

Herrmann's syndrome — an inherited disorder of the nervous

Herrmann's syndrome (*continued*)
    system beginning in childhood, characterized by deafness, diabetes mellitus, progressive dementia, pyelonephritis and glomerulonephritis

Herrmannsdorfer's diet

Hers's disease — glycogen storage disease

Hershell's culture medium

Hersman's disease — idiopathic progressive enlargement of the hands

Hertel's exophthalmometer

Herter's disease — same as *Herter-Heubner disease*

Herter's infantilism, test

Herter-Foster method

Herter-Heubner disease — the infantile form of nontropical sprue

Hertig-Rock ova

Hertwig's sheath

Hertwig-Magendie syndrome — dissociation of gaze, marked by downward and inward rotation of the eyes on the side of a cerebellar lesion and upward and outward deviation on the contralateral side

Hertwig-Magendie phenomenon, sign

Hertwig-Weyers syndrome — aplasia of the ulna with abnormalities of the sternum, kidneys, spleen, and jaws

Herxheimer's disease — a chronic, progressive disease of the extremities, marked by visibility of blood vessels through a bluish, atrophic, wrinkled skin resembling tissue paper

Herxheimer's fever, fibers, reaction, spirals

Heryng's sign

Herz's triad

Herzberg's test

Heschl's convolution, gyrus

Hess's capillary test, forceps, scoop, spoon

Hess-Barraquer forceps

Hess-Gill forceps

Hess-Horwitz forceps

Hesselbach's hernia, ligament, triangle

Hesseltine's umbiliclip

Heublein's method

Heubner's disease — syphilitic endarteritis of the cerebral vessels

Heubner's specific endarteritis

Heubner-Herter disease — the infantile form of nontropical sprue, or celiac disease

Heuser's membrane

Hey's operation — separation of the metatarsus from the tarsus with removal of part of the medial cuneiform bone

Hey's amputation, derangement, hernia, ligament, saw

Heyd's syndrome — renal disorder associated with diseases of the biliary tract or the liver

Heyer-Schulte prosthesis

Heyman's capsules, forceps, law

Heyman-Paparella scissors

Heyns's decompression

Heynsius' test

Hibbs's operation — fracturing the spinous processes of the vertebrae in Pott's disease

Hibbs's chisel, curet, forceps, frame, mouth gag, osteotome, retractor

Hibbs-Spratt curet
Hickey's method
Hickey-Hare test
Hicks's syndrome — familial perforating ulcers of the foot
Hicks's contractions, sign, version
Hicks-Pitney test
Higbee's speculum
Higgins's catheter, incision
Highman's Congo red stain
Highmore's antrum, body
Higouménakis's sign
Hikojima antigen
Hildebrandt's test
Hildenbrand's disease — typhus
Hildreth's cautery
Hilger's syndrome — pain in the head and neck regions caused by vasodilation of the carotid artery and its branches
Hilger's stimulator, tube
Hill's cell, reaction, sign
Hill-Ferguson retractor
Hillis's perforator, retractor
Hilsinger's knife
Hilton's law, muscle, sac, white line
Himmelsteins's retractor, valvulotome
Hinckle-James speculum
Hindenlang's test
Hines-Anderson pyeloureteroplasty
Hines-Bannick syndrome — intermittent attacks of low temperature
Hines-Brown test
Hinman's reflux
Hinton's test
Hippel's disease —same as von Hippel's disease
Hippel's trephine

Hippel-Lindau disease — retinocerebral angiomatosis. Also called von Hippel-Lindau disease
Hippocrates's bandage
Hirsch's syndrome — oseitis fibrosa of the ribs, sternum and metacarpus
Hirsch-Pfeiffer stain
Hirschberg's magnet, method, reflex, sign
Hirschfeld's disease — acute diabetes mellitus
Hirschfeld's canals
Hirschfeld-Klinger reaction
Hirschfelder's tuberculin
Hirschfeldt's test
Hirschman's anoscope, forceps, proctoscope
Hirschman-Martin proctoscope
Hirschowitz's fiberscope, gastroscope
Hirschsprung's disease — congenital megacolon
Hirschtick's splint
Hirst's test
Hirst-Emmet forceps
Hirst-Hare test
His's disease — same as His-Werner disease
His's band, bundle, bundle electrogram, bursa, canal, duct, isthmus, space, spindle, tubercle, zones
His-Werner disease — a self-limited, louse-borne, rickettsial disease with intermittent fever, generalized aches and pains, vertigo, malaise and multiple relapses
Hiss's capsule stain, serum water
Hitchens-Hansen antigen
Hittorf's number, tube

Hitzig's syndrome — unintentional movement of the orbicularis and other muscles innervated by the seventh cranial nerve

Hitzig's girdle, test

Hoboken's nodules, valves

Hoche's bandelette

Hochenegg's operation — for rectal cancer

Hochenegg's ulcer

Hochsinger's phenomenon, sign

Höchst's peptone

Hodara's disease — trichorrhexis of the scalp

Hodge's forceps, maneuver, pessary, planes

Hodgen's apparatus, method, splint

Hodgkin's disease — a malignant neoplasm of transformed lymphocytes, marked by painless, progressive enlargement of the lymph nodes, spleen and general lymphoid tissue

Hodgkin's cells, cycle, granuloma, sarcoma

Hodgson's disease — aneurysmal dilatation of the aorta

Hodgson's hypospadias repair

Hoehne's sign

Hoen's elevator, forceps, hook, raspatory, scissors

Hoet-Abaza syndrome — postpartum diabetes mellitus and obesity

Hofacker-Sadler law

Hofbauer's cells

Hoff's law

Hoffa's disease — traumatic proliferation of fatty tissue in the knee joint

Hoffa's operation — same as *Lorenz's operation*

Hoffa-Kastert syndrome — chronic synovitis of the knee joint resulting in tumor-like lesions and adhesions that restrict joint motility

Hoffa-Lorenz operation — same as *Lorenz's operation*

Hoffmann's syndrome — muscular hypertrophy, painful spasms, pseudomyotonia and hypothyroidism in adults

Hoffmann's anodyne, atrophy, drops, duct, forceps, phenomenon, reflex, serum, sign, test

Hoffmann-Werdnig syndrome — a hereditary, progressive form of muscular atrophy resulting from degeneration of the anterior horn cells of the spinal cord, usually followed by death in infancy or childhood

Hoffmann-Zurhelle syndrome — a lipomatous nevus of the gluteal region, marked by yellowish nodules that may become large plaques

Hofmann's bacillus, violet

Hofmeister's gastrectomy, gastroenterostomy, series, test

Hofmeister-Billroth gastrectomy

Hoguet's maneuver

Högyes's treatment

Hohmann's retractor

Hoke's incision, osteotome

Holden's curet, line

Holinger's applicator, bougie, bronchoscope, esophagoscope, forceps, laryngoscope, needle, telescope, tube

Holinger-Garfield laryngoscope

Holinger-Hurst bougie

Holinger-Jackson bronchoscope

Hollenhorst's plaques

Holman's retractor

Holman-Mathieu cannula

Holmblad's method

Holmes's disease — progressive familial ataxia with cerebello-olivary degeneration

Holmes's operation — excising the os calcis

Holmes's syndrome — space perception disorders caused by brain injuries, marked by inability to recognize the position, distance and size of objects in space, impaired fixation and absence of the blinking reflex

Holmes's degeneration, forceps, method, nasopharyngoscope, phenomenon, sign

Holmes-Adie syndrome — same as *Adie's syndrome*

Holmes-Stewart phenomenon

Holmgren's skeins, test

Holmgren-Golgi canals

Holt-Oram syndrome — hereditary heart disease, usually an atrial or ventricular septal defect

Holten's test

Holter's monitor, shunt, tube, valve

Holtermüller-Wiedemann syndrome — a rare, congenital form of hydrocephalus

Holth's operation — excision of the sclera by punch operation

Holth's cystotome, forceps, sclerectomy

Holthouse's hernia

Holtz's curet, machine

Holz's phlegmon

Holzer's stain

Holzknecht's chromoradiometer, space, stomach, unit

Homans's sign

Homén's syndrome — a genetically determined disease of the nervous system, marked by vertigo, ataxia, dysarthria, increasing dementia and rigidity of the body

Honore-Smathers tube

Hood's dermatome

Hood-Graves speculum

Hood-Kirkland incision

Hooft's syndrome — familial hypolipidemia

Hooper's scissors

Hoorweg's law

Hoover's sign

Hope's resuscitator, sign

Hopf's keratosis

Hopkins's clamp, forceps, raspatory, telescope, thiophene test

Hopkins-Cole test

Hopmann's papilloma, polyp

Hopp's blade, laryngoscope

Hoppe-Goldflam disease — myasthenia gravis

Hoppe Seyler's test

Horgan's blade

Hörlein-Weber disease — chronic familial methemoglobinemia

Horn's degeneration, sign

Horner's syndrome — same as *Bernard-Horner syndrome*

Horner's law, muscle, ptosis, pupil, sign, teeth

Horner-Bernard syndrome — same as *Bernard-Horner syndrome*

Horner-Trantas spots

Horsley's operation — excision of an area of motor cortex for relief of convulsive movements of the upper extremities

Horsley's elevator, forceps, putty, pyloroplasty, sign, sutures, test, trephine, wax

Hortega's cell, cell tumor, method

Horton's disease — migrainous neuralgia

Horton's syndrome(s) — temporal arteritis; migrainous neuralgia

Horton's arteritis, headache, neuralgia

Hosford's dilator, spud

Hosford-Hicks forceps

Hotchkiss's operation — resection of part of the mandible and maxilla for epithelioma of the cheek, with plastic restoration of the defect

Hotchkiss-McManus technique

Hotis's test

Hottentot apron, veil

Hotz's curet, probe

Hotz-Anagnostakis procedure

Hough's forceps, hoe, method, osteotome

Houghton's law of fatigue, test

Hounsfield's numbers

Hourin's needle

House-Barbara needle

House-Bellucci scissors

House-Dieter nipper

House-Metzenbaum scissors

House-Paparella curet

House-Rosen needle

House-Wullstein forceps

Houses' bur, dissector, excavator, forceps, hammer, irrigator, knife, prosthesis, retractor, scissors, stapedectomy, wire

Houssay's syndrome — amelioration of diabetes mellitus by a destructive lesion of the pituitary gland

Houssay's animal, phenomenon

Housset-Debray gastroscope

Houston's muscle, valves

Houtz's curet

Hovius's canal, circle, membrane, plexus

Howard's abrader, forceps, method, stone basket, test

Howell's bodies, method, test

Howell-Jolly bodies

Howorth's elevator, osteotome, retractor

Howship's lacuna

Howship-Romberg syndrome — neuralgic pain in the leg caused by obturator hernia

Hoxworth's forceps

Hoyle's medium

Hoyne's sign

Hoyt's forceps

Hryntschak's catheter

Hsieh's method

Hubbard's bolt, electrode, forceps, tank

Hubbenet's spots

Hubell's meatoscope

Hübl number

Huchard's disease — continued arterial hypertension—a possible cause of arteriosclerosis

Huchard's sign, symptom

Hucker-Conn crystal violet

Huddleson's test

Hudgins's cannula

Hudson's brace, clamp, drill, forceps, lactone rule, line, rongeur

Hudson-Stähli line

Huebener-Thomsen-Friedenreich phenomenon

Hueck's ligament

Huët-Pelger nuclear anomaly

Hueter's bandage, line, maneuver,
sign
Huey's scissors
Huffman's speculum, vaginoscope
Huffman-Graves speculum
Hufnagel's clamp, forceps, pros-
thesis, valve
Huggins's operation — castration
for cancer of the prostate
Huggins's test
Hugh-Leifson medium
Hughes's eye implant, reflex
Hughes-Stovin syndrome — pul-
monary arterial thrombosis,
pulmonary arterial aneurysm
and peripheral venous throm-
bosis
Hughes-Young adrenalectomy,
incision
Hughston's method
Huguenin's edema
Huguier's canal, circle, sinus
Huguier-Jersild syndrome —
lymphedema of the rectal and
external genital regions, often
with stricture of the anus and
introitus vaginae, caused by
syphilis, gonorrhea, ulcers or
lymphogranuloma venereum
Huhner's test
Huldshinsky's radiation
Human's sign
Humby's knife
Hume's clamp
Humphrey's tubercle
Humphries's clamp
Humphry's ligament
Hünermann's disease — a heredit-
ary condition marked by
multiple opacities of the
epiphyses, dwarfism, cataract,

Hünermann's disease (*continued*)
shortened digits, dulled mentation and general debility. Usually a cause of death in the
first year of life
Hunner's stricture, ulcer
Hunt's disease — generalized
tremor due to disturbance of
muscle tone and of muscular
coordination associated with
myoclonic epilepsy
Hunt's syndrome — facial paralysis
accompanied by otalgia and
vesicular eruption of the external canal of the ear, caused
by herpes zoster virus infection
Hunt's atrophy, clamp, epilepsy,
forceps, method, neuralgia,
paralysis, phenomenon, reaction, sound, test, tremor, trocar
Hunt-Transley procedure
Hunter's operation — ligation of
an artery for aneurysm
Hunter's syndrome — same as
Hunter-Hurler syndrome
Hunter's canal, chancre, curet,
glossitis, gubernaculum, ligament, line, separator
Hunter-Given method
Hunter-Hurler syndrome — an
error of mucopolysaccharide
metabolism, similar to *Hurler's
syndrome* but distinguished
by less severe skeletal effects
Hunter-Schreger bands
Huntington's disease — a rare,
hereditary disease marked by
chronic, progressive chorea
and severe mental deterioration

Huntington's operation — replacement of a chronically inverted uterus through an opening in the abdominal wall below the umbilicus

Huntington's chorea, sign

Hupp's retractor

Huppert's test

Huppert-Cole test

Hurd's dissector, elevator, forceps, retractor

Hurler's syndrome — a defect of mucopolysaccharide metabolism, with accumulation of abnormal cellular material in the urine and with severe abnormalities of skeletal bone and cartilage, including dwarfism, and marked by deformity of limbs and mental retardation

Hurler's polydystrophy

Hurler-Pfaundler syndrome — same as *Hurler's syndrome*

Hurler-Scheie compound

Hurst's disease — an acute, fatal disease marked by cerebral hemorrhage, leukocytic infiltrations and vascular degeneration

Hurst's bougie, dilator

Hürthle cell adenoma, cell carcinoma, cell tumor

Hurtig's dilator

Hurtley's test

Hurwitz's clamp, trocar

Huschke's auditory teeth, canal,

Huschke's (*continued*) foramen, ligaments, valve

Huse's cannula

Husks's rongeur

Hutch's diverticulum, evacuator

Hutchins's needle

Hutchinson's disease — a papular form of polymorphous benign eruption

Hutchinson's facies, freckle, incisor, mask, patch, prurigo, pupil, sign, teeth, triad, type

Hutchinson-Boeck disease/syndrome — sarcoidosis

Hutchinson-Gilford disease/syndrome — progeria

Hutchison's syndrome — neuroblastoma with cranial metastases

Hutinel's disease(s) — tuberculous pericarditis with cirrhosis of the liver in children; erythema due to an infection

Huxley's layer, membrane

Hyams's clamp

Hyde's disease — an eruption of hard nodules in the skin, accompanied by intense itching

Hyde's syndrome — a form of severe, pruritic, nodular and verrucous skin eruption consisting of lesions of the back, extremities and thighs, usually in adult women

Hynes's pharyngoplasty

Hyrtl's anastomosis, loop, recess, sphincter

Ide's reaction, test
Iglesias's resectoscope
Ihle's paste
Ilfeld-Gustafson splint
Ilfeld-Holder deformity
Ilheus encephalitis, virus
Iliff's trephine
Ilimow's test
Ilosvay's reagent, test
Imerslund-Gräsbeck syndrome —
    a chronic, relapsing, familial
    form of megaloblastic anemia
    in children, with onset between
    the ages of five months and
    four years. Principal symptoms
    are pallor, weakness, irritabil-
    ity, dyspnea, fever, gastroin-
    testinal disorders with diarrhea
    and vomiting, lack of appetite,
    glossitis, jaundice, heart mur-
    murs, proteinuria and other
    disorders
Imerslund-Najman-Gräsbeck syn-
    drome — same as *Imerslund-
    Gräsbeck syndrome*
Imhoff's tank
Imlach's fat plug
Immergut's tube
Inaba antigen
Ingals's speculum
Inge's procedure
Ingersoll's curet, needle
Ingrassia's apophysis, process,
    wings
Inikawa-Ogura method

Ionescu's method
Ionescu-Shiley valve
Irvine's syndrome — macular
    edema that occasionally
    follows cataract surgery
Irvine's scissors
Irving's sterilization operation —
    tubal ligation in which the
    uterine tubes are ligated and
    severed
Isaacs' syringe
Isaacs-Ludwig arteriole
Isambert's disease — acute miliary
    tuberculosis of the larynx and
    pharynx
Isherwood's methods
Ishihara's plate, test
Israel's dissector, retractor
Israéls-Wilkinson anemia
Israelson's reaction, test
Itard's catheter
Itard-Cholewa sign
Itô's nevus
Ito-Reenstierna reaction, test
Itsenko-Cushing syndrome — same
    as *Cushing's syndrome*
Ivalon's implant, patch, sutures
Ivemark's syndrome — imperfect
    splenic development and
    cardiac malformation
Iverson's dermabrader
Ives's speculum
Ivy's method, rongeur
Iwanoff's (Iwanow's) cysts
Izar's reagent

J ─────────────────────────────────────

Jaboulay's operation — interpelvi-abdominal amputation

Jaboulay's amputation, button

Jaccoud's syndrome — chronic arthritis occurring after rheumatic fever

Jaccoud's fever, sign

Jackson's syndrome — paralysis of the 10th, 11th, and 12th cranial nerves, soft palate, larynx and one half of the tongue and the sternomastoid and trapezius muscles

Jackson's bronchoscope, clamp, dilator, epilepsy, forceps, incision, laryngoscope, law, membrane, rule, safety triangle, scissors, sign, tube, veil

Jackson-MacKenzie syndrome — same as *Jackson's syndrome*

Jackson-Moore shears

Jackson-Mosher dilator

Jackson-Plummer dilator

Jackson-Pratt drain

Jackson-Trousseau dilator

Jacob's disease — permanent constriction of the mandible, with inability to open the mouth

Jacob's clamp, forceps, membrane, ulcer

Jacobaeus's operation — thoracoscopy and cauterization for treatment of adhesions

Jacobi's disease — a form of poikiloderma characterized by telangiectasia, pigmentation and atrophy of the skin and oral mucosa

Jacobs's syndrome — a deficiency disease characterized by ex-

Jacobs's syndrome (*continued*) foliating dermatitis of the scrotum, stomatitis and conjunctivitis

Jacobs-Palmer laparoscope

Jacobson's anastomosis, canal, cartilage, clamp, forceps, nerve, organ, plexus, retinitis, retractor, scissor, sulcus

Jacobsthal's test

Jacoby's test

Jacod's syndrome — complete paralysis of the eye muscles, blindness and trigeminal neuralgia

Jacod's triad

Jacquart's angle

Jacquemin's test

Jacquet's biokinetic treatment, dermatitis, erythema

Jadassohn's disease — a skin disorder marked by slightly elevated, red papules that appear first at the elbow area and later spread to other parts of the arm and forearm and hand

Jadassohn's macular atrophy, sebaceous nevus, test

Jadassohn-Bloch test

Jadassohn-Lewandowsky syndrome — a rare congenital disorder, marked by abnormal thickening of the nails that progresses to hyperkeratosis of the palms, soles, knees and elbows and leukoplakia of the oral mucous membranes

Jadassohn-Tièche nevus

Jadelot's furrows, lines

Jaeger's keratome, knife, lid retractor, test type
Jaeger-Whiteley catheter
Jaffé's reaction, test
Jaffe-Lichtenstein disease/syn-
drome — fibrous dysplasia
Jaffe-Lichtenstein-Uehlinger syndrome — same as *Jaffe-Lichtenstein disease/syndrome*
Jahnke's syndrome — congenital
angiomas of the leptomeninges
and choroid, often associated
with intracranial calcification,
hemiplegia and epilepsy. A
variant of the *Sturge-Weber
syndrome* without glaucoma
Jahnke-Cook-Seeley clamp
Jako's knife, laryngoscope
Jakob's disease — same as *Creutz-
feldt-Jakob disease*
Jakob's pseudosclerosis
Jakob-Creutzfeldt disease — same
as *Creutzfeldt-Jakob disease*
Jaksch's disease — deficiency of
hemoglobin, poikilocytosis,
erythroblastosis, severe leukocytosis and hepatomegaly in
infants and children
Jaksch's anemia, test
Jaksch-Hayem syndrome — same
as *Jaksch's disease*
Jaksch-Hayem-Luzet syndrome —
same as *Jaksch's disease*
Jalaguier's incision
Jamar's dynamometer
James's fiber
James-Lange theory
Jameson's forceps, hook, needle
Jamshidi's needle
Janbon's syndrome — a gastroin-
testinal syndrome resembling
cholera, produced by oxytet-
racycline

Janet's disease(s) — functional
neurosis marked by morbid
fears, obsessions and a sense
of inadequacy and self-accusa-
tion; feelings of unreality and
depersonalization
Janet's test
Janeway's gastroscope, lesion,
pills, sphygmomanometer,
spots
Janin's tetanus
Jannetta's retractor
Janosik's embryo
Jansen's disease — metaphyseal
dysostosis
Jansen's operation — for disease
of frontal sinus
Jansen's forceps, periosteotome,
raspatory, retractor, test
Jansen-Gifford retractor
Jansen-Gruenwald forceps
Jansen-Middleton forceps
Jansen-Newhart probe
Jansen-Struycken forceps
Jansen-Wagner retractor
Janský's classification
Jansky-Bielschowsky disease —
juvenile form of cerebral
sphingolipidosis
Janus's syndrome — same as
Bret's syndrome
Jaquet's apparatus
Jarcho's syndrome — metastatic
carcinoma of the bone mar-
row associated with thrombo-
cytopenia and purpura
Jarcho's cannula, pressometer
Jarisch-Herxheimer reaction
Jarjavay's muscle
Jarotzky's (Jarotsky's) treatment
Jarvis's operation — removal of a
portion of the lower turbinate
bone

Jarvis's clamp, snare
Javal's ophthalmometer
Javid's clamp, shunt, tube
Jaworski's bodies, corpuscles, test
Jayle-Ourgaud syndrome — ataxic nystagmus
Jeanselme's nodules
Jeddah ulcer
Jefferson's syndrome — aneurysm of the internal carotid artery with involvement of the visual pathways
Jefferson's retractor
Jegher's syndrome — same as *Peutz-Jeghers syndrome*
Jelanko's splint
Jelks's operation — incision of fibrous tissue around the rectum performed for stricture of the rectum
Jellinek's sign, symptom
Jelm's catheter
Jendrassik's maneuver, sign
Jenner's stain
Jenner-Giemsa blood-smear staining
Jenner-Kay test
Jenning's mouth gag, test
Jennings-Skillern mouth gag
Jensen's disease — a small area of inflammation on the fundus of the eye in otherwise healthy persons
Jensen's classification, retinitis, sarcoma, tumor
Jergesen's reamer, tube
Jersild's syndrome — same as *Huguier-Jersild syndrome*
Jervell and Lange-Nielsen syndrome — attacks of syncope and sudden death in persons congenitally deaf and with cardiac anomalies

Jesberg's bronchoscope, esophagoscope, forceps, tube
Jesionek's lamp
Jesse-Stryker saw
Jeune's syndrome — asphyxiating thoracic dystrophy
Jewett's nail, prosthesis, sound
Jirásek-Zuelzer-Wilson syndrome — congenital neurogenic ileus
Job's syndrome — a chronic granulomatous disease affecting girls with red hair and fair skin, marked by recurrent staphylococcal abscesses and eczema
Jobert's fossa, sutures
Jobert de Lamballe sutures
Jocasta complex
Jochmann's test
Joel-Baker anastomosis, tube
Joest's bodies
Joffroy's reflex, sign
Johne's disease — a lethal form of chronic enteritis caused by *Mycobacterium paratuberculosis,* usually affecting mammals other than humans
Johne's bacillus
Johnson's syndrome — pseudoparalysis of lateral or superior rectus muscles
Johnson's forceps, knife, modification method, retractor, stone basket, test, twin wire appliance
Johnson-Kerrison punch
Johnson-Stevens disease — a severe form of erythema multiforme, with involvement of the oronasal and anogenital mucosa, eyes and viscera
Johnson-Tooke knife
Johnston's clamp, dilator

Jolles's test

Jolliffe's syndrome — an almost always fatal condition thought to be caused by nicotinic acid deficiency, characterized by clouding of consciousness, cogwheel rigidity of the extremities and uncontrollable grasping and sucking reflexes

Jolly's bodies, reaction

Jonas's symptom

Jonas-Graves speculum

Jonell's splint

Jones's disease — familial fibrous dysplasia of the jaws

Jones's albumosuria, clamp, cylinder, dilator, forceps, nasal splint, position, protein, scissors

Jones-Cantarow test

Jones-Mote reaction

Jonge's position

Jonnesco's operation — sympathectomy

Jonnesco's fold, fossa

Jonston's arc

Joplin's forceps, toe prosthesis

Jordan's tartrate culture medium

Jordan-Day bur, drill

Jorgenson's retractor, scissors

Jorissen's test

Joseph's syndrome — an inborn defect of amino acid metabolism, characterized by a high protein level in the cerebrospinal fluid, excessive amounts of glycine, proline and hydroxyproline in the urine and convulsions

Joseph's clamp, elevator, periosteotome, raspatory, scissors

Joseph-Killian elevator

Joseph-Maltz saw, scissors

Josephs-Diamond-Blackfan anemia

Joule's equivalent

Jourdain's disease — suppurative inflammation of the gums and alveolar processes

Judd's clamp, forceps, method, trocar

Judd-Allis clamp, forceps

Judd-DeMartel forceps

Judd-Masson retractor

Judet's dissector, prosthesis

Juers's forceps

Juers-Derlacki holder

Juers-Lempert forceps, rongeur

Juhel-Rénoy's syndrome — bilateral renal cortical necrosis

Jukes family

Julian's forceps, needle holder

Julian-Fildes clamp

Jung's method, muscle

Jungbluth's vessels

Jüngling's disease — sarcoidosis

Jüngling's polycystic osteitis

Junin virus

Junker's apparatus, bottle, inhaler

Junod's boot

Jurasz's forceps

Jürgen's syndrome — hemorrhagic diathesis

Jürgensen's sign

Juster's reflex

Justus's test

Jutte's tube

Juvara's fold

juvenile Paget's disease — a hereditary condition marked by abnormally high serum alkaline phosphatase levels and abnormal enlargement of the skull

K

Kabatschnik's test

Kader's operation — same as *Kader-Senn operation*

Kader's needle

Kader-Senn operation — gastrostomy, allowing a feeding tube to be introduced through a valvelike flap that closes when the tube is withdrawn

Kaes's feltwork, line

Kaes-Bekhterev layer

Kafka's reaction, test

Kahlbaum's disease — catatonic schizophrenia

Kahler's disease — multiple myeloma

Kahler's forceps, law

Kahn's albumin A reaction, cannula, dilator, scissors, tenaculum, test

Kahn-Graves speculum

Kaiser's nuclei

Kaiserling's fixative, fluid, method, solution

Kalischer's disease — same as *Dimitri's disease*

Kallikak family

Kallmann's syndrome — hypogonadism with olfactory anesthesia

Kalmuk idiocy, type

Kalt's forceps, needle, sutures

Kaminer's reaction

Kammerer's incision

Kanavel's cannula, cock-up splint, conductor, sign, triangle

Kandel's method

Kane's clamp

Kanner's syndrome — a severe emotional disturbance of childhood, marked by inability to form meaningful interpersonal relationships

Kantor's clamp, forceps, sign

Kantor-Geis test

Kantrowicz's clamp, forceps

Kaplan's lymphoma, needle, test

Kaposi's disease(s) — a skin disease marked by numerous whitish punctiform papules and brownish macules arranged in a necklace-like pattern; a chronic, exfoliative disease of the skin marked by dry, acuminate papules surrounding the hair follicles; a rare variant of lichen planus

Kaposi's angiomatosis, dermatitis, dermatosis, sarcoma, varicelliform eruption, xeroderma

Kaposi-Irgang disease — a variation of discoid lupus erythematosus

Kapp's clamp

Kapp-Beck clamp

Kappeler's maneuver

Kapsinow's test

Kara's erysiphake

Karell's cure, diet, treatment

Karnovsky's stain

Karplus's sign

Karr's method

Karras's needle

Kartagener's disease — a mild form of pulmonary infiltration occurring in eosinophilia

Kartagener's syndrome — a hereditary disorder of dextrocardia, bronchiectasis and sinusitis

Kartagener's triad

Kasabach's method

Kasabach-Merritt syndrome — giant hemangiomas of the skin and spleen in infants

Kasai's operation — surgical anastomosis of the jejunum to a decapsulated area of liver and to the duodenum

Kashida's sign

Kashin-Beck disease — a slowly progressive, chronic, disabling, degenerative disease of the peripheral joints and spine, occurring chiefly in children

Kashiwado's test

Kaslow's tube

Kast's syndrome — enchondromatosis associated with multiple cutaneous or visceral hemangiomas. Usually called *Maffucci's syndrome*

Kastle's test

Kastle-Meyer test

Katayama's test

Kathrein's test

Kato's test

Katsch's chisel

Katz's formula

Katzin's scissors

Katzin-Barraquer forceps

Kaufman's forceps, pneumonia, prosthesis, syringe, vitrector

Kaup's index

Kawasaki disease — an erythematous febrile disease of unknown etiology accompanied by conjunctivitis, pharyngitis, cervical lymphadenopathy, vasculitis and other signs of toxic systemic involvement

Kay-Shiley valve prosthesis

Kay-Suzuki valve prosthesis

Kayser's disease — hepatolenticular degeneration

Kayser-Fleischer ring

Kazanjian's operation — surgical extension of the buccal vestibular sulcus of edentulous ridges

Kazanjian's forceps, scissors, splint, T bar

Kazanjian-Cottle forceps

Kearns's syndrome — pigmentary retinal dystrophy and cardiomyopathy

Kearns's dilator

Keating-Hart fulguration, method, treatment

Kedani disease — scrub typhus

Keegan's operation — a modification of the Indian rhinoplasty for reconstructing the nose

Keeler's cryophake

Keeley's cure, vein stripper

Keen's operation — omphalectomy

Keen's point, sign

Kehr's incision, sign, tube

Kehrer's reflex

Keidel's tube

Keith's bundle, drain, low ionic diet, needle, node, scissors

Keith-Flack node

Keith-Wagener retinopathy

Keith-Wagener-Barker classification

Keitzer's urethrotome

Kell blood group

Keller's bunionectomy, cresyl echt violet stain

Keller-Blake splint

Keller-Killian reaction

Kelley's gouge

Kelling's gastroscope, test

Kellock's sign

Kelly's operation(s) — for correction of urinary incontinence in women; surgical fixation of arytenoid cartilage or muscle

Kelly's adenotome, cystoscope, endoscope, forceps, hemostat, proctoscope, sigmoidoscope, sign, speculum, sphincteroscope, sutures

Kelly-Gray curet

Kelly-Murphy forceps

Kelly-Sims retractor

Kelman's cryostylet, cystotome, extractor, forceps

Kelsey's clamp

Kelvin's scale, thermometer

Kemerova virus

Kemp Harper method

Kempf's disease — acute homosexual panic

Kempner's diet

Ken's plate

Kendall's compound A., B., E. and F., culture medium, method

Kennedy's syndrome — same as *Foster Kennedy syndrome*

Kennedy's bar, classification, forceps

Kenny's syndrome — a familial syndrome marked by intrauterine dwarfism, late closure of the anterior fontanel, thickening of the tubular bones, myopia and transient hypocalcemia and hyperphosphatemia

Kenny's method, treatment

Kent's bundle, forceps

Kent-His bundle

Kentmann's test

Kerandel's sign, symptom

Kerckring's folds, nodules, ossicles, valves

Kergaradec's sign

Kerley's lines

Kern's forceps, plasma relation theory

Kernan-Jackson bronchoscope

Kernechtrot's method

Kerner's test

Kernig's sign

Kerr's cesarean section, rongeur, sign, splint

Kerrison's forceps, retractor, rongeur

Kershner-Adams syndrome — chronic, nonspecific, suppurative pneumonitis

Kessel's plate

Kessler's sutures

Kestenbach-Anderson procedure

Kestenbaum's sign

Kety-Schmidt method

Kevorkian's curet, forceps

Kevorkian-Young curet, forceps

Key's operation — the lateral operation of lithotomy done with a straight staff

Key's elevator

Key-Retzius connective tissue sheath, foramen

Keyes's chisel, lithotrite, punch

Kezerian's chisel, curet, gouge, osteotome

Kidd's blood group, cystoscope, tube

Kidde-Robbins tourniquet

Kiel's graft

Kielland's (Kjelland) forceps

Kielland-Luikart forceps

Kienböck's disease — slowly progressive osteochondrosis of the carpal lunate bone

Kienböck's atrophy, dislocation, luxation, phenomenon, syringomyelia, unit

Kienböck-Adamson points

Kiernan's spaces

Kiesselbach's area, space

Kilian's line, pelvis

Killgren's treatment

Killian's operation — excision of the anterior wall of the frontal sinus, with removal of diseased tissue and formation of a permanent communication with the nose

Killian's bronchoscope, forceps, incision, knife, speculum, test, tube

Killian-Eichen cannula

Killian-King retractor

Killian-Reinhard chisel

Kilner's hook, scissors

Kilner-Dott mouth gag

Kiloh-Nevin syndrome — ocular myopathy in persons with ptosis and paralysis of the external ocular muscles

Kimball's catheter, hook

Kimmelstiel-Wilson syndrome — glomerulosclerosis associated with diabetes, albuminuria, hypertension and nephrotic edema

Kimpton-Brown tube

Kimura's disease — angiolymphoid hyperplasia

Kinberg's test

King's operation — surgical fixation of arytenoid cartilage or muscle

King's brace, retractor, traction, unit

King-Armstrong unit

King-Hurd dissector, retractor

King-Prince forceps

King-Steelquist amputation

Kingsley's forceps, splint

Kinnier Wilson disease — hepatolenticular degeneration

Kinsbourne syndrome — myoclonic encephalopathy of childhood

Kinsella's elevator

Kinsella-Buie clamp

Kinyoun's staining method

Kirby's keratome, knife, scissors, sutures

Kirby-Bauer agar diffusion test

Kirchhoff's law

Kirchner's diverticulum

Kirk's amputation, mallet

Kirkland's disease — acute infection of the throat with regional lymphadenitis

Kirkland's knife, retractor

Kirkpatrick's forceps

Kirmisson's operation — transplantation of the Achilles tendon to the peroneus longus muscle in clubfoot

Kirmisson's elevator, raspatory

Kirschner's apparatus, wire, wire splint

Kirstein's method

Kisch's reflex

Kisselbach's area

Kistner's button, dissector, probe, tube

Kitasato's broth, filter, glucoseformate gelatin

Kite's method

Kitner's dissector, forceps

Kittel's treatment

Kitzmiller's test

Kiwisch's bandage

Kjeldahl's method, test
Klaff's speculum
Klapp's creeping treatment
Klatskin's needle
Klauder's syndrome — congenital maldevelopment of organs of ectodermal derivation—nervous system, retina, eyeball and skin
Klebs's disease — glomerulonephritis
Klebs's tuberculin
Klebs-Löffler bacillus
Kleihauer's technique
Klein's punch, reaction, test
Klein-Gumprecht nuclei
Klein-Waardenburg syndrome — embryonic fixation syndrome
Kleine-Levin syndrome — periodic somnolence, morbid hunger and motor unrest, often associated with psychosis
Kleinert's sutures
Kleinschmidt's syndrome — influenzal infection resulting in laryngeal stenosis, suppurative pericarditis, pleuropneumonia and, sometimes, suppurative meningitis
Kleinschmidt's technique
Kleist's apraxia, sign
Klemm's sign, tetanus
Klemme's hook, retractor
Klemperer's disease — disease of the spleen secondary to portal hypertension. Also called *Banti's disease*
Klemperer's tuberculin
Kliger's iron agar
Klimow's test
Kline's test
Kline-Young test

Klinefelter's syndrome — a chromosomal anomaly in which males are masculine in development but have seminiferous tubule dysgenesis, elevated urinary gonadotropins and eunuchoid characteristics
Klippel's disease — arthritic general pseudoparalysis
Klippel-Feil syndrome — a congenital defect marked by fusion of the cervical vertebrae and abnormalities of the brain stem and cerebellum
Klippel-Feil sign
Klippel-Feldstein syndrome — simple familial cranial hypertrophy
Klippel-Trenaunay syndrome — a rare condition affecting only one extremity, marked by hypertrophy of bone and soft tissues, large cutaneous hemangiomas and varices
Klippel-Trenaunay-Weber syndrome — same as *Klippel-Trenaunay syndrome*
Kloepfer's syndrome — complete blindness beginning at two months of age, with blistering after exposure to sunlight, cessation of growth at the age of five or six years and progressive mental retardation
Klondike bed
Klotz's syndrome — primary amenorrhea, genital infantilism, aplasia of the labia minora, small nonovulating ovaries and progressive sclerosis, male chromosomal sex, slight mongoloid facies and, sometimes, hypertrichosis

Klumpke's palsy, paralysis

Klumpke-Déjérine syndrome — atrophic paralysis of the muscles of the arm and hand from a lesion of the eighth cervical and first dorsal nerves. Called also *Klumpke's paralysis*

Klüver-Barrera method

Klüver-Bucy syndrome — bizarre behavioral disturbances following bilateral temporal lobectomy

Knapp's operation — the formation of a peripheral opening in the capsule behind the iris, without iridectomy

Knapp's cystotome, forceps, knife, law, retractor, scissors, speculum, streaks, striae, test

Kneist syndrome — a type of dwarfism marked by short limbs, round face, stiffness of joints, contracture of fingers and often cleft palate, scoliosis and deafness

Knie's sign

Knight's brace, forceps, scissors

Knight-Sluder forceps

Knoepfelmacher's butter meal

Knoop hardness number

Knott's test

Knowles's pin, scissors

Kobak's needle

Kobelt's tubes, tubules

Kober's test

Kobert's test

Köbner's response

Koby's cataract

Kobyashi's hook

Koch's bacillus, law, lymph, node, phenomenon, postulates, reaction, test, tuberculin

Koch-Mason dressing

Koch-McMeekin method

Koch-Weeks bacillus, hemophilus

Kocher's operation(s) — a method of excising the ankle joint; a method of reducing a subcoracoid dislocation of the humerus; excision of the tongue; a method of mobilizing the duodenum; a method of pylorectomy

Kocher's syndrome — leukopenia resulting from granulocytopenia, occasionally accompanying thyrotoxicosis

Kocher's clamp, dilatation ulcer, forceps, incision, maneuver, point, reflex, retractor, sign, spoon, symptom

Kocher-Crotti retractor

Kocher-Debré-Sémélaigne syndrome — same as *Debré-Sémélaigne syndrome*

Kocks's operation — shortening of the base of the broad ligament by the vaginal route for uterine retroversion or prolapse

Koeberlé's forceps

Koebner's phenomenon

Koenecke's reaction, test

Koenig's syndrome — alternating attacks of constipation and diarrhea, sometimes symptomatic of cecal tuberculosis

Koenig-Wichman disease — chronic pemphigus

Koeppe's disease(s) — epithelial punctate keratitis; corneal dystrophy with a clearly defined grayish-white band on the cornea, visible to the naked eye

Koeppe's lens, nodules

Koerber-Salus-Elschnig syndrome
— irregular oscillation of the
eyeballs, either horizontal,
lateral or rotatory, with retraction of the eye backward
into the orbit when the direction of sight changes

Kofferath's syndrome — obstetric
diaphragmatic paralysis

Koffler's forceps

Koffler-Lillie forceps

Koga's treatment

Kogan's endospeculum

Kogoj's pustule

Köhler's bone disease — either
osteochondrosis of the tarsal
navicular bone in children or
a disorder of the second metatarsal bone with thickening of
its shaft and changes about its
articular head, the latter often
called *Kohler's second bone
disease*

Köhler's illumination

Köhler-Pellegrini-Stieda disease —
semilunar bone formation in
the upper portion of the
medial lateral ligament of the
knee. Called also *Pellegrini's
disease*

Köhlmeier-Degos disease — a
cutaneovisceral syndrome
characterized by pathogno-
monic papules followed by
development of intestinal
ulcers that perforate, causing
peritonitis

Kohlrausch's folds, valves, veins

Kohn's needle, pores

Kohnstamm's phenomenon

Kokka disease — epidemic hemorrhagic fever

Kolb's forceps, trocar

Koler's reaction

Kölliker's column, interstitial
granules, membrane, nucleus

Kollmann's dilator

Kolmer's test

Kolodny's forceps, hemostat

Kolomnin's operation — cauterization of the diseased tissues in
hip joint disease by ignipunc-
ture

Kondo's test

Kondoleon's operation — treatment of elephantiasis by
removal of strips of subcutaneous tissue

Konew's test

König's disease — osteochondroly-
sis

König's operation — for congenital
dislocation of hip

König's syndrome — local infection of the cecum and terminal
ileum, associated with abdominal distention, hyper-
peristalsis, intermittent constipation and diarrhea, colic
simulating intestinal obstruction, and intestinal spasms

König's rods

Konjetzny's gastritis

Kono's procedure

Konsuloff's reaction, test

Kopetzky's bur

Koplik's sign, spots

Kopp's asthma

Korányi's auscultation, percussion,
sign, treatment

Korányi-Grocco triangle

Korff's fibers

Körner's septum

Korotkoff's method, sounds, test

Korovnikov's disease — splenomegaly with thrombocytosis and gastrointestinal hemorrhage, beginning between the ages of 20 and 37

Korsakoff's (Korsakov's) disease — a syndrome encountered in chronic alcoholics, characterized by confusion and severe impairment of memory. Delirium tremens may often precede onset of the syndrome

Korsakoff's (Korsakov's) psychosis

Körte-Ballance operation — anastomosis of the facial and hypoglossal nerves

Kortzeborn's operation — relief of ape hand caused by median nerve paralysis

Kos's cannula

Koser's citrate broth

Koshevnikoff's (Koschewnikow's, Kozhevnikov's disease/syndrome — continuous clonic movements of a part of the body

Koshevnikoff's (Koschewnikow's, Kozhevnikov's) epilepsy

Kossel's test

Köster's nodule

Kostmann's syndrome — infantile genetic agranulocytosis

Koszewski's syndrome — congenital osteosclerosis

Kottmann's reaction, test

Kovács's method

Kovalevsky's canal

Kowarsky's test

Koyter's muscle

Kozowski's degeneration

Krabbe's disease — infantile familial sclerosis—a metabolic

Krabbe's disease (*continued*) leukoencephalopathy with progressive cerebral degeneration

Krabbe's syndrome — a congenital form of generalized muscular hypoplasia beginning in infancy with irritability and rigidity

Krabbe's leukodystrophy

Kraepelin's classification

Kraft's point

Krämer's disease — suppurative scleritis

Kramer's speculum, telescope

Kramer-Gittleman method

Kramer-Pollnow disease — sudden onset of progressive hyperkinesia between the ages of one and four years, reaching a peak at age six years, followed by mental retardation, retrogression of speech ability and anxiety

Kramer-Tisdall method

Kraske's operation — removal of the coccyx and part of the sacrum for access to a carcinoma of the rectum

Kraske's approach, position, retractor

Krause's operation — extradural excision of the gasserian ganglion for trigeminal neuralgia

Krause's syndrome — a retinopathy associated with prematurity and combined with cerebral dysplasia

Krause's bulbs, cannula, corpuscles, forceps, glands, ligament, line, membrane, suture, valve

Krause-Wolfe graft

Krawitz's technique

Krebs's 2 carcinoma, cycle, leukocyte index, 2 tumor
Krebs-Henseleit cycle
Kreibig's opticomalacia
Kreischer's chisel
Kreiselman's incubator
Kreissl's knife
Kretschmann's space
Kretschmer's syndrome — semicoma following unconsciousness of several days or weeks in patients with acute brain injuries
Kretschmer's types
Kretz's granules, paradox
Kreuscher's scissors
Kreutzmann's cannula, trocar
Kreysig's sign
Krimer's operation — plastic reconstruction of the palate, in which mucoperiosteal flaps from each side of the palatal cleft are sutured together at the median line
Krishaber's disease — a neurosis characterized by tachycardia, insomnia, vertigo and hyperesthesia. Also called *cerebrocardiac syndrome*
Krisovski's (Krisowski's) sign
Kristeller's expression, method, retractor, speculum, technique
Kristiansen's screw
Kroener's fimbriectomy
Krogh's method
Krokiewicz's test
Kromayer's burn, lamp, treatment
Krompecher's carcinoma, tumor
Kron's dilator, probe
Kronecker's center, needle, puncture
Kroner's tubal ligation

Kronfeld's electrode, forceps, retractor
Krönig's area, cesarean section, field, isthmus, percussion
Krönlein's operation(s) — exposure of the third branch of the trigeminal nerve for facial neuralgia; resection of the outer wall of the orbit for removal of orbital tumor without excising the eye
Krönlein's hernia
Krönlein-Berke orbital decompression
Krueger-Schmidt method
Krukenberg's amputation, arm, hand, spindle, tumor, veins
Krull's knife
Krumwiede's triple sugar agar
Kruse's brush
Krwawicz's cryoextractor, extractor
Kuchendorf's method
Kufs's disease — a juvenile form of sphingolipidosis
Kugel-Stoloff syndrome — congenital idiopathic hypertrophy of the heart
Kugelberg-Welander disease — a hereditary, juvenile form of muscular atrophy affecting the proximal muscles of the lower extremities
Kuhlman's brace, traction
Kuhlmann's test
Kuhn's mask, tube
Kühne's methylene blue, muscular phenomenon, spindle, terminal plates
Kuhnt's forceps, gouge, illusion, intermediary tissue, meniscus, postcentral vein

Kuhnt-Junius disease — macular degeneration

Kulchitsky's cell carcinoma, cells

Kulenkampff's anesthesia

Kulenkampff-Tarnow syndrome — spasmodic tension of the muscles of the neck, tongue, floor of the mouth and pharynx, respiratory disorders, speech disorders, tachycardia and hypertension, following the first few days of chlorpromazine therapy

Kulp's culture medium

Kulvin-Kalt forceps

Külz's cast, cylinder, test

Kumba virus

Kümmell's disease — vertebral compression fracture, characterized by spinal pain, intercostal neuralgia and motor disturbances

Kümmell's kyphosis, spondylitis

Kümmell-Verneuil disease — same as *Kümmell's disease*

Kundrat's disease — lymphosarcoma

Kunkel's syndrome — lupoid hepatitis

Küntscher's nail, pin, rod

Kupffer's cells, cell sarcoma

Kupressoff's center

Kurloff's (Kurlov's) bodies

Kurnick's methyl green–pyronine Y method

Kurten's vein stripper

Kurz's syndrome — congenital blindness, with a high degree of axial hypermetropia, enoph-

Kurz's syndrome (*continued*) thalmos, pupillary areflexia and searching eye movements

Kurzbauer's method

Kurzrok-Miller test

Kushner-Tandatnick curet

Küss's disease — stenosis of the rectum and sigmoid from inflammatory processes

Küss's experiment

Kussmaul's disease — same as *Kussmaul-Maier disease*

Kussmaul's aphasia, breathing, coma, paralysis, pulse, respiration, sign, symptom

Kussmaul-Kien respiration

Kussmaul-Landry paralysis

Kussmaul-Maier disease — periarteritis nodosa

Küster's hernia

Küstner's operation — replacement of an inverted uterus through an incision made in the cervix and uterus

Küstner's incision, law, sign

Kutler's amputation

Kutlik's ferric iron method

Küttner's ganglion

Kveim antigen, test

Kwilecki's method

Kyasanur Forest disease virus

Kyle's applicator, knife, speculum

Kyoto-Barrett-Boyes technique

Kypher's sutures

Kyrle's disease — a rare follicular disease characterized by discrete, keratotic patches in the hair follicles and eccrine ducts

L

La Porte's treatment

La Roque's sign, sutures, technique

Laband's syndrome — gingival fibromatosis associated with lysis of the distal phalanges

Labarraque's solution

Labbé's syndrome — intermittent hypertension associated with adrenal tumors

Labbé's neurocirculatory syndrome — an anxiety neurosis associated with tachycardia

Labbé's triangle, vein

Laborde's forceps, method, sign, test

Ladd's syndrome — congenital obstruction of the duodenum caused by peritoneal bands

Ladd's caliper, knife, raspatory

Ladd-Franklin theory

Ladd-Gross syndrome — icterus neonatorum associated with atresia of the bile ducts

Ladendorff's test

Ladin's sign

Laennec's disease(s) — cirrhosis of the liver associated with chronic excessive intake of alcohol; dissecting aneurysm

Laennec's catarrh, cirrhosis, pearls, sign, thrombus

Lafora's disease — myoclonic epilepsy

Lafora's bodies, sign

Laforce's adenotome, tonsillectomy

Laforce-Grieshaber adenotome

Laforce-Stevenson adenotome

Lagrange's operation — sclerecto-iridectomy

Lahey's drain, forceps, osteotome, scissors, tube

Lahey-Babcock forceps

Lahey-Péan forceps

Lahore ulcer

Laidley's cystoscope

Laimer-Haeckerman area

Lake's pigment

Laki-Lorand factor

Lallemand's bodies

Làllemand-Trousseau bodies

Lalouette's pyramid

Lamarck's theory

Lamaze's method

Lambda's pacemaker

Lambert's cosine law, treatment

Lambert-Berry raspatory

Lambert-Eaton syndrome — same as *Eaton-Lambert syndrome*

Lambert-Lowman clamp

Lambl's excrescences

Lambling's syndrome — postgastrectomy malabsorption associated with extreme thinness, anemia, hypoproteinemia, edema and diarrhea

Lambotte's clamp, forceps, osteotome, treatment

Lambotte-Henderson osteotome

Lambrinudi's splint

Lamm's incision

Lamont's rasp, saw

Lancaster's keratome, magnet, sclerotome

Lancaster-O'Connor speculum

Lancefield's classification, precipitation test

Lancereaux's diabetes, nephritis

Lancereaux-Mathieu disease — leptospiral jaundice

Lancet coefficient

Lancisi's nerves, stria

Landau's color test, reaction, reflex

Landeker-Steinberg light

Landing-Oppenheimer syndrome — ceroid storage disease

Landolfi's caustic

Landolt's operation — formation of a lower eyelid with a bridge flap of eyelid skin taken from the upper lid

Landolt's bodies, keratome

Landouzy's disease — infectious jaundice

Landouzy's syndrome — muscular atrophy associated with sciatica

Landouzy's dystrophy, purpura, type

Landouzy-Déjérine atrophy, dystrophy, type

Landouzy-Grasset law

Landry's disease/syndrome — acute, febrile polyneuritis

Landry's palsy, paralysis

Landsteiner-Miller method

Landström's muscle

Landzert's fossa

Lane's disease — small bowel obstruction in chronic constipation

Lane's operation — dividing the ileum near the cecum, closing the distal portion and anastomosing the proximal end with the upper part of the rectum or lower part of the sigmoid

Lane's bands, dissector, kink,

Lane's (*continued*)
method, mouth gag, plates, raspatory

Lang's dissector, fluid, knife, solution, speculum, test

Langat virus

Langdon Down's disease — same as *Down's syndrome*

Lange's operation — artificial tendon transplantation with strands of silk

de Lange's syndrome — same as *Brachmann–de Lange syndrome*

Lange's position, reaction, solution, speculum, test

Langenbeck's amputation, incision, pedicle mucoperiosteal flap, triangle

Langenbeck-O'Brien raspatory

Langer's axillary arch, lines, muscle

Langerhans's cells, corpuscles, granules, islets, islands, layer

Langhans's cells, layer, stria

Langley's ganglion, granules, nerves

Langoria's sign

Lansing's virus

Lantermann's clefts, incisures

Lantermann-Schmidt incisures

Lanz's operation — for elephantiasis of the leg

Lanz's point, tube

Lapicque's constant, law

Lapides's catheter, needle, procedure

Laplace's forceps, law, retractor

Laquerriere-Pierquin method

Larat's treatment

Larcher's sign

Lardennois's button

LaRocca's tube

Larrey's operation — disarticulation of the humerus at the shoulder joint

Larrey's amputation, bandage, cleft, dressing, spaces

Larrey-Weil disease — infectious jaundice caused by a species of *Leptospira*

Larry's director, probe

Larsen's disease — same as *Larsen-Johansson disease*

Larsen's syndrome — cleft palate and flattened facies, with multiple congenital dislocations and foot deformities

Larsen-Johansson disease — presence of an accessory center of ossification in the lower pole of the patella

Larsen-Johansson syndrome — juvenile osteopathia patellae

Lasègue's disease — persecution mania

Lasègue's sign

Lash-Löffler implant

Lassa fever virus

Lassar's betanaphthol paste, plain zinc paste

Lassueur–Graham Little triad

Latham's circle

Lathbury's applicator

Latino virus

Latrobe's retractor

Latzko's operation(s) — cesarean section; a method of repairing a vesicovaginal fistula

Latzko's cesarean section, colpocleisis, radical hysterectomy

Lauber's disease — a disorder in which gray mottling of the fundus of the eyes is associated with night blindness

Laubry-Soulle syndrome — abnormal accumulations of gas in the colon and stomach following acute myocardial infarction

Lauenstein's method

Laufe-Barton-Kielland forceps

Laufe-Piper forceps

Laugier's hernia, sign

Laumonier's ganglion

Launois's syndrome — same as *Launois-Cléret syndrome*

Launois-Cléret syndrome — adiposogenital dystrophy caused by adenohypophyseal tumor. Also called *Fröhlich's syndrome*

Lauren's operation — a plastic operation for closure of a cicatricial opening following mastoid operation

Laurence-Biedl syndrome — same as *Biedl's disease*

Laurence-Moon syndrome — same as *Biedl's disease*

Laurence-Moon-Bardet-Biedl syndrome — same as *Biedl's disease*

Laurence-Moon-Biedl syndrome — same as *Biedl's disease*

Laurer's canal

Lauth's canal, ligament, sinus, violet

Lautier's test

Lavdovski's nucleoid

Laveran's bodies, corpuscles

Law's method, position

Läwen-Roth syndrome — dwarfism with thyroid deficiency and usually cretinism

Lawford's syndrome — a form of *Dimitri's disease,* consisting of angiomas of face and

Lawford's syndrome (*continued*)
choroid only, with late glaucoma

Lawrence's syndrome — lipoatrophic diabetes

Lawrence's forceps, method

Lawrence-Seip syndrome — loss of subcutaneous fat, associated with hepatomegaly, excessive bone growth and insulin-resistant diabetes

Lawson-Thornton plate

Lawton's forceps, scissors

Le Dentu's suture

Le Dran's sutures

Le Fort's operation — same as *Le Fort-Neugebauer operation*

Le Fort's amputation, bougie, fracture, osteotomy, sound, suture

Le Fort-Neugebauer operation — repair of prolapse of the uterus

Le Grand–Geblewics phenomenon

Le Nobel's test

Leach's test

Leadbetter-Politano ureteroneocystotomy

Leader's forceps, hook

Leader-Kollmann dilator

Lear complex

Lebbin's test

Leber's disease(s) — a hereditary disorder of males, characterized by bilateral progressive optic atrophy; congenital amaurosis

Leber's congenital amaurosis, corpuscles, optic atrophy, plexus

Leboyer's method, technique

Lebsche's forceps, knife, raspatory, shears

Lecat's gulf

Lechini's test

Leclanché's cell

Ledbetter's maneuver

Ledderhose's syndrome — plantar aponeurositis and fibrous nodules of the flexor tendons, resulting in clawfoot

Lederberg's replica plating technique

Lederer's anemia

Leduc's current

Lee's polyp

Lee-Cohen elevator, knife

Lee-White whole blood clotting time method

Leede-Rumpel phenomenon

Lees's clamp, ganglion, test

Leff's stethoscope

Leffmann-Beam test

Legal's disease — a disease affecting the pharyngotympanic region, marked by headache and localized inflammation

Legal's test

Legg's disease — same as *Legg-Calvé-Perthes disease*

Legg's osteotome

Legg-Calvé-Perthes disease — osteochondritis of the capitular epiphysis of the femur

Legg-Calvé-Waldenström disease — same as *Legg-Calvé-Perthes disease*

Legueu's retractor

Lehman's catheter, syringe

Leichtenstern's encephalitis, phenomenon, sign, type

Leifson's staining method

Leigh's disease — necrotizing encephalomyelopathy

Leighton's tube technique

Leinbach's osteotome, prosthesis

Leiner's disease — a condition affecting chiefly newborn breast-fed infants, characterized by generalized exfoliative dermatitis and marked erythroderma

Leiner's dermatitis, test

Leipert's method

Leishman's anemia, cells, nodules, stain

Leishman-Donovan bodies

Leiter's cystoscope, tube

Leitner's syndrome — pulmonary tuberculous eosinophilic syndrome

Lejeune's syndrome — cri du chat (crying cat syndrome)

Lejeune's forceps, scissors

Leksell's forceps, rongeur

Leland-Jones forceps

Lell's esophagoscope, tube

Leloir's disease — discoid lupus erythematosus

Lem-Blay clamp

Lembert's suture

Lemmon's retractor, spreader

Lempert's fenestration operation — for otosclerosis

Lempert's excavator, incision, perforator, retractor, rongeur

Lempert-Colver retractor, speculum

Lempka's vein stripper

Lenard's rays

Lendrum-McFarlane-Mayer hemalum

Lenegre's disease — acquired complete heart block due to primary degeneration of the conduction system

Lennarson's tube

Lennhoff's index, sign

Lennox syndrome — a childhood epileptic encephalopathy

Lenoble-Aubineau syndrome — hereditary congenital nystagmus associated with tremor of the head and arms, fasciculation of the muscles, vasomotor disorders, and overactive reflexes

Lente's probe

Lentulo's drill

Lenz's syndrome — a hereditary syndrome marked by abnormal smallness of the eyes, digital and skeletal anomalies and sometimes urogenital and cardiovascular defects

Leo's sugar, test

Leonard's forceps, tube

Leonard-George method

Leonardo's band

Leopold's law, maneuvers

Léopold-Lévi's syndrome — paroxysmal thyroid instability

Leotta's syndrome — perivisceritis on the right side in the subhepatic area

Lepehne-Pickworth benzidine technique

Lepley-Ernst tube

Lerch's percussion

Leredde's syndrome — severe dyspnea on exertion, combined with emphysema and bronchiectasis

Leri's disease — thickening of the shafts of the long bones, with hyperostoses protruding into the medullary canal and from the external surface of the bone

Léri's pleonosteosis, sign
Léri-Weill syndrome − a form of dyschondroplasia
Lerich's treatment
Leriche's disease − post-traumatic osteoporosis
Leriche's syndrome − obstruction of the terminal aorta causing fatigue, absence of pulse in the femoral artery and impotence
Leriche's forceps
Lermoyez's syndrome − labyrinthine angiospasm
Lermoyez's punch
Leroy's disease − mucolipidosis
Les's culture medium
Lesch-Nyhan syndrome − a rare hereditary disorder of purine metabolism, marked by self-mutilation, spastic cerebral palsy and excessive urinary secretion of uric acid
Leschke's syndrome − congenital pigmentary dystrophy
Leser-Trélat sign
Lesgaft's space, triangle
L'Esperance's erysiphake
Lespinasse's sutures
Lesser's test, triangle
Letterer-Siwe disease − heritable reticuloendotheliosis of early childhood, marked by hemorrhagic tendency, hepatosplenomegaly and progressive anemia
Leuckhart's embedding irons
Leudet's bruit, sign, tinnitus
Leunbach's paste
Lev's disease − acquired complete heart block caused by sclerosis of the cardiac skeleton

Levaditi's stain
Levant's stone dislodger
Levasseur's sign
LeVeen's shunt
Lever's adenoacanthoma
Lévi's syndrome − paroxysmal hyperthyroidism
Levi-Lorain dwarf, infantilism, type
Levin tube
Levine's eosin-methylene blue (EMB) agar
Levinson's test
Levinthal-Coles-Lillie bodies
Levis's splint
Levitt's eye implant
Levret's forceps, law
Lévy-Roussy syndrome − progressive neuropathic muscular atrophy, with scoliosis and cerebral ataxia
Levy-Rowntree-Marriott method
Lewandowsky's nevus, periporitis, tuberculid
Lewandowsky-Lutz disease − a viral disease marked by numerous warts that have a tendency to become malignant
Lewin's dissector, forceps
Lewin-Stern splint
Lewis's disease − familial congenital hepatic glycogenosis caused by a deficiency in hepatic glycogen synthetase, associated with convulsions and hypoglycemia following overnight fasting
Lewis's blood group, carcinoma, cystometer, hemostat, leukotome, loupe, method, mouth gag, phenomenon, reaction, secretor status, tube

Lewis-Benedict method
Lewis-Lobban modified Schultz reaction
Lewis-Pickering test
Lewisohn's method
Lewkowitz's forceps
Lewy's bodies, laryngoscope
Lewy-Rubin needle
Lexer's chisel, scissors
Leyden's disease — periodic vomiting of uncertain cause
Leyden jar
Leyden's ataxia, crystals, neuritis, paralysis
Leyden-Möbius syndrome — a slowly progressive form of muscular dystrophy in the shoulder or pelvic girdle, marked by wasting
Leydig's cell tumor, cells, cylinders, duct
Leyro-Diaz forceps
Lhermitte's syndrome — oculomotor paralysis, with nystagmus and paralysis of abduction during attempted lateral deviation of the eye
Lhermitte's sign
Lhermitte-Cornil-Quesnel syndrome — progressive pyramidopallidal degeneration
Lhermitte-McAlpine syndrome — disease of combined pyramidal and extrapyramidal systems
Lhermitte-Trelles syndrome — lymphoblastic infiltrations of the peripheral nervous system, with paresis and amyotrophia
Lian-Siguier-Welti syndrome — diaphragmatic hernia or eventration with venous thrombosis
Libman's sign

Libman-Sacks disease/syndrome — atypical vegetative endocarditis
Lichtenberg's keratome, trephine
Lichtenstern's syndrome — pernicious anemia in tabes dorsalis
Lichtheim's disease/syndrome — subacute degeneration of the spinal cord
Lichtheim's aphasia, plaques, sign, test
Lichtwicz's needle, trocar
Liddel-Sherrington reflex
Lieben's reaction, test
Lieben-Ralfe test
Lieberkühn's ampulla, crypts, follicles, glands
Lieberman's proctoscope, sigmoidoscope
Liebermann's test
Liebermann-Burchardt reaction, reagent, test
Liebermeister's furrows, grooves, rule
Liebig's test, theory
Liebreich's symptom
Liepmann's disease — apraxia
Liesegang's phenomenon, rings, striae, waves
Lieutaud's body, luette, triangle, uvula
Liga's clip
Ligat's test
Light-Veley apparatus, drill, headrest
Lightwood's syndrome — renal tubular acidosis
Lightwood-Albright syndrome — rickets with renal tubular acidosis
Lignac's syndrome — cystinosis
Lignac-Fanconi disease — same as *Lignac's syndrome*

Lignières's reation, test
Liley's three-zone chart
Lilienfeld's method
Lilienthal's guillotine, incision, probe
Lilienthal-Sauerbruch retractor
Lillie's alcoholic lead nitrate formalin, Biebrich scarlet picro-aniline blue, method, procedure, retractor, scissors, speculum
Lillie-Killian forceps
Lillie Mayer hemalum
Lincoff's eye implant
Lincoln's scissors
Lindau's disease — same as *von Hippel–Lindau disease*
Lindau's tumor
Lindau–von Hippel disease — same as *von Hippel–Lindau disease*
Lindbergh's pump
Lindblom's method
Linde's walker
Lindeman's hysteroflator
Lindeman-Silverstein tube
Lindemann's cannula, method, test
Linder's sign
Lindner's initial bodies, sign, spatula, test
Lineweaver-Burk plot for enzyme reaction
Links's test
Linnartz's clamp, forceps
Linser's method
Linton's incision, retractor, tourniquet, tube
Linton-Blakemore needle
Lippes's loop
Lippman's hip prosthesis
Lipps's test

Lipschütz's disease — a nonvenereal, rapidly progressing lesion of the vulva, possibly due to *Bacillus crassus,* a normally nonpathogenic organism
Lipschütz's bodies, cell, erythema, ulcer
Li-Rivers's culture medium
Lisfranc's amputation, dislocation, joint, ligament, tubercle
Lissauer's atrophy, column, dementia, marginal zone, paralysis, tract
Lister's antiseptic, dressing, forceps, scissors, tubercle
Lister-Burch speculum
Listing's law, plane
Liston's operation — for excision of the upper jaw
Liston's forceps, knives, scissors, splint
Liston-Stille forceps
Littauer's forceps, scissors
Littauer-Liston forceps
Litten's diaphragm phenomenon, sign
Little's disease — spastic paralysis of corresponding parts on both sides of the body
Little's syndrome — a skin disorder marked by a follicular, spinous eruption involving the scalp, trunk and extremities
Little's area, retractor, scissors
Littlewood's amputation
Littman's agar
Littre's operation — inguinal colostomy
Littre's crypts, foramina, glands, hernia, sutures
Littre-Richter hernia
Litwak's scissors
Litwin's scissors

Litzmann's obliquity
Livermore's trocar
Livi's index
Livierato's reflex, sign
Livingston's bar, forceps, triangle
Lizars's operation — excision of
the upper jaw
Lloyd's syndrome — adenoma of
the pituitary, with adenoma-
toid enlargements of the para-
thyroid glands and islands of
Langerhans
Lloyd's catheter, reagent, sign,
tube
Lobo's disease — a chronic, local-
ized mycosis of the skin, re-
sulting in fibrous nodules or
keloids
Lobstein's disease — an inherited
condition in which bones are
abnormally brittle and subject
to fracture
Lobstein's ganglion
Locke's fluid, solution
Locke-Ringer's solution
Lockwood's clamp, forceps, ligament
Lockwood-Allis forceps
Loeb's decidual reaction, decidu-
oma
Loebisch's coefficient, formula
Loevit's cell
Loewe's test
Loewenthal's purpura
Loewi's reaction, symptom, test
Löffler's disease — transient infiltrations of the lungs associated
with increased eosinophilic
leukocytes in the blood
Löffler's agar, blood serum, endo-
carditis, eosinophilia, medium,
method, methylene blue,
pneumonia, stains, sutures

Löfgren's syndrome — bilateral
hilar lymphoma syndrome
Logan's bow
Löhlein's diameter, nephritis
Löhlein-Baehr lesion
Lohmann's reaction
Lohnstein's saccharimeter
Löhr-Kindberg syndrome — eo-
sinophilic pneumopathy
Lombard's test
Lombard-Beyer forceps, rongeur
Lombard-Boies rongeur
Lombardi's sign
Long's coefficient, formula
Long-Lukens animal
Longdwel's catheter, needle
Longmire's valvulotome
Longuet's operation — extraserous
transplantation of the testicle
for varicocele and hydrocele
Longuet's incision
Looser's transformation zones
Looser-Milkman syndrome — a
generalized bone disease
marked by multiple stripes of
absorption in the long and flat
bones
Lorain's disease — idiopathic in-
fantilism
Lorain's infantilism, type
Lorain-Lévi syndrome — pituitary
dwarfism
Lord-Blakemore tube
Lordan's forceps, hook
Lore's forceps, tube
Lore-Lawrence tube
Lorenz's operation — for con-
genital dislocation of the
hip, with reduction of dis-
location
Lorenz's method, osteotomy, sign,
tube
Lorenzo's prosthesis

Loreta's operation — gastrotomy, with distal dilatation of the pylorus

Loreta's method

Lorfan's anesthesia

Lorie's retractor, trephine

Loring's ophthalmoscope

Lorrain Smith blood serum, stain

Lortat-Jacob disease — benign mucosal pemphigoid

Lortet's lamp

Lorthiore's method

Loschmidt's number

Lossen's law, rule

Lostorfer's bodies, corpuscles

Lotheissen's herniorrhaphy

Lothrop's dissector, forceps, retractor

Lottes's nail, pin, reamer

Loughnane's hook

Louis's angle, law

Louis-Bar syndrome — familial progressive cerebellar ataxia with oculocutaneous telangiectases

Lounsbury's curet

Loutit's anemia

Love's leukotome, retractor, splint

Love-Adson elevator

Love-Gruenwald forceps, rongeur

Love-Kerrison forceps, rongeur

Lovelace's forceps

Lovén's reflex

Lovset's maneuver, method

Low's preactivated papain technique

Löw-Beer method, projection

Lowe's disease — a hereditary disorder occurring only in males, characterized by vitamin D-resistant rickets, congenital

Lowe's disease (*continued*) glaucoma and cataracts, mental retardation and tubule reabsorption dysfunction

Lowe's syndrome — oculocerebrorenal syndrome

Löwe's ring

Lowe-Breck knife

Lowe-Terrey-MacLachlan syndrome — same as *Lowe's disease*

Lowell's knife

Löwenberg's canal, forceps, scala

Löwenstein's culture medium, lithotrite, ointment

Löwenstein-Jensen culture medium

Löwenthal's sclerosis, test, tract

Lower's forceps, rings, sacs, tubercle

Löwitt's bodies, lymphocytes

Lowman's balance board, clamp

Lown-Ganong-Levine syndrome — a short P-R interval (atrial activity) and normal duration of the QRS complex (ventricular activity), often associated with paroxysmal tachycardia

Lowsley's operation — repair of epispadias

Lowsley's forceps, nephropexy, tractor, urethroscope

Lowsley-Peterson cystoscope

Lowy's test

Loyez's myelin stain

Lubarsch's syndrome — primary systematized amyloidosis, marked by macroglossia and large deposits of amyloid in the skin, tongue, heart, stomach, intestine and skeletal muscle

Lubarsch's crystals

Lubs's syndrome — a familial form of male pseudohermaphroditism

Luc's operation — same as *Caldwell-Luc operation*

Lucae's forceps, probe

Lucas's sign

Lucas-Championnière disease — fibrinous bronchitis

Lucatello's sign

Lucey-Driscoll syndrome — retention jaundice occurring in infants as a result of bilirubin dysfunction

Lucherini's syndrome — juvenile rheumatoid arthritis associated with iridocyclitis

Lucherini-Giacobini syndrome — familial endocrine osteochondropathy

Luciani's triad

Lucio's phenomenon

Luck's fasciotome, saw

Lucké's renal adenocarcinoma, test, tumor

Luder-Sheldon syndrome — a familial, congenital disorder of renal tubular reabsorption of glucose and amino acids associated with dwarfism

Ludloff's operation — osteotomy of the first metatarsal bone for correction of hallux valgus

Ludloff's incision, osteotomy, sign

Ludovici's angulus

Ludwig's angina, angle, ganglion, labyrinths, plane, theory

Luebert's test

Luedde's exophthalmometer

Luer's syringe

Luer-Hartman rongeur

Luer-Korte scoop

Luer-Lok syringe

Luer-Whiting forceps

Luetscher's syndrome — secondary hyperaldosteronism associated with heart, kidney and liver diseases

Luft's disease — a disorder of striated muscle characterized by excessive mitochondria, abnormally increased basal metabolic rate and debility

Lugol's caustic, solution

Luikart's forceps

Luikart-Bill traction handle

Luikart-Kielland forceps

Luikart-McLane forceps

Luikart-Simpson forceps

Lukens's aspirator, enterotome, retractor, tube

Lumsden's center

Lund's operation — removal of the astragalus for correction of talipes

Lundsgaard's blade, knife, sclerotome

Lundsgaard-Burch knife, rasp, sclerotome

Lundvall's blood crisis

Lundy's laryngoscope, needle

Lundy-Irving needle

Lunyo virus

Luongo's cannula, elevator, needle, retractor

Luschka's body, bursa, cartilage, crypts, ducts, fibers, foramen, fossa, ganglion, gland, joints, ligaments, muscles, nerve, tonsil, tubercle

Lusskin's drill

Lust's phenomenon, reflex, sign

Lutembacher's syndrome — a congenital abnormality of the heart, consisting of interatrial septal defect, mitral stenosis and right atrial hypertrophy

Lutembacher's complex

Lütkens's sphincter

Lüttke's test

Lutz's forceps

Lutz-Jeanselme nodules

Lutz-Miescher disease — a skin disease usually affecting males in their twenties, marked by keratotic papules forming an eruption on the neck near the hairline

Lutz-Splendore-Almeida disease — South American blastomycosis

Luys's body syndrome — a violent form of motor restlessness, involving only one side of the body, caused by a lesion of the hypothalamic nucleus

Luys's body, nucleus, segregator, separator

Lyell's disease/syndrome — an exfoliative skin disease in infants and children that rapidly spreads over the entire body and is followed by skin scaling and separation

Lyle's syndrome — blindness with normal fundus oculi, often resulting from hysteria and neurasthenia

Lyle-Curtman test

Lyman's method, rays

Lyman-Smith brace

Lyme arthritis

Lynch's dissector, incision, laryngoscope, scissors

Lyon's forceps, hypothesis, method, test, tube

Lyser's trapezoid bone

Lysholm's method

Lyster's bag, tube

Lytle's splint

Macalister's ethmoidal spine, ligament, process, triangular fascia, valve

MacAusland chisel, retractor

MacAusland-Kelly retractor

MacCallum's patch

Macchiavello's stain

MacConkey's agar, broth, medium

MacDonagh's test

Macdonald's index, test

MacDougal's theory

Macdowel's frenum

Macewen's operation(s) — supracondylar division of the femur for genu valgum; for the radical cure of hernia

Macewen's osteotomy, sign, triangle

MacFee's incision

Mach's syndrome — hyperaldosteronism with adrenal hyperplasia, retention of sodium chloride and edema affecting the extremities and sometimes the brain, larynx and eyes

Machado's reaction, test

Machado-Guerreiro reaction, test

Mache's unit

Macht's test

Machupo virus

MacIntosh's laryngoscope, prosthesis

Mack's tonsillectome

Mackay's retractor

MacKay-Marg electronic tonometer

Mackenrodt's operation — vaginal fixation of the round ligaments for retrodisplacement of the uterus

Mackenrodt's incision, ligament

MacKenty's forceps, scissors, tube

Mackenzie's disease — a complex of symptoms of unknown cause, consisting of malaise with sensitivity to cold, dyspepsia, intestinal disorder and disturbances of respiration and heart action

MacKenzie's syndrome — associated paralysis of the tongue, soft palate and vocal cord on the same side

MacKenzie's amputation

Mackenzie's point

Mackler's prosthesis

MacLachlan's method, process

Maclagan's thymol turbidity test

Maclay's scissors

MacLean's test

MacLean-de Wesselow test

MacLean-Maxwell disease — a chronic condition of the heel bone marked by enlargement and pain on pressure

Macleod's syndrome — a syndrome of unknown cause in which an affected lung is underventil-

Macleod's syndrome (*continued*) ated and underperfused with blood and in which associated obstruction of the bronchioles occurs

MacLeod's capsular rheumatism

MacMunn's test

MacQuarrie's test

MacWilliam's test

Madden's clamp, hook

Maddox's prism, rods

Madelung's disease — abnormal deposits of fatty tissue on the upper back, shoulder and neck

Madelung's deformity, neck, subluxation

Madlener's operation — female sterilization

Maeder-Danis dystrophy

Maffucci's syndrome — same as *Kast's syndrome*

Magendie's foramen, law, phenomenon, sign, solution, space, symptom

Magendie-Hertwig sign

Magielski's curet, forceps, needle

Magill's forceps, laryngoscope, tube

Magitot's disease — osteoperiostitis of the dental alveoli

Magnan's movement, sign, symptom

Magnus-de Kleijn neck reflexes

Magnuson's saw, splint, valve

Magovern's prosthesis

Magovern-Cromie prosthesis

Magpie's test

Magrassi-Leonardi syndrome — eosinophilic pneumopathy marked by monocytic-histiocytic cells in the blood, followed by eosinophilia

Mahaim's fibers

Maher's disease — inflammation of the vaginal tissues

Mahler's sign

Mahoney's dilator, speculum

Maier's forceps, sinus

Maillard's coefficient

Maingot's hemostat

Maisler's treatment

Maisonneuve's amputation, bandage, sign, urethrotome

Maissiat's band, ligament, tract

Maixner's cirrhosis

Majocchi's disease — a rare, purpuric eruption beginning on the lower extremities and becoming generalized, often followed by atrophy of the affected skin and loss of hair

Majocchi's granuloma, purpura

Makeham's hypothesis

Makka's operation — for ectopia of the bladder, using the cecum as a bladder and the appendix as a ureter

Makonde virus

Malabar ulcer

Malacarne's antrum, pyramid, space

Malassez's disease — testicular cyst

Malassez's rest

Malecot's catheter

Malerba's test

Malfatti's method

Malgaigne's amputation, apparatus, fossa, fracture, hook, luxation, pad, triangle

Malherbe's disease — a benign tumor of the skin and subcutis resembling basal cell carcinoma

Malherbe's calcifying epithelioma, tumor

Malherbe-Chenantais epithelioma

Malibu disease — surfers' nodules

Malin's syndrome — anemia in which red blood cells are ingested by leukocytes. Also called *autoerythrophagocytosis*

Malis's forceps, scissors

Mall's formula, ridge

Mallory's acid fuchsin, bodies, orange G and aniline blue stain, phosphotungstic acid–hematoxylin stain, triple stain

Mallory-Weiss syndrome — laceration of the lower end of the esophagus, usually caused by severe retching or vomiting

Malm-Himmelstein valvulotome

Maloney's bougies

Malot's test

Malpighi's pyramids, vesicles

Maltz's knife, retractor, saw

Maltz-Lipsett rasp

Maly's test

Manchester brown

Manchester's operation — same as *Fothergill's operation*

Manchester's colporrhaphy, uterine suspension

Mandelin's reagent

Mangoldt's epithelial grafting

Mangus's sign

Mankowsky's syndrome — familial dysplastic osteopathy, marked by clubbing of the fingers and toes secondary to various chronic diseases

Mann's syndrome — contusion of the brain accompanied by generalized disorders of coordination

Mann's forceps, sign

Mann-Bollman fistula

Mann-Williamson ulcer

Mannkopf's sign, symptom

Mannkopf-Rumpf sign

Manoiloff's (Manoilov's) reaction

Manson's disease — infection with flukes of *Schistosoma mansoni* living in the mesenteric veins but depositing their eggs in venules of the large intestine

Manson's hemoptysis, schistosomiasis, test

Mantoux's conversion, reaction, reversion, test

Mantz's dilator

Manz's glands

Manzullo's test

Maragliano's tuberculin

Marañon's syndrome — scoliosis with ovarian insufficiency

Marañon's lipomatosis, reaction, sign

Marburg disease — a severe, often fatal, virus disease characterized by skin lesions, conjunctivitis, enteritis, hepatitis, encephalitis and renal failure

Marburg's virus

March's disease — same as *Graves's disease*

Marchal's bodies

Marchand's adrenals, adventitial cell, organ

Marchesani's syndrome — a hereditary syndrome of abnormally small lens, short stature and brachydactyly

Marchi's balls, globules, reaction, stain, tract

Marchiafava's hemolytic anemia

Marchiafava-Bignami disease — progressive degeneration of

Marchiafava-Bignami disease (*continued*) the corpus callosum, marked by intellectual deterioration, emotional disturbances, hallucinations, tremor, rigidity and convulsions

Marchiafava-Micheli disease — an uncommon form of hemolysis of unknown cause, marked by episodic hemoglobinuria and often associated with leukopenia or thrombocytopenia

Marchiafava-Micheli anemia

Marcks's knife

Marcus Gunn's syndrome — same as *Gunn's syndrome*

Marcus Gunn's pupillary phenomenon, sign

Marcy agent

Maréchal's test, tuberculin

Maréchal-Rosin test

Marey's law

Marfan's syndrome — a congenital disorder of connective tissue, marked by abnormal length of extremities, cardiovascular abnormalities and other deformities

Marfan's abiotrophy, epigastric puncture, method, sign

Marfan-Madelung syndrome — a combination of *Marfan's syndrome* and *Madelung's deformity*

Margolis's syndrome — sex-linked deaf-mutism with albinism

Margulles's coil

Marian's operation — for stone in the bladder

Marie's disease(s) — acromegaly; hypertrophic pulmonary osteoarthropathy

Marie's syndrome — a hereditary
disease of the nervous system
beginning in young adulthood
or middle age with spastic-
ataxic gait, poor coordination,
tremor, impaired deep sensi-
bility, pain, cramps, paresthesia
and dysarthric speech

Marie's anarthria, ataxia, hypertrophy, quadrilateral space,
sclerosis, sign, three-paper test

Marie-Bamberger disease/syn-
drome — hypertrophic pul-
monary osteoarthropathy

Marié-Davy cell

Marie-Foix sign

Marie-Léri syndrome — osteolysis
of the articular surfaces of the
fingers, resulting in mobility
of the joints so that the fingers
can be elongated or shortened

Marie-Robinson syndrome — mel-
ancholia, insomnia and impotence associated with the
presence of fructose in the
urine

Marie-Sée syndrome — a benign
type of hydrocephalus in infants, caused by large doses of
vitamin A

Marie-Strümpell disease — rheumatoid spondylitis

Marie-Tooth disease — progressive
neuropathic muscular atrophy

Marín Amat's syndrome — closure
of the eye when the mouth is
widely or forcibly opened

Marinesco's sign, succulent hand

Marinesco-Garland syndrome — a
rare, hereditary disorder
marked by degeneration of
tissues of the brain and lens
with mental retardation

Marinesco-Radovici reflex

Marinesco-Sjögren's syndrome —
same as *Marinesco-Garland
syndrome*

Marion's disease — congenital obstruction of the posterior
urethra due to muscular
hypertrophy of the bladder
neck or absence of the dilator
fibers in the urinary tract

Mariotte's blind spot, experiment,
law

Marjolin's ulcer

Markham-Meyerding retractor

Markoe's abscess

Marlow's test

Marme's reagent

Marochetti's blisters

Maroteaux-Lamy syndrome — an
error of mucopolysaccharide
metabolism, marked by growth
retardation and hepatosplenomegaly but without mental
retardation

Marquardt's test

Marquis's reagent, test

Marriott's method

Marsden's paste

Marsh's disease — same as *Graves's
disease*

Marsh's factor, test

Marsh-Bendall factor

Marshall's syndrome — a rare syndrome of hypoplasia, cataract
and sensorineural hearing loss

Marshall's fold, method, oblique
vein, test

Marshall Hall's facies

Marshall-Marchetti operation —
for the correction of stress
incontinence

Marshall-White syndrome —
chronic vasoconstrictor spots

Marshall-White syndrome (*continued*)
   associated with insomnia and tachycardia
Marshik's forceps
Martel's clamp
Martin's disease — periosteoarthritis of the foot, usually due to prolonged walking
Martin's operation — for cure of hydrocele
Martin's bandage, broth, depilatory, speculum
Martin-Albright syndrome — familial pseudohypoparathyroidism
Martin-Davy speculum
Martin du Pan–Rutishauser disease — laminar osteochondritis that occurs during adolescence, marked by pain, ankylosis and destruction of cartilage
Martinotti's cells
Martius-scarlet-blue stain
Martorell's syndrome — progressive obliteration of the brachiocephalic trunk and left carotid arteries, leading to loss of pulse in both arms and carotids and to transient hemiplegia, transient blindness, retinal atrophy and muscular atrophy of the arms
Marwedel's gastrostomy
Maryan's forceps
Maschke's test
Masini's sign
Mason's incision, splint
Mason-Allen splint
Mason-Auvard speculum
Masselon's spectacles
Masset's test

Masshoff's syndrome — abscess-forming reticulocytic lymphadenitis of the mesentery, thought to be caused by *Pasteurella pseudotuberculosis*
Massie's nail
Massier's solution
Masson's bodies, stain
Masson-Fontana stain
Masson-Judd retractor
Master's "2-step" exercise test
Masterson's clamp
Mastin's clamp
Masuda-Kitahara disease — an exudative disorder of the macula lutea seen in Japan and Indonesia, probably caused by a virus
Masugi's nephritis
Matas's operation — for aneurysm by opening the aneurysmal sac and closing the internal orifices
Matas's band, test, treatment
Matchett-Brown prosthesis
Mateer-Streeter ovum
Mátéfy's reaction, test
Mathes's mastitis
Mathews's speculum, test
Mathieu's disease — leptospiral jaundice
Mathieu's forceps, retractor
Matson's elevator, raspatory
Mattioli-Foggia and Raso syndrome — a progressive, recurrent, muscular disorder marked by the presence of hard, painless tumors
Mattis's scissors
Matuhasi-Ogata phenomenon
Matzenauer's speculum
Matzenauer-Polland syndrome — a skin disease marked by in-

Matzenauer-Polland syndrome
(*continued*)
flammatory lesions and followed by attacks of erythema
and urticarial edema
Mauchart's ligaments
Maugeri's syndrome — mediastinal
silicotic lesions causing laryngeal and respiratory disturbances
Maumené's test
Maumenee's erysiphake, forceps
Maumenee-Park speculum
Maunier-Kuhn disease — slackness
of the eyelids and ears in
childhood, followed by trach-
eomegaly and bronchomegaly
Maunoir's hydrocele, scissors
Maunsell's sutures
Maurer's clefts, dots, spots, stippling
Mauriac's syndrome(s) — an erythematous, nodular eruption on
the legs, and sometimes on
other parts of the body, seen
in syphilis; hepatomegaly,
dwarfism and obesity with
juvenile diabetes mellitus
Mauriceau's lance, maneuver
Mauriceau-Levret maneuver
Mauriceau-Smellie-Veit maneuver
Mauthner's cell, fiber, membrane,
sheath, test
Maxcy's disease — a rickettsial
infection endemic in south-
eastern United States
Maximow's fixative, staining
method
Maxwell's ring, spot
Maxwell-Boltzmann distribution
law
May's method, spore stain

May-Grünwald stain
May-Grünwald-Giemsa stain
May-Hegglin anomaly
Mayaro virus
Maydl's operation(s) — colostomy;
insertion of the ureters into
the rectum for exstrophy of
the bladder
Maydl's hernia
Mayer's albumin, glycerin-albumin
mixture, hemalum, ligament,
method, muchematein, pes-
sary, position, reagent, reflex,
stain, test
Mayer-Gross apraxia
Mayer-Rokitansky-Küster syn-
drome — lack of development
of the embryonic tubes from
which the vagina and uterus
are derived, with consequent
lack of vagina and rudimentary
development of the uterus
Mayerhofer's test
Mayfield's forceps, osteotome,
spatula
Maylard's incision
Mayo's operation(s) — excision of
the pyloric end of the stom-
ach; radical cure of umbilical
hernia; removal of varicose
veins
Mayo's anemic spot, sign
Mayo-Adams retractor
Mayo-Blake forceps
Mayo-Boldt inverter
Mayo-Collins retractor
Mayo-Guyon clamp
Mayo-Harrington forceps, scissors
Mayo-Kelly inverter
Mayo-Lovelace retractor
Mayo-Ochsner forceps
Mayo-Péan forceps, hemostat

Mayo-Robson forceps, incision, position

Mayo-Simpson retractor

Mayor's hammer, scarf

Mazzini's test

Mazzoni's corpuscles

McAllister's scissors

McArdle's disease — same as *McArdle-Schmid-Pearson disease*

McArdle-Schmid-Pearson disease — glycogen-storage disease with hepatophosphorylase deficiency

McArthur's incision, method

McAtee's apparatus

McBride's bunionectomy

McBride-Moore prosthesis

McBurney's operation — for the radical cure of inguinal hernia

McBurney's incision, point, sign

McCarthy's cystoscope, electrotome, panendoscope, reflex, resectoscope

McCarthy-Alcock forceps

McCarthy-Campbell cystoscope

McCarthy-Peterson cystoscope

McCaskey's catheter

McCleery-Miller clamp

McClintock's soap

McClure's scissors

McClure-Aldrich test

McCollum's tube

McConckey's cocktail

McCormac's reflex

McCoy's forceps

McCrea's cystoscope

McCrudden's method

McCullough's forceps

McCune-Albright syndrome — sexual precocity, fibrous dysplasia and patchy pigmentation of the skin

McCurdy's needle

McDermott's clip

McDonald's cerclage, clamp, maneuver, rule

McDowall's reflex

McDowell's mouth gag

McElroy's curet

McEwen's point

McGannon's forceps, retractor

McGee's forceps

McGee-Caparosa wire crimper

McGhan's eye implant, prosthesis

McGill's operation — suprapubic transvesical prostatectomy

McGill's forceps, retractor

McGinn-White sign

McGivney's ligator

McGoey-Evans cup

McGraw's ligature, sutures

McGuire's forceps, scissors

McHenry's forceps

McIndoe's colpocleisis, forceps, scissors

McIntire's splint

McIntosh's forceps

McIvor's mouth gag

McKay's forceps

McKee-Farrar prosthesis

McKeever's knife, prosthesis

McKenzie's clamp, drill, forceps, leukotome

McKinnon's test

McKissock's incision, sutures

McKittrick-Wheelock syndrome — adenoma of the colon and rectum, associated with electrolyte imbalance

McLane's forceps

McLane-Tucker-Luikart forceps

McLaughlin's incision, nail, speculum

McLean's formula, index, tonometer

McLean-VanSlyke method
McLetchie-Aikens disease — fever followed by tumors of the thigh and, several months later, of the biceps
McManus method
McMurray's maneuver, sign, test
McNaught's prosthesis
McNealy-Glassman-Babcock forceps
McNeer's classification
McNeill-Goldmann scleral ring
McPheeters's treatment
McPherson's forceps, scissors, speculum
McPherson-Castroviejo scissors
McPherson-Vannas scissors
McPherson-Wheeler knife
McPherson-Ziegler knife
McQuigg's clamp
McReynolds's keratome, knife, scissors
McVay's herniorrhaphy, incision
McWhinnie's electrode
McWhirter's technique
McWhorter's hemostat
Mead's rongeur
Means's sign
Mecke's reagent
Meckel's syndrome — same as *Meckel-Gruber syndrome*
Meckel's band, cartilage, cavity, diverticulum, ganglion, ligament, plane, rod, space, tubercle
Meckel-Gruber syndrome — a malformation syndrome, lethal in the perinatal period, marked by intrauterine growth failure, ocular anomalies, cleft palate, polydactyly, polycystic kidney and other defects. Called also *Gruber's syndrome*

Medin's disease — acute anterior poliomyelitis
Medinger-Craver irradiation
Meeh's formula
Meeker's forceps
Mees's lines, stripes
Meesmann's dystrophy
Méglin's point
Mehlis's gland
Méhu's test
Meige's disease — congenital hereditary lymphedema of the legs, caused by lymphatic obstruction
Meigs's syndrome — fibromyoma of the ovary
Meigs's capillaries, test
Meinicke's reaction, test
Meirowsky's phenomenon
Meissner's corpuscles, ganglion, plexus
Meleney's ulcers
Melkersson's syndrome — same as *Melkersson-Rosenthal syndrome*
Melkersson-Rosenthal syndrome — a rare, hereditary triad of recurrent facial paralysis, facial edema and fissured tongue
Meller's operation — excision of the tear sac
Meller's retractor, spatula
Mellinger's speculum
Melnick-Needles syndrome — a probably hereditary disease marked by generalized skeletal dysplasia and constrictions of the ribs and tubular bones
Melnick-Needles osteodysplasty
Melotte's metal
Meltzer's anesthesia, law, method, nasopharyngoscope, sign

Meltzer-Lyon method, test
Mencière's mixture, solution
Mende's syndrome — a congenital familial disorder combining abnormalities of pigmentation with mongoloid characteristics and deaf mutism
Mendel's law, reflex, test
Mendel-Bekhterev reflex, sign
Mendeléeff's (Mendeléev's) law, table, test
Mendelsohn's test
Mendelson's syndrome — acid pulmonary aspiration syndrome, occurring during labor under general anesthesia
Ménétrier's disease — giant hypertrophic gastritis
Menge's pessary
Mengert's shock syndrome — a condition in the late antepartum period, resembling shock, from pressure of the uterus on the vena cava
Mengert's index
Menghini's needle
Mengo encephalomyelitis, virus
Ménière's disease — hearing loss, tinnitus and vertigo resulting from nonsuppurative disease of the labyrinth
Menkes's syndrome(s) — a congenital metabolic defect, manifest in sparse, kinky hair, associated with mental and physical retardation and progressive deterioration of the brain; an inborn error of leucine, isoleucine, and valine metabolism, associated with gross mental deficiency
Mennell's sign

Menzel's disease — genetically transmitted, progressive ataxia of young adults
Mercier's operation — prostatectomy
Mercier's bar, catheter, valve
Mercurio's position
Merindino's procedure
Merkel's cells, corpuscles, disks, filtrum, muscle, tactile cells
Merkel-Ranvier cells
Merrifield's knife
Merseburg triad
Merseburger triad
Merz's serum
Merzbacher-Pelizaeus disease — familial, centrolobar sclerosis
Messinger-Huppert method
Mester's test
Metchnikoff's (Mechnikov's) law, phenomenon, theory
Mett's method, test tubes
Metzenbaum's forceps, knife, scissors
Metzenbaum-Lipsett scissors
Metzenbaum-Tydings forceps
Meulengracht's diet, icterus, method
Meunier's sign
Meyenburg's disease — same as *Meyenburg-Altherr-Uehlinger syndrome*
Meyenburg's complexes
Meyenburg-Altherr-Uehlinger syndrome — relapsing polychondritis
Meyer's disease — adenoid vegetations of the pharynx
Meyer's hockey stick incision, law, line, loop, method, organ, reagent, sign, sinus, test

Meyer-Betz disease — a rare, familial disease marked by the presence of myoglobin in the urine, resulting in tenderness, swelling, paralysis, muscular pain and weakness and sometimes renal failure

Meyer-Halsted incision

Meyer-Schwickerath and Weyers syndrome — anomalies of the iris, associated with malformed teeth and deformities of the fingers, including syndactyly or absent phalanges

Meyerding's curet, gouge, osteotome, retractor

Meyerding-Deaver retractor

Meyhoeffer's curet, knife

Meynert's amentia, bundle, cells, commissure, decussation, fasciculus, layer, tract

Meynet's nodes

Mezei's granules

Mibelli's disease — a rare dermatosis marked by progressive thickening of the corneal epidermis and progressive atrophy

Mibelli's porokeratosis

Michaelis's constant, rhomboid, stain, veronal acetate buffer

Michaelis-Gutmann bodies

Michaelis-Menten equation, law

Michailow's test

Michel's clamp, deafness, forceps

Michelson's bronchoscope

Michelson-Weiss sign

Middeldorpf's splint, triangle, tumor

Middlebrook-Cohn agar medium

Middlebrook-Dubos hemagglutination test

Middleton's curet

Miehlke-Partsch syndrome — thalidomide-induced ear deformity and facial paralysis

Mielke's template method

Mierzejewski's effect

Miescher's disease — degeneration of elastic tissue, occurring alone or in association with other disorders such as *Down's syndrome* or *Marfan's syndrome*

Miescher's cheilitis, corpuscles, elastoma, trichofolliculoma, tubes, tubules

Miescher-Leder granulomatosis

Mignon's eosinophilic granuloma

Migula's classification

Mikulicz's disease — a benign, self-limited, lymphocytic infiltration of the lacrimal and salivary glands, usually affecting older women. Similar to *Sjögren's syndrome*

Mikulicz's operation(s) — removal of the sternocleidomastoid muscle for torticollis; pyloroplasty; tarsectomy; enterectomy

Mikulicz's angle, aphthae, cells, clamp, drain, incision, pack, pad, pyloroplasty

Miles's operation — abdominoperineal resection for cancer of the lower sigmoid and rectum, which includes permanent colostomy

Miles's clamp, proctosigmoidectomy

Milian's erythema, sign

Milkman's syndrome — same as *Looser-Milkman syndrome*

Milkman-Looser syndrome — same as *Looser-Milkman syndrome*

Millar's asthma

Millard's test

Millard-Gubler syndrome — same as *Gubler's syndrome*

Millard-Gubler paralysis

Miller's disease — osteomalacia

Miller's syndrome — a hereditary disorder marked by vitamin D-resistant rickets, hydrophthalmia, congenital glaucoma, mental retardation and tubule reabsorption dysfunction

Miller modification of Welin's technique

Miller's collutory, curet, forceps, laryngoscope, method, ovum, speculum

Miller-Abbott tube

Miller-Kurzrok test

Miller-Senn retractor

Milligan's trichrome stain

Millikan's rays

Millikan-Siekert syndrome — intermittent insufficiency of the basilar arterial system

Millin's clamp, forceps, retractor, tube

Millin-Bacon retractor

Millin-Read operation — correction of stress incontinence

Millipore filter

Millon's reaction, reagent, test

Millonig's fixative

Mills's disease — ascending hemiplegia, eventually developing into quadriplegia

Mills's forceps, test

Mills-Reincke phenomenon

Milroy's disease — congenital hereditary lymphedema of the legs, caused by lymphatic obstruction

Milroy's edema

Milton's disease — angioneurotic edema

Milton's edema, urticaria

Minamata disease — a severe, neurologic disorder caused by alkyl mercury poisoning, leading to critical permanent neurologic and mental disabilities or death

Miner's osteotome

Minerva cast, jacket

Mingazzini-Förster operation — same as *Förster's operation*

Minin's light

Minkowski's figure, method

Minkowski-Chauffard syndrome — congenital hemolytic jaundice

Minor's disease — hemorrhage into the spinal cord, usually caused by trauma, marked by sudden onset of flaccid paralysis with sensory disturbances

Minor's sign, triangle

Minot's law

Minot-Murphy diet, treatment

Minot–von Willebrand syndrome — a congenital tendency to hemorrhage, characterized by a deficiency of coagulation and prolonged bleeding

Minsky's circles

Mira's photocoagulator, unit

Mirchamp's sign

Mirizzi's syndrome — hepatic duct stenosis

Miskiewicz's method

Mitchell's disease — a disease affecting the extremities of the body, marked by paroxysmal vasodilatation with burning pain and increased skin temperature

Mitchell's fluid, knife, stone basket, treatment

Mitchell-Diamond forceps

Mitscherlich's test

Mitsuda's antigen, reaction, test

Mittelmeyer's test

Mittendorf's dot

Mixter's clamp, forceps, tube

Mixter-McQuigg forceps

M'Naghten (McNaughten) rule

Moberg's arthrodesis

Mobin-Uddin filter

Mobitz's block, heart block

Möbius's disease — periodic oculomotor paralysis

Möbius's syndrome — developmental bilateral facial paralysis, usually associated with other neurological disorders

Möbius's sign

Moe's plate

Moehle's forceps

Moeller's glossitis, reaction

Moeller-Barlow disease — subperiosteal hematoma in rickets

Moerner-Sjöqvist method, test

Moersch's bronchoscope, esophagoscope, forceps

Moersch-Woltmann syndrome — prodromal tightness of the axial muscles progressing to generalized stiffness and paroxysmal attacks of agonizing pain and tachycardia

Mohr's method, test

Mohrenheim's fossa, space

Molisch's reaction, test

Moll's glands

Mollaret's meningitis

Möller's fluid, glossitis

Möller-Barlow disease — infantile scurvy

Mollison's retractor

Moloney's leukemia, reaction, test, virus

Molt's guillotine, mouth gag

Moltz-Storz tonsillectome

Monakow's syndrome — hemiplegia on the side opposite the lesion in occlusion of the anterior choroidal artery

Monakow's bundle, fasciculus, nucleus, theory, tract

Monaldi's drainage

Mönckeberg's arteriosclerosis, calcification, degeneration, mesarteritis, sclerosis

Moncrieff-Wilkinson syndrome — a combination of sucrosuria, mental retardation and hiatus hernia

Moncrieff's cannula, irrigator

Mondini's deafness, malformation

Mondonesi's reflex

Mondor's disease — inflammation of the subcutaneous veins of the chest wall and breast

Monge's disease — chronic mountain sickness

Monias-Shapiro's method

Monks-Esser flap

Monneret's pulse

Monro's abscesses, bursa, fissure, foramen, line, sulcus

Monro-Kellie doctrine

Monro-Richter line

Monroe-Kerr incision

Monsel's solution

Monson's curve

Monsur's agar

Montague's abrader, proctoscope, sigmoidoscope

Montefiore's tube

Monteggia's dislocation, fracture

Montenegro reaction, test

Monteverde's sign

Montevideo's units

Montgomery's cups, follicles, glands, straps, tapes, tubercles

Montigne's test

Moon's molars, teeth

Moore's operation — introduction of a coil of wire into the sac of an aortic aneurysm for co-agulation

Moore's syndrome — paroxysmal abdominal pain expressing an abnormal neuronal discharge from the brain, sometimes causing convulsions

Moore's button, extractor, for-ceps, fracture, osteotome, prosthesis, retractor, test, thoracoscope

Moore-Blount driver, extractor

Moore-Corradi operation — Moore's operation in which a strong galvanic current is passed through the wire

Moorehead's clamp, dissector, periosteotome, retractor

Mooren's ulcer

Moorhead's foreign body locator

Mooser's bodies, cell

Moots-McKesson ratio

Morand's foot, foramen, spur

Morawitz's theory

Morax's diplobacillus

Morax-Axenfeld bacillus, conjunc-tivitis, diplococcus, hemoph-ilus

Morch's tube

Morel's syndrome — thickening of the inner table of the frontal bone

Morel's ear

Morel-Fatio blepharoplasty

Morel-Kraepelin disease — schizo-phrenia

Morel-Wildi syndrome — dissem-inated nodular dysgenesis of the frontal cerebral cortex

Morelli's reaction, test

Moreno's clamp

Moreschi's phenomenon

Morestin's operation — disarticu-lation of the knee with intra-condyloid division of the femur

Morestin's method

Moretti's test

Morgagni's disease/syndrome — thickening of the inner table of the frontal bone

Morgagni's appendix, caruncle, columns, crypt, foramen, fos-sa, fovea, frenula, frenum, glands, globules, hernia, hy-datid, hyperostosis, lacunae, liquor, nodules, prolapse, sinus, sphere, tubercle, valves, ventricle

Morgagni-Adams-Stokes syndrome — sudden attacks of syncope in severe bradycardia or pro-longed asystole accompany-ing heart block, with or with-out convulsions

Morgagni-Stewart-Morel syndrome — same as *Morgagni's syn-drome*

Morgan's bacillus, line

Morison's incision, method, paste, pouch

Morita's therapy
Moritz's reaction, test
Moritz-Schmidt forceps
Morley's peritoneocutaneous re-
flex
Mörner's body, reagent, test
Moro's embrace reflex, reaction,
test, tuberculin
Moro-Heisler diet
Morquio's disease(s) — congenital
atrioventricular block assoc-
ciated with a septal defect of
the heart; infantile hereditary
chondrodysplasia
Morquio's sign
Morquio-Ullrich disease — same as
Morquio's disease
Morquio-Ullrich syndrome — same
as *Brailsford-Morquio disease*
Morris's syndrome — a form of
male pseudohermaphroditism
characterized, when complete,
by female external genitalia
Morris's catheter, hepatoma, retractor
Morrison-Hurd dissector, retractor
Morrow-Brooke syndrome — a
skin disease resembling keratosis follicularis, in children
Morse-Andrews suction tube
Morse-Ferguson suction tube
Morson's forceps
Mortensen's disease — a hemato-
logic disorder marked by prolonged bleeding time despite a
permanent increase in blood
platelet count
Mortimer's disease — a skin disease
marked by raised, red patches
that spread into a symmetrical
pattern
Mortimer's malady

Morton's syndrome — a congenital
insufficiency of the first metatarsal segment of the foot,
causing pain and often associated with some degree of syn-
dactylism
Morton's cough, current, fluid,
foot, metatarsalgia, neuralgia,
plane, test, toe
Morvan's syndrome — edema and
cyanosis with recurring felons
of the hands, a condition seen
in syringomyelia and sometimes in *Hansen's disease*
Morvan's chorea
Moschcowitz's disease — thrombotic thrombocytopenic purpura
Moschcowitz's operation — repair
of femoral hernia by the inguinal approach
Moschcowitz's sign, test
Mosenthal's test
Moser's serum
Mosetig-Moorhof bone wax
Mosher's drain, esophagoscope,
forceps, speculum, tube
Mosler's diabetes, sign
Mosny-Beaufume lipomatosis
Moss's classification
Mossbauer's spectrometer
Mosse's syndrome — polycythemia
rubra vera with cirrhosis of
the liver
Mossé-Marchand-Mallory cirrhosis
Mosso's ergograph, plethysmo-
graph, sphygmomanometer
Mossuril virus
Motais's operation — for ptosis,
by transplanting the middle
portion of the tendon of the
superior rectus muscle of the
eyelid into the upper lid

Mott's bodies, cell, law of anticipation

Mouchet's syndrome — remote paralysis of the cubital nerve caused by fracture of the external condyle of the humerus

Moult's curet

Mounier-Kuhn's syndrome — dilatation of the trachea and bronchi, associated with chronic respiratory infection

Mount's syndrome — a hereditary disorder marked by attacks similar to those of *Huntington's chorea*

Mount-Mayfield forceps

Moure's esophagoscope

Moyer's line

Moynihan's clamp, cream, forceps, gastrojejunostomy, position, test

Moynihan-Navratil forceps

Mozambique ulcer

Mozart's ear

Mozer's disease — adult myosclerosis

Much's granules, reaction

Much-Holzmann reaction

Mucha's disease — same as *Mucha-Habermann disease*

Mucha-Habermann disease/syndrome — a cutaneous disease marked by vesicles, papules and crusted lesions that are self-limiting but likely to recur and to leave smallpox-like scars

Muck's forceps

Muckle-Wells syndrome — familial amyloidosis involving the kidneys, marked by progressive hearing loss and periods of febrile urticaria

Mueller's arteries, prosthesis, speculum, tonometer, trephine

Mueller-Balfour retractor

Mueller-Frazier tube

Mueller-Hinton agar medium

Mueller-Laforce adenotome

Mueller-Pynchon tube

Mueller-Yankauer tube

Muer's anoscope

Muir's clamp

Muirhead's treatment

Mulder's angle, test

Muldoon's dilator, tube

Mules's operation — evisceration of the eyeball and insertion of artificial vitreous

Mules's eye implant, scoop

Müller's operation(s) — vaginal hysterectomy; cesarean section; resection of the sclera for detachment of the retina

Müller's canal, capsule, cells, duct, dust, experiment, fibers, fluid, ganglion, law, liquid, maneuver, muscle, radial cells, reaction, sign, test, tubercle

Müller-Haeckel law

Müller-Hillis maneuver

Müller-Jochmann test

Müller-Weiss disease — malacia of the navicular bone

Mulligan's prosthesis

Mumford-Gigli saw guide

Munchausen's syndrome — habitual presentation by a patient for medical treatment of an apparent acute illness, clinically convincing but all false

Münchmeyer's disease — a probably hereditary, uncommon disorder of children in which muscle cells are replaced by collagenous tissue

Mundie's forceps
Munk's disease — lipid nephrosis
Munro's microabscess, point
Munro Kerr maneuver
Munsell's colors
Munson's sign
Münzer-Rosenthal syndrome — a
    combination of hallucinations,
    anxiety and catalepsy
Murat's sign
Murchison-Pel-Ebstein fever
Murchison-Sanderson syndrome —
    same as *Hodgkin's disease*
Murdock-Wiener speculum
Murphy's button, drip, kidney
    punch, method, percussion,
    sign, test, treatment
Murphy-Sturm lymphosarcoma
Murray Valley encephalitis virus
Murri's disease — intermittent
    hemoglobinuria
Museholdt's forceps
Musken's tonometer
Musset's sign

Mussy's point
Mustard's operation — correction
    of a hemodynamic fault in
    transposition of the great
    vessels
Mustarde's otoplasty
Myà's disease — congenital dilata-
    tion of the colon
Myers's method, punch, retractor
Myers-Fine test
Myers-Wardell method
Myerson's electrode, forceps,
    punch, sign
Myhrman-Zetterholm disease —
    an infectious renal disease
    marked by sudden onset of
    chills, fever, headache, ab-
    dominal symptoms and
    vomiting
Myles's adenotome, clamp, curet,
    forceps, speculum, tonsillec-
    tome
Mylius's test

N

Nabatoff's vein stripper
Naboth's cysts, follicles, glands,
    ovules, vesicles
Nachlas's tube
Naegeli's syndrome — a hereditary
    disorder in which early vesicu-
    lar and later bizarre pigmented
    lesions of the skin are associ-
    ated with developmental de-
    fects of the eyes, bones and
    nervous system
Naegeli's culture medium, incon-
    tinentia pigmenti, law, leu-

Naegeli's (*continued*)
    kemia, macroblast, solution
Naffziger's operation — excision
    of the superior and lateral
    walls of the orbit for exoph-
    thalmos
Naffziger's syndrome — pain over
    the shoulder and extending to
    the arm, due to compression
    of nerves between a cervical
    rib and an anterior scalene
    muscle
Naffziger's test

Naffziger–Poppen Crain orbital decompression

Nagamatsu's incision

Nagel's test

Nägele's obliquity, pelvis, rule

Nägeli's maneuver, method, treatment

Nageotte's bracelets, cells

Nager's acrofacial dysostosis

Nager–de Reynier syndrome – hypoplasia of the mandible, with abdominal implantation of the teeth, deformities of the pinna and atresia of the external auditory meatus

Nagler's effect, reaction, test

Nakayama's test

Nakiwogo virus

Nance's leeway space

Napier's serum test

Narath's operation – to establish collateral circulation in portal obstruction by fixing the omentum to the subcutaneous tissue of the abdominal wall

Narath's omentopexy

Narsaroff's phenomenon

Nasmyth's membrane

Natelson's pipette

Nathan's pacemaker, test

Nauheim's bath, treatment

Naunyn-Minkowski method

Neal's cannula, catheter

Nebécourt's syndrome – diabetes mellitus, pituitary dwarfism and genital infantilism

Nebenthau's factor

Neef's hammer

Neer's prosthesis

Neftel's disease – a burning sensation of the head and neck and extreme discomfort except in a recumbent position

Nègre antigen

Negri bodies

Negro's phenomenon, sign

Negus's bronchoscope, telescope

Neill's medium

Neill-Dingwall syndrome – a familial syndrome allied to progeria and characterized by dwarfism

Neill-Mooser body, reaction

Neisser's diplococcus, reaction, staining method, syringe

Neisser-Doering phenomenon

Neisser-Wechsberg leukocidin, phenomenon, test

Neivert's knife, retractor

Neivert-Eves snare

Nélaton's disease – a central tumor of bone

Nélaton's operation – excision of the shoulder joint

Nélaton's catheter, dislocation, fibers, fold, line, probe, sphincter, tumor, ulcer

Nelson's syndrome – hyperpigmentation and nerve damage caused by development of a pituitary tumor after adrenalectomy

Nelson's ascites, forceps, method, scissors, trocar

Nelson-Bethune rib shears

Nelson-Roberts stripper

Nencki's test

Neri's sign

Neri-Barré syndrome – same as *Barré-Lieou syndrome*

Nernst's equation, law

Nesbit's cystoscope, resectoscope

Nessler's reagent, solution, test

Netherton's syndrome – a hereditary syndrome consisting of lamellar ichthyosis and atopic dermatitis, associated with

Netherton's syndrome (*continued*)
fracturing and splitting of the cortex of hair shafts

Nettleship's syndrome — a chronic skin disease of early childhood characterized by pigmented macules or nodules

Nettleship-Wilder dilator

Neubauer's artery, hemocytometer

Neubauer-Fischer test

Neubeiser's splint

Neuber's operation — filling a cavity in bone with skin flaps taken from the sides of the wound

Neuber's treatment, tubes

Neuberg's ester

Neuendorf's treatment

Neufeld's nail, phenomenon, plate, reaction, screw, test

Neuhauser-Berenberg syndrome — cardioesophageal relaxation resulting in vomiting in infants, marked by nonfunction of the cardioesophageal sphincter, dilatation of the esophagus and lack of gastric contractions

Neukomm's test

Neumann's disease — a condition in which vegetations develop on the eroded surfaces of ruptured bullae and new bullae develop

Neumann's syndrome — a benign, tender, pedunculated tumor of newborn infants, usually attached to the oral mucosa

Neumann's aphthosis, cells, law, method, pemphigus, sheath

Neusser's granules

Neve's cancer

Nevin's syndrome — subacute encephalopathy occurring between the ages of 50 and 70, marked by blindness, motor paralysis, speech disorders, cerebellar symptoms, mental disorders and myoclonus epilepsy

New's forceps, needle, scissors, tube

Newcastle disease virus

Newcastle-Manchester bacillus

Newland's law

Newman's forceps, knife, proctoscope, tenaculum

Newton's alloy, disk, law, rings

Nezelof's syndrome — cellular immunodeficiency with abnormal immunoglobulin synthesis

Nichols's clamp, speculum

Nickerson-Kveim test

Nicklès test

Nicol prism

Nicola's clamp, gouge, raspatory

Nicoladoni's sign

Nicolas-Favre disease — lymphogranuloma venereum

Nicolas-Moutot-Charlet syndrome — a familial, congenital, pemphigoid mucocutaneous disease, marked by a single bulla or vesicle followed by ulcerovegetative lesions

Nicolau-Hoigne syndrome — a nonallergic reaction to drugs introduced into an artery, resulting in hearing and visual disorders, vertigo, paresthesia and anxiety

Nicolau's septineuritis

Nidoko disease — epidemic hemorrhagic fever

Niebauer's prosthesis

Nieden's syndrome — multiple telangiectases of the face, arms and hands, with cataract and aortic stenosis

Niedner's clamp, forceps, knife, valvulotome

Nielsen's syndrome — weakness and muscular atrophy and fascicular twitching caused by extreme exhaustion

Niemann's disease — same as *Niemann-Pick disease*

Niemann's splenomegaly

Niemann-Pick disease — a hereditary disease marked by massive hepatosplenomegaly, nervous system involvement, and presence in the liver, spleen, lung and bone marrow of phospholipid-storing histiocytes

Niemann-Pick cells

Nierhoff-Hübner syndrome — a variant of dysostosis enchondralis, marked by faulty ossification of the skull, vertebrae, ribs and long bones in newborn infants

Nievergelt's syndrome — hereditary malformation of an extremity

Nievergelt-Erb syndrome — same as *Nievergelt's syndrome*

Niewenglowski's rays

Nikiforoff's method

Nikolsky's sign

Nimeh's method

Nippe's test

Nirenstein-Schiff method

Nisbet's chancre

Nissen's forceps, gastrectomy, sutures

Nissl bodies, degeneration, granules, stain, substance

Nitabuch's layer, stria, zone

Nithsdale's neck

Noack's syndrome — hereditary acrocephalosyndactyly with polydactyly

Nobel's test

Nobis's aortic occluder

Noble's forceps, position, scissors

Nocard's bacillus

Noguchi's culture medium, leutin reaction, reagent, test

Noland-Budd curet

Nolke's method

Nonne's syndrome — hereditary cerebellar ataxia

Nonne's test

Nonne-Apelt phase, reaction, test

Nonne-Froin syndrome — same as *Froin's syndrome*

Nonne-Marie syndrome — same as *Marie's syndrome*

Nonne-Milroy syndrome — same as *Nonne-Milroy-Meige syndrome*

Nonne-Milroy-Meige syndrome — a familial form of dilatation of the lymphatic vessels associated with edema, spongy or honeycomb changes, susceptibility to infection and cellulitis

Nonne–Pierre Marie syndrome — same as *Marie's syndrome*

Nonnenbruch's syndrome — oliguric kidney disease without organic renal changes

Noonan's syndrome — a symptom complex of short stature, webbed neck, low-set ears, low nuchal hairline and

Noonan's syndrome (*continued*)
deviated elbow with valvular
pulmonary stenosis
Noorden treatment
Nordach's treatment
Nordau's disease — a general term
for a condition of deterioration of the powers of mind
and body
Norman-Wood syndrome — a
congenital form of amaurotic
idiocy
Norrie's disease — a hereditary disorder consisting of bilateral
blindness, mental retardation
and deafness, transmitted as
an X-linked trait
Norris's corpuscles
Norum's disease — a genetic disorder, transmitted as an autosomal recessive trait, in which
an absolute enzyme deficiency
leads to hemolytic anemia in
young adulthood, as well as
liver and kidney failure, vascular degeneration and lens
opacities
Norwalk agent
Norwood's forceps
Nothnagel's syndrome — dizziness,
staggering, irregular oculomotor paralysis and often

Nothnagel's syndrome (*continued*)
nystagmus—the symptoms of
a midbrain tumor
Nothnagel's acroparesthesia,
bodies, type
Nott's speculum
Nott-Guttmann speculum
Nourse's syringe
Novak's curet
Novikoff's hepatoma
Noyes's forceps, rongeur, scissors,
speculum
Noyes-Shambaugh scissors
Nuck's canal, diverticulum, hydro-
cele
Nuel's spaces
Nugent's forceps, hook
Nugent-Gradle scissors
Nugent-Green-Dimitry erysiphake
Nuhn's glands
Nunez's clamp, tube
Nunez-Nunez knife
Nunn's gorged corpuscles
Nürnberg's gold
Nussbaum's bracelet, clamp, ex-
periment, narcosis
Nuttall's retractor
Nygaard-Brown syndrome — es-
sential thrombophilia
Nyiri's test
Nylander's reagent, test
Nysten's law

Oakley-Fulthorpe test
Obal's syndrome — amblyopia in
severe malnutrition, associated
with retrobulbar neuritis, scotoma and visual disturbances

O'Beirne's experiment, sphincter,
tube, valve
Ober's operation — division of a
joint capsule
Ober's sign, tendon passer, test

Oberhill's retractor
Obermayer's reagent, test
Obermüller's test
Oberst's method
Obersteiner-Redlich area, space, zone
O'Brien's akinesia, block, cataract, forceps
Obwegeser's incision, osteotomy, retractor
Ochsner's clamp, forceps, muscle, position, ring, scissors, treatment
Ochsner-Dixon forceps
Ockerblad's clamp
O'Connor's clamp, forceps, hook, retractor
O'Connor-O'Sullivan retractor
O'Conor's nephropexy
Oddi's muscle, sphincter
Odelberg's disease — same as *Van Neck's disease*
Odman-Ledin catheter
O'Donaghue's splint
O'Dwyer's tube
Oedipus complex
Oehler's symptom
Oertel's treatment
Oertli's knife
Oestreicher's reaction
Ogata's method
Ogawa antigen
Ogilvie's syndrome — persistent contraction of intestinal musculature without evidence of organic disease of the colon, but simulating colonic obstruction and occurring as a result of a defect in the sympathetic nerve supply. Also called *false colonic obstruction*
Ogilvie's herniorrhaphy

Ogino-Knaus method
Ogston's operation(s) — removal of the inner condyle of the femur for knock knee; excision of the wedge of the tarsus for restoring the arch in flat feet
Ogston's line
Ogston-Luc operation — for frontal sinus disease
Oguchi's disease — a form of congenital night blindness occurring principally in Japan
O'Hanlon's forceps
Ohara's disease — occurring chiefly in Japan, probably identical with tularemia
O'Hara's forceps
O'Higgins's disease — an anicteric condition associated with leukopenia, blood platelet deficiency with retarded blood coagulation, hypocholesterolemia, hypocalcemia, capillaritis and equilibrium disturbances
Ohm's law
Oken's body, canal, corpus
Oldberg's dissector, forceps, retractor
Oliver's retractor, sign, test
Ollier's disease/syndrome — the presence of irregular fragments of nonossified cartilage in the metaphyses and diaphyses of the long bones
Ollier's incision, law, layer, raspatory, retractor
Ollier-Klippel-Trenaunay syndrome — same as *Klippel-Trenaunay syndrome*
Ollier-Thiersch graft
Olmer's disease — endemic in the

Olmer's disease (*continued*)
Mediterranean area, caused by *Rickettsia conorii* and marked by chills, fever and skin lesions

Olshausen's operation — for the cure of retroversion by suturing the uterus to the abdominal wall

Olshevsky's tube

O'Malley's knife

Ombrédanne's operation(s) — for hypospadias; transscrotal orchiopexy

Ombrédanne's syndrome — postoperative hyperthermia and pallor in children, caused by anesthesia

Ombrédanne's method

Omeliansky's nutritive culture medium

Omodei-Zorini syndrome — bronchial dilatation caused by a broncholith

Omsk hemorrhagic fever virus

Ondine's curse

O'Neill's clamp, scissors

O'nyong-nyong fever, virus

Oort's bundle

Opalski's syndrome — a combination of hypoesthesia of pain and temperature in the face and paralysis of the extremities on one side of the body, associated with hypoesthesia of pain and temperature in the trunk and extremities

Opie's paradox

Opitz's disease — enlargement of the spleen due to thombosis of the splenic vein

Oppenheim's disease — a pseudoparalysis of congenital origin,

Oppenheim's disease (*continued*)
observed principally in children, characterized by deficiency in tone of muscles innervated by the spinal nerves

Oppenheim's syndrome — sclerosis of the spinal cord and tumor of the pituitary

Oppenheim's brace, gait, reflex, sign

Oppenheim-Urbach syndrome — a skin disorder observed in female diabetic patients, with multiple red or yellowish papules that later develop into round or oval scleroderma-like plaques

Orbeli's effect, phenomenon

Orbinsky's syndrome — abdominal muscle deficiency

Ord's operation — for breaking up joint adhesions

Ordóñez's melanosis

Ormond's disease/syndrome — retroperitoneal fibrosis

Oropouche virus

Oroya fever

Orr's incision, method, technique, treatment

Orsi-Grocco method

Orth's solution

Orthmann's tumor

Ortner's syndrome — heart disease associated with laryngeal paralysis

Ortolani's click, sign

Ortved's stone dislodger

Osborne-Folin method

Osgood-Haskins test

Osgood-Schlatter disease — osteochondrosis of the tuberosity of the tibia

O'Shaughnessy's clamp, forceps

Osler's disease(s) — polycythemia vera; hereditary hemorrhagic telangiectasia

Osler's syndrome(s) — the presence in the diverticulum of Vater of a free-moving gallstone that blocks the outflow of bile from the common duct; multiple telangiectatic lesions of the face and body

Osler's nodes, phenomenon, sign, triad

Osler-Libman-Sacks disease — same as *Libman-Sacks syndrome*

Osler-Vaquez disease — polycythemia vera

Osler-Weber-Rendu disease — hereditary hemorrhagic telangiectasia

Osterberg's test

Österreicher's syndrome — same as *Österreicher-Turner syndrome*

Österreicher-Turner syndrome — a hereditary syndrome transmitted as a dominant trait and marked by anomalies of the patellae, nails and elbows and by iliac horns

Ostrum-Furst syndrome — congenital abnormal union of adjacent bones of the neck, deformity of the occipital bone and upper end of the

Ostrum-Furst syndrome (*continued*) cervical spine and elevation of the scapula

Ostwald's viscosimeter

O'Sullivan's retractor

O'Sullivan-O'Connor retractor, speculum

Ota's nevus

Ott's test

Ottenheimer's dilator

Otto's disease — osteoarthritic protrusion of the acetabulum

Otto's syndrome — same as *Guérin-Stern syndrome*

Otto's pelvis

Otto-Chrobak syndrome — protrusion of the acetabulum

Ottonello's method

Ouchterlony line, technique, test

Oudin current, resonator, test

Overholt's elevator, forceps, raspatory, retractor

Overholt-Finochietto rib spreader

Overholt-Jackson bronchoscope

Overstreet's forceps

Owen's lines, position, spaces, sutures

Owren's disease — deficiency of calcium, with consequent impairment of coagulation

Owren's syndrome(s) — hemolytic crisis; labile factor deficiency

Owren's crisis

Ozzard's filariasis

Paas's disease — a familial disorder marked by skeletal deformities, such as shortening of phalanges, scoliosis and spondylitis

Pacchioni's foramen

Pace's knife

Pachon's test

Paci's operation — a modification of Lorenz's operation for congenital dislocation of the hip

Pacini's corpuscles

Padgett's dermatome, graft

Padgett-Hood electrodermatome

Pagano's reaction

Page's syndrome — hypertensive diencephalic syndrome

Page's forceps, knife

Pagenstecher's circle, linen thread, ointment, scoop, sutures

Paget's disease(s) — increased bone resorption resulting in weakened and deformed bones; inflammatory cancerous affection of the areola and nipple, usually associated with carcinoma of the lactiferous ducts

Paget's disease, extramammary — a counterpart of Paget's disease of the breast, usually involving the vulva and sometimes the perianal and axillary regions

Paget's disease, juvenile — a bowing deformity of the legs, with elevated levels of blood alkaline phosphatase, cortical thickening of all bones and muscular weakness

Paget's abscess, cancer, carcinoma, cells, nipple, quiet necrosis of bone, test

Paget-Schroetter syndrome — intermittent venous claudication

Pai's culture medium

Paine's syndrome — microcephaly, arthrogryposis, spastic diplegia, convulsions, mental retardation, aminoaciduria, irregular dental arches, abnormal skin ridges and congenital heart defects

Pajot's hook, law, maneuver, method

Pal's stain

Palade's buffered fixative

Palfyn's sutures

Palmer's dilator

Paltauf's dwarf, nanism

Panas's operation — for ptosis, by attaching the upper eyelid to the occipitofrontalis muscle

Panas's technique

Pancoast's syndrome — tumor of the apex of the lung as shown by roentgenographic shadow, with neuritic pain and muscle weakness of the upper extremity caused by tumor pressure on the brachial plexus

Pancoast's suture, tumor

Pander's islands, layer, nucleus

Pándy's reaction, test

Paneth's cells

Pang's forceps

Panizza's plexuses

Panner's disease — osteochondrosis of the distal end of the

Panner's disease (*continued*) lateral epicondyle of the humerus

Pansch's fissure

Panton-Valentine (P-V) leukocidin

Panum's areas, casein

Panzer's scissors

Pap's silver method

Papanicolaou's smear, stain, test

Paparella's catheter, curet, fenestrometer, retractor, scissors, tube

Papillon-Léage and Psaume syndrome — orodigitofacial dysostosis

Papillon-Lèfevre syndrome — a congenital hyperkeratosis of the palms and soles, with progressive destruction of alveolar bone about the teeth

Papin's digester

Pappenheim's lymphoid hemoblast, stain

Pappenheimer's bodies

Paquelin's cautery

Paré's suture

Parenti's disease — a type of osteogenesis imperfecta marked by absence of normal ossification and abnormal smallness of limbs

Parhad-Poppen needle

Parham's band

Parham-Martin band, clamp

Parietti's broth

Parinaud's syndrome — a general term for conjunctivitis, usually unilateral and follicular, often caused by infection from a leptothrix or associated with other infections

Parinaud's conjunctivitis, conjunctivoadenitis, ophthalmoplegia

Parish's reaction

Park's aneurysm

Park-Guyton speculum

Park-Maumenee speculum

Park-Williams chocolate culture medium

Parker's fluid, incision, method, retractor

Parker-Heath cautery

Parker-Kerr forceps, stitch, sutures

Parker-Mott retractor

Parkinson's disease — a disease of the central nervous system of unknown etiology, characterized by masklike facies, tremor of the muscles, decreased motor power and control, postural instability and muscular rigidity

Parkinson-dementia complex

Parkinson's facies, mask, position, sign

parkinsonian syndrome — a form of parkinsonism resulting from idiopathic degeneration of the striate body of the basal ganglia. It is slowly progressive and marked by masklike facies, tremor, slowing of voluntary movement, short accelerating steps in walking, uncertain posture and muscle weakness

Parnum's test

Parona's space

Parrot's disease(s) — pseudoparalysis of one or more extremities of an infant, caused by syphilitic osteochondritis; short-limb dwarfism transmitted as an autosomal dominant trait

Parrot's atrophy of the newborn, cicatrix, node, pseudoparalysis, sign, ulcer

Parry's disease — same as *Graves's disease*

Parry-Romberg syndrome — facial hemiatrophy

Parson's disease — same as *Graves's disease*

Parsonage-Turner syndrome — severe pain across the shoulder and upper arm with atrophic paralysis of muscles of the shoulder girdle, usually following infection or minor surgery

Partipilo's clamp

Partsch's operation — marsupialization of a dental cyst

Pascal's law

Pascheff's conjunctivitis, folliculoma

Paschen's bodies, corpuscles, granules

Paschutin's degeneration

Pasini's syndrome — a type of epidermolysis bullosa, occurring at an early age and characterized by bullae that rupture, leaving scars and areas of pigmentation

Pasini-Pierini syndrome — progressive idiopathic atrophy of the skin, usually occurring in young women

Pasqualini's syndrome — eunuchoidism with spermatogenesis and normal secretion of follicle-stimulating hormone

Passavant's bar, cushion, pad, ridge

Passow's syndrome — essentially the same as *Bernard-Horner syndrome* but with color

Passow's syndrome (*continued*) difference in the irides

Pasteur's culture medium, effect, fluid, liquid, method, reaction, solution, therapy

Pasteur-Chamberland filter

Pastia's lines, sign

Patau's syndrome — failure of cleavage of the prosencephalon, due to an extra chromosome 13, in which central nervous system defects are associated with mental retardation, cleft lip, polydactyly and abnormalities of the heart, viscera and genitalia

Patein's albumin

Patella's disease — pyloric stenosis in tuberculosis

Paterson's syndrome — same as *Plummer-Vinson syndrome*

Paterson's bodies, cannula, corpuscles, forceps, nodules

Paterson-Brown-Kelly syndrome — dysphagia with glossitis, anemia, splenomegaly and atrophy of the mouth, pharynx and esophagus. Called also *Plummer-Vinson syndrome*

Paterson-Kelly syndrome — same as *Paterson-Brown-Kelly syndrome*

Paterson-Kelly webs

Paton's forceps, knife, spatula, trephine

Patrick's sign, test

Patterson's test

Patton's dilator, speculum

Paufique's knife, trephine

Paul's test, treatment

Paul-Bunnell reaction, test

Paul-Bunnell-Barrett test

Paul-Bunnell-Davidsohn differential test

Paul-Mixter tube

Pauly's point

Paunz's test

Pautrier's abscess, microabscess

Pautrier-Woringer syndrome — lipomelanotic deposits in enlarged lymph nodes in association with various types of skin disease

Pauzat's disease — periostitis of the metatarsal bones

Pavlov's method, pouch, stomach

Pavy's disease — cyclic proteinuria

Pavy's test

Pawlik's triangle, trigone

Pawlow's method

Paxton's disease — same as *Beigel's disease*

Payne-Ochsner forceps

Payne-Péan forceps

Payne-Rankin forceps

Payr's disease — constipation, with upper quadrant pain from kinking of an adhesion between the transverse and descending colon with obstruction

Payr's clamp, method

Peabody's splint

Péan's operation(s) — vaginal hysterectomy bit by bit; hip joint amputation with ligation of vessels

Péan's amputation, forceps, hysterectomy, incision, position

Pearsall's sutures

Pearson's method

Pecquet's cistern, duct, reservoir

Pedersen's speculum

Pel's crisis

Pel-Ebstein disease — same as *Hodgkin's disease*

Pel-Ebstein fever, pyrexia, symptom

Pelger's nuclear anomaly

Pelger-Huët nuclear anomaly, phenomenon

Pelizaeus-Merzbacher disease — familial centrolobar sclerosis

Pellegrini's disease — same as *Pellegrini-Stieda disease*

Pellegrini-Stieda disease — formation of a semilunar body in the upper portion of the medial lateral ligament of the knee, resulting from trauma

Pellizzi's syndrome — precocious development of external genitalia and sexual function, linked with abnormal growth of long bones and signs of internal hydrocephalus

Pélouse-Moore test

Pemberton's clamp, forceps, retractor

Pende's syndrome — thymic hyperfunction associated with adiposity, genital dystrophy and retarded mental and physical development

Pende's sign

Pendinski ulcer

Pendred's syndrome — a hereditary syndrome of congenital bilateral nerve deafness associated with goiter

Penfield's syndrome — epilepsy caused by a tumor pressing on the hypothalamus

Penfield's clip, elevator, forceps, modification of Rio-Hortega's method

Penjdeh sore, ulcer

Penn's seroflocculation reaction
Pennington's forceps, speculum
Penrose drain, tube
Penzoldt's reagent, test
Penzoldt-Fisher test
Pepper's disease — neuroblastoma of the adrenal gland, with metastases to the liver
Percy's cautery, forceps, retractor
Percy-Wolfson retractor
Perdrau's staining method
Perenyi's solution
Pereyra's bladder suspension, cannula, needle
Perez's sign
Peria's test
Perkins's tractor
Perlia's nucleus
Perlmann's tumor
Perls's anemia bodies, reaction, stain, test
Perrin-Ferraton disease —a condition marked by slippage of the hip joint with an audible snap
Perritt's forceps
Perroncito's apparatus, spirals
Perry's bag
Persian ulcer
Perthes's disease — osteochondrosis of the femoral epiphyses
Perthes's incision, test
Perthes-Calvé-Legg-Waldenström syndrome — same as *Calvé-Legg-Perthes syndrome*
Perthes-Jüngling disease — a progressive form of polycystic osteitis involving the surrounding soft tissue
Pertik's diverticulum
Peterman's test
Peters's anomaly, method, ovum
Petersen's operation — modification of high lithotomy

Petersen's bag
Petges-Cléjat syndrome — poikiloderma marked by extensive telangiectasia, pigmentation, atrophy of the skin and muscles and myositis
Petit's syndrome — an oculopupillary syndrome caused by irritation of the sympathetic nervous system
Petit's canal, hernia, law, ligament, sinus, triangle
Petragnani's culture medium
Petrén's diet, treatment
Pétrequin's ligament
Petri's dish, plate, reaction, test
Petroff's synthetic culture medium
Petroff-Hauser counting chamber
Petruschky's culture medium, litmus whey, spinalgia
Pette-Döring disease — subacute sclerosing inflammation of the brain
Pette-Döring encephalitis, panencephalitis
Pettenkofer's test, theory
Petz's clamp
Petzetakis's reaction, test
Petzetakis-Takos syndrome — superficial keratitis, edema of the eyelids and bulbar conjunctiva, hypoesthesia of the cornea, diminished reflexes of the iris, xerophthalmia and lesions of the corneal and precorneal layers
Peutz's syndrome — same as *Peutz-Jeghers syndrome*
Peutz-Jeghers syndrome — generalized multiple polyposis of the intestinal tract

Peyer's follicles, glands, insulae, patches, plaques

Peyronie's disease — of unknown cause, marked by formation of dense fibrous tissue about the corpus cavernosum of the penis, causing deformity and painful erection

Peyrot's thorax

Peyton's brain spatula

Pezzer's catheter

Pfannenstiel's syndrome — hemolytic anemia of the neonate

Pfannenstiel's incision

Pfau's forceps, punch

Pfaundler-Hurler syndrome — same as *Hurler-Pfaundler syndrome*

Pfeiffer's disease — infectious mononucleosis

Pfeiffer's syndrome — craniostenosis with polydactyly

Pfeiffer's bacillus, glandular fever, law, phenomenon, reaction

Pfeiffer-Comberg method

Pfiffner-Myers method

Pfister-Schwartz stone basket

Pflüger's cords, law, tubes

Pfuhl's sign

Pfuhl-Jaffé sign

Phalen's maneuver, sign

Phaneuf's clamp, forceps

Pheifer-Young retractor

Phelps's operation — an incision through the sole and inner side of the foot for talipes

Phelps's splint

Phelps-Gocht osteoclast

Phemister operation — onlay graft of cancellous bone without internal fixation, for treatment of ununited fracture

Phemister's bone graft, incision, punch, reamer

Philip's glands

Philippe-Gombault tract

Philippson's reflex

Phillips's bougie, catheter, muscle

Phipps-Bird water bath

Phocas's disease — chronic glandular mastitis

Physick's operation — removal of a circular piece of iris to create an artificial pupil

Physick's pouches

Piazza's fluid, reaction, test

Picchini's syndrome — a form of polyserositis caused by presence of a trypanosome

Pick's disease(s) — lobar atrophy of the brain with progressive intellectual deterioration, loss of memory, disorientation and apathy; ascites and fibrotic liver disease associated with pericarditis

Pick's cells, cirrhosis, convolutional atrophy, hallucinations, retinitis, vision

Pickerill's imbricating lines

Pickrell's method, solution, spray

pickwickian syndrome — obesity, somnolence, hypoventilation and erythrocytosis

Picot's retractor, speculum

Pictet's chloroform

Pierce's cannula, elevator, forceps, syringe, tube

Pierce-Hoskins forceps

Pierre Robin syndrome — micrognathia and abnormal smallness of the tongue, with cleft palate and often with bilateral eye defects

Piersol's point

Pietrantoni's syndrome — mucosal and cutaneous areas of anesthesia and neuralgia of the face and oral cavity

Piffard's curet, paste

Pignet's formula, index, standard

Pike's streptococcal broth

Pilcher's catheter, hemostatic bag

Pillat's dystrophy

Pilling's bronchoscope, tube

Piltz's reflex, sign

Piltz-Westphal phenomenon

Pinard's maneuver

Pinaud's triangle

Pincus's test

Pinel's system

Pinkerton-Moorer reaction

Pinkus's disease — a rare skin eruption marked by minute, flat, sharply marginated, discrete papules barely raised above the skin surface

Pinkus's epithelioma, tumor

Pins's sign

Piotrowski's sign, test

Piper's forceps

Piria's test

Pirie's bone, method

Piringer's lymphadenitis

Piringer-Kuchinka's syndrome — benign cervical lymphadenitis marked by epithelioid reticulum cells in the lymph nodes

Pirogoff's amputation, angle, edema, triangle

Pirquet's cutireaction, index, reaction, test

Piry virus

Pischel's electrode, elevator, forceps

Piskacek's sign

Pitfield's fluid

Pitha's forceps

Pitkin's needle, solution

Pitres's sections, sign

Piulachs-Hederich syndrome — acute dilatation of the colon

Placido's disk

Planck's constant, theory

Platner's crystallized bile, crystals

Plaut's angina, ulcer

Plaut-Vincent stomatitis

Playfair's treatment

Plesch's percussion, test

Pley's forceps

Plimmer's bodies, salt

Plimmer-Skelton method

Plugge's test

Plummer's disease — toxicity in adenoma of the thyroid

Plummer's adenoma, sign

Plummer-Vinson syndrome — dysphagia with glossitis, anemia, splenomegaly and atrophy of the mouth, pharynx and esophagus

Plummer-Vinson applicator, dilator

Plunket's caustic

Poehl's test

Pohl's mark

Poirier's glands, line

Poiseuille's equation, law, space

Poisson-Pearson formula

Poitou's colic

Poland's syndrome — unilateral absence of the sternocostal head of the greater pectoral muscle. Also called *Poland's deformity*

Poland's anomaly, deformity, syndactyly

Polenske number

Polhemus-Schafer-Ivemark syndrome — same as *Ivemark's syndrome*

Polisar-Lyons tube

Politzer's operation(s) — creation of an artificial opening in the membrana tympani; division of the anterior ligament of the malleus

Politzer's bag, cone, otoscope, speculum, test, treatment

Pollacci's test

Polley-Bickel trephine

Pollock's operation — amputation at the knee joint, preserving the patella

Polya's operation — anastomosis of the transected end of the stomach to the side of the jejunum following subtotal gastrectomy

Pomeroy's operation — female sterilization

Pompe's disease — glycogen storage disease

Poncet's disease — tuberculous rheumatism

Poncet's operation(s) — lengthening of the Achilles tendon for talipes equinus; perineotomy; perineal urethrostomy

Poncet's rheumatism

Pond's splint

Ponfick's shadow

Pongola virus

Pool's phenomenon, tube

Pool-Schlesinger sign

Poppen's coagulator, forceps, rongeur

Poppen-Blalock clamp

Porak-Durante syndrome — same as *Vrolik's syndrome*

Porcher's method

Porges-Hermann-Perutz reaction

Porges-Meier reaction, reagent, test

Porges-Salomon test

Porret's phenomenon

Porro's cesarean section

Porter's syndrome — a form of benign pericarditis that does not belong to the rheumatic, bacterial or uremic group

Porter's sign, test

Porter-Silber chromogens, reaction

Porteus's maze test

Porzett's splint

Posada-Wernicke disease — coccidioidomycosis

Posada's mycosis

Posada-Wernicke disease — coccidiomycosis

Posey's belt

Posner's reaction, test

Posner-Schlossman syndrome — benign paroxysmal ocular hypertension

Post-Harrington erysiphake

Potain's apparatus, sign

Poth's keratosis

Pott's disease — tuberculosis of the spine

Pott's abscess, aneurysm, caries, clamp, curvature, fracture, gangrene, paralysis, paraplegia, puffy tumor

Pottenger's sign

Potter's syndrome — a rare lethal disease of infancy, marked by renal agenesis or hypoplasia with skeletal abnormalities and characteristic facies

Potter's facies, treatment, version

Potter-Bucky diaphragm, grid

Potts's anastomosis, dissector, periosteotome, valvulotome

Potts-Neidner clamp

Potts-Riker dilator, valvulotome

Potts-Satinsky clamp

Potts-Smith scissors, tenaculum, valvulotome

Potts-Smith-Gibson operation — anastomosis between the aorta and the pulmonary artery in congenital pulmonary stenosis

Poulet's disease — rheumatic osteoperiostitis

Poupart's ligament, line

Poutasse's clamp, forceps

Pouteau's fracture

Powassan's encephalitis, virus

Power's operation — removal of a corneal leukoma, followed by insertion of a rabbit's cornea

Power-Wilder method

Pozzi's senile pseudorickets, tenaculum

Prader's orchidometer

Prader-Willi syndrome — a congenital disease of unknown etiology, marked by short stature, marked obesity, mental retardation, severe muscle hypotonia and sexual infantilism

Prague's maneuver

Pratesi's syndrome — intermittent claudication of the lower extremities, with cold feet

Pratt's anoscope, director, forceps, sign, sound speculum, symptom, test

Pratt-Smith forceps

Prausnitz-Küstner antibodies, reaction, test

Pregl's test

Prehn's sign

Preiser's disease — osteoporosis and atrophy of the carpal

Preiser's disease (*continued*) scaphoid from trauma or from fracture that has not been kept immobilized

Preisz-Nocard bacillus

Prendergast's test

Preshaw's clamp

Prévost's law, sign

Preyer's reflex, test

Price-Jones curve, method

Price-Thomas clamp, forceps

Priessnitz's bandage, compress

Priestley's mass

Prieur-Trénel syndrome — the association of monilethrix and cataract

Prigge's toxin

Prince's cautery, forceps, rongeur, scissors

Prince-Potts scissors

Pringle's disease — a cutaneous malformation or benign tumorlike nodule of the face, involving blood vessels and connective tissue

Pringle's incision

Prinzmetal's angina

Prinzmetal-Massumi syndrome — pain and tenderness of the anterior chest wall, which may occur weeks or months after myocardial infarct but may also occur in the absence of history of coronary disease

Pritchard's cannula, syringe

Pritikin's punch

Prochownick's diet, method

Proctor's elevator, retractor

Proetz's position, test, treatment

Profeta's immunity, law

Profichet's syndrome — growth of calcareous nodules in the

Profichet's syndrome (*continued*) subcutaneous tissues, especially about the joints, with a tendency to ulceration

Proneze's pad

Proskauer-Beck medium

Proust's law

Prowazek's bodies

Prowazek-Greeff bodies

Prower's factor

Pruitt's anoscope, proctoscope

Prussak's fibers, pouch, space

Pryor-Péan retractor

Pudenz's shunt, tube, valve

Pugh's nail

Purcell's retractor

Purdy's method, test

Purkinje's cells, corpuscles, fibers, figures, images, layer, network, phenomenon, shadows, shift, vesicle

Purkinje-Sanson mirror images

Purmann's method

Purtscher's disease — angiopathy of the retina, with edema and hemorrhage, usually following crush injuries of the chest

Purtscher's angiopathic retinopathy

Pusey's emulsion

Pusto's dilatation

Putnam's acroparesthesia

Putnam-Dana syndrome — subacute degeneration of the spinal cord

Putti's syndrome — sciatica from arthrosis of the posterior vertebral joints

Putti's approach, gouge, splint

Putti-Chavany syndrome — unilateral sciatica with severe attacks of pain followed by foot paralysis

Putti-Platt director

Puusepp's operation — splitting of the central canal of the spinal cord for treatment of syringomyelia

Puusepp's reflex

Pyle's disease — familial metaphyseal dysplasia

Pynchon's applicator, speculum, tube

Pynchon-Lillie tongue depressor

Q

Quaglino's operation — sclerotomy

Quain's ambiguous nucleus, degeneration, fatty heart, triangular fascia

Quant's sign

Quaranfil virus

Quarelli's syndrome — striatopallidal syndrome with parkinsonian tremor, seen in carbon disulfide poisoning

Quatrefages's angle

Queckenstedt's phenomenon, sign, test

Quénu-Mayo operation — excision of the rectum and lymph glands for cancer

Quénu-Muret sign

Quervain's disease — same as *de Quervain's disease*

Quervain's forceps, fracture

Quervain-Sauerbruch retractor

Quesada's method
Quetelet's rule
Quevedo's forceps
Quevenne's iron
Queyrat's erythroplasia
Quick's test, tourniquet test
Quincke's disease — angioneurotic edema
Quincke's edema, meningitis, pulse, puncture, sign

Quincke-Tirmann-Schmelzer method
Quinlan's test
Quinquaud's disease — papular or pustular inflammation of the hair follicles of the scalp, with hair loss and scarring
Quinquaud's sign
Quinton's tube
Quisling's hammer

Raabe's test
Rabe-Salomon syndrome — congenital afibrinogenemia
Rabuteau's test
Racine's syndrome — swelling of the salivary glands and breasts four or five days premenstrually
Rademacher's disease — diminished immunity resulting in frequent infections, associated with hypogammaglobulinemia
Rademacher's system
Radovici's sign
Raeder's paratrigeminal syndrome — a form of *Bernard-Horner syndrome* with cranial nerve disturbance caused by involvement of the carotid sympathetic plexus
Raimiste's sign
Rainey's corpuscles, tubes, tubules
Raiziss-Dubin method
Ralfe's test
Ralks's applicator, drill, forceps, magnet, mallet
Ralks-Davis mouth gag

Raman's effect
Ramdohr's sutures
Ramirez's dermatosis, shunt
Ramon's anatoxin, flocculation, flocculation test
Ramond's point, sign
Ramsay Hunt syndrome — same as *Hunt's syndrome*
Ramsay Hunt paralysis
Ramsbotham's hook, knife, sickle
Ramsden's eyepiece
Ramstedt's operation — same as *Fredet-Ramstedt operation*
Ramstedt's dilator, pyloromyotomy, pyloroplasty
Randall's curet, forceps, plaques, solution
Randolph's cannula, test
Raney's clip, drill, forceps, punch, retractor, rongeur
Raney-Crutchfield tongs
Raney Gigli-saw guide
Ranke's angle, complex, formula, stages
Rankin's clamp, forceps, retractor, tractor
Rankin-Crile forceps

Rankine's scale, thermometer
Ranson's pyridine silver stain
Rantzman's test
Ranvier's constrictions, crosses, internode, membrane, nodes, segment, tactile disks
Ranzewski's clamp
Raoult's law
Rapaport's dilator
Raschkow's plexus
Rasin's sign
Rasmussen's aneurysm, nerve fibers, olivocochlear bundle
Rastelli's operation − to correct cardiac anomalies
Rathbun's syndrome − a congenital deficiency of alkaline phosphatase in the blood, marked by lack of calcification and abnormal cartilage maturation, with the cranial vault being nearly devoid of calcium
Rathke's columns, cysts, duct, folds, pocket, pouch, trabeculae, tumor
Ratliff-Blake forceps
Ratliff-Mayo forceps
Rau's apophysis, process
Rauber's layer, ligament, spinal crest
Rauchfuss's sling, triangle
Rauscher's leukemia virus
Ravich's cystoscope, lithotriptoscope
Ray's angulation method, curet, forceps, mania, speculum
Ray-Parsons-Sunday elevator
Rayer's disease − biliary xanthomatosis
Raygat's test
Raymond's apoplexy, type

Raymond-Céstan syndrome − same as *Céstan-Raymond syndrome*
Raynaud's disease(s) − idiopathic paroxysmal cyanosis of the digits, caused by arterial contraction either from cold or emotional disturbance; paralysis of the throat muscles following parotiditis
Raynaud's gangrene, phenomenon, sign
Rayner-Choyce eye implant
Read's formula
Réaumur's scale, thermometer
Reaves's punch
Rebuck's skin window technique, test
Recamier's curet
Rechcigl-Sidransky hepatoma
Recklinghausen's disease(s) − neurofibromatosis; osteitis with fibrous degeneration and formation of cysts and fibrous nodules on affected bones
Recklinghausen's canals, tonometer, tumor
Recklinghausen-Applebaum disease − hemochromatosis
Reclus's disease(s) − painless, cystic enlargement of the mammary glands; cellulitis with induration
Redlich's encephalitis
Redlich-Fisher miliary plaques
red Robinson catheter
Reed's cells
Reed-Hodgkin disease − same as *Hodgkin's disease*
Reed-Muench method
Reed-Sternberg cells
Reenstierna's antiserum
Rees's test

Rees-Ecker diluting fluid, solution

Reese's syndrome — retinal dysplasia, congenital and always bilateral, usually associated with microphthalmia, cerebral agenesis and other abnormalities

Reese's dermatome, dysplasia, forceps, knife

Refetoff's syndrome — goiter and an elevated serum level of thyroid hormones but without true thyrotoxicosis

Refsum's disease — a hereditary disease of lipid metabolism, characterized by chronic polyneuritis, retinitis, cerebellar ataxia and persistent elevation of protein in the cerebrospinal fluid

Regan's isoenzyme

Regaud's fluid

Regnaud's residual body

Regnoli's operation — excision of the tongue

Rehberg's test

Rehfuss's method, test, tube

Reich-Nechtow clamp, dilator, forceps

Reichel's syndrome — synovial osteochondromatosis

Reichel's cloacal duct

Reichert's syndrome — neuralgia of the glossopharyngeal nerve

Reichert's canal, cartilages, membrane, recess, scar, substance

Reichert-Meissl number

Reichl's test

Reichmann's disease/syndrome — excessive and continuous secretion of gastric juice

Reichmann's rod

Reichstein's substance

Reid's base line

Reid Hunt's reaction, test

Reifenstein's syndrome — a male form of pseudohermaphroditism, marked by ambiguous genitalia or hypospadias and by infertility due to sclerosis of the seminiferous tubules, sometimes accompanied by cryptorchidism and impotence

Reil's ansa, band, insula, island, ribbon, sulcus, triangle, trigone

Reilly's bodies, granulations, phenomenon

Reimann's periodic disease — familial paroxysmal polyserositis

Reinecke's acid

Reiner's curet, knife, rongeur

Reiner-Beck snare

Reiner-Knight forceps

Reinhoff-Finochietto rib spreader

Reinke's crystals, edema

Reinsch's test

Reis-Bücklers disease — annular corneal dystrophy

Reisinger's forceps

Reisseisen's muscles

Reissner's fiber, membrane

Reiswig's reamer

Reiter's disease/syndrome — a triad of urethritis, iridocyclitis and arthritis

Rejchman's disease — same as *Reichmann's disease*

Rekoss's disk

Reliquet's lithotrite

Relton-Hall frame

Remak's band, fibers, ganglion, paralysis, plexus, reflex, sign, symptom, type

Remont's test

Renaut's bodies

Rendu's tremor

Rendu-Osler-Weber disease/syndrome — hereditary hemorrhagic telangiectasia

Renikhet disease — an acute, febrile disease of fowl caused by a paramyxovirus, marked by respiratory and nervous system symptoms. It is transmissible to humans, causing severe but transient conjunctivitis

Rénon-Delille syndrome — thyroovarian insufficiency, hypophyseal hyperfunction and acromegaly, associated with hypotension, tachycardia, hyperhidrosis, oliguria, insomnia and intolerance to heat

Renpenning's syndrome — familial X-linked mental retardation

Renshaw's cells

Renver's funnel

Replogle's tube

Retan's treatment

Retter's needle

Retzius's body, cavity, fibers, foramen, gyrus, lines, space, striae, stripes, veins

Reuber's hepatoma

Reuss's color charts, formula, tables, test

Reuter's button, tube

Reverdin's operation — transplanting an epidermic graft to a defect

Reverdin's graft, method, needle

Revilliod's sign

Revol's disease — same as *Mortensen's disease*

Reye's syndrome — sudden loss of consciousness in children following a premonitory, severe infection, marked by cerebral edema and fatty change in the liver, often followed by death

Reynold's clamp, number, scissors, test, tube

Rezek's forceps

Rhein's picks

Rheinberg's microscope

Rheinhard's myocarditis

Rheinstaedter's curet

Rhese's method

Rhinelander's clamp

Rhoton's punch

Riba's meatotome

Ribas-Torres disease — a mild form of smallpox

Ribbert's theory, thrombosis

Ribbing's syndrome — hereditary multiple diaphyseal sclerosis

Ribble's bandage

Ribes's ganglion

Ricard's amputation

Ricco's law

Richard's forceps

Richards's clamp, nail, prosthesis, screw

Richards-Rundle syndrome — a congenital nervous system disorder marked by progressive sensorineural hearing loss, ataxia, muscle wasting, nystagmus, mental retardation and failure to develop secondary sexual characteristics

Richardson's elevator, retractor, sign, sutures

Richardson-Eastman retractor

Richet's aneurysm, bandage, fascia

Richner-Hanhart syndrome — a familial syndrome consisting

Richner-Hanhart syndrome (*continued*)
of keratosis of the palms and soles, growth retardation and mental retardation, transmitted as a recessive trait

Richter's syndrome — histiocytic lymphoma developing in chronic lymphocytic leukemia

Richter's forceps, hernia, sutures

Richter-Monro line

Rickham's reservoir

Ricord's treatment

Riddoch's syndrome — visual disorientation resulting from unilateral lesions of the parietal lobe

Riddoch's mass reflex

Rideal-Walker coefficient

Ridell's operation — excision of the anterior and inferior walls of the frontal sinus for chronic inflammation

Ridgway's osteogenic sarcoma

Ridley's sinus

Ridlon's knife

Ridpath's curet

Rieckenberg's test

Riecker's bronchoscope

Riedel's disease — a rare, fibrous induration of the thyroid, with adhesion to adjacent structures that may cause tracheal compression

Riedel's lobe, struma, thyroiditis

Rieder's cell, cell leukemia, lymphocyte, paralysis

Riegel's pulse, symptoms, test

Rieger's syndrome — iridocorneal mesodermal dysgenesis

Rieger's anomaly, malformation, phenomenon

Riegler's test

Riehl's melanosis

Rienhoff's dissector, forceps

Riesman's pneumonia, sign

Rietti-Greppi-Micheli syndrome — hemolytic jaundice, with increased red cell fragility

Rieux's hernia

Rifkind's sign

Riga's aphthae, papilloma

Riga-Fede disease — granuloma of the lingual frenum in children that occurs after abrasion by the lower central incisors

Rigal's sutures

Rigaud's operation — a plastic operation for urethral fistula

Rigby's retractor

Riggs's disease — compound periodontitis

Riley's needle

Riley-Day syndrome — familial dysfunction of the autonomic nervous system

Riley-Shwachman syndrome — osseous changes and hyperreflexia, with a peculiar gait marked by stiff legs, ankle clonus and calcaneal limp

Riley-Smith syndrome — macrocephaly without hydrocephalus

Rimbaud-Passouant-Vallat syndrome — febrile encephalitis with coma, convulsions, hemiplegia, headache, vertigo, Cheyne-Stokes respiration and deglutition disorders

Rimini's test

Rindfleisch's cells, folds

Ringenberg's electrode

Ringer's injection, irrigation, lactate, mixture, solution

Rinne's test

Rio-Hortega method
Riolan's anastomosis, arch, bone, muscle, nosegay, ossicles
Ripault's sign
Risdon's approach, incision, wire
Rish's chisel, knife
Risley's prism
Ritchie's formol-ether method, tenaculum
Ritgen's maneuver, method
Ritisch's sutures
Ritter's disease — exfoliative dermatitis supervening in bullous impetigo of the neonate
Ritter's dermatitis, dilator, fiber, forceps, law, rasp, sound, tetanus
Ritter-Rollet phenomenon, sign
Ritter-Valli law
Riva-Rocci sphygmomanometer
Rivalta's reaction, test
Riverius's alum curd, draft
Rivers's cocktail
Rivière's potion
Riviere's sign
Rivinus's canals, ducts, foramen, gland, incisure, notch, segment
Rizzo's retractor
Rizzoli's osteoclast
Rizzuti's lens expressor, retractor
Rizzuti-McGuire scissors
Roaf's syndrome — a nonhereditary craniofacial-skeletal disorder marked by early retinal detachment, cataracts, myopia, shortened long bones and mental retardation
Roaf's method
Robb's cannula, forceps, syringe
Robert's syndrome — a hereditary syndrome marked by defective development of the long

Robert's syndrome (*continued*)
bones and cleft palate and other anomalies
Robert's ligament, pelvis
Robert Jones dressing
Roberts's applicator, esophagoscope, forceps, laryngoscope, speculum, test
Roberts-Nelson rib shears, tourniquet
Robertson's syndrome — a symptom of neurosyphilis, especially tabes dorsalis, and of other diseases of the central nervous system
Robertson's culture medium, pupil, sign
Robin's syndrome — same as *Pierre Robin syndrome*
Robin's spaces
Robinow's syndrome — dwarfism associated with malaligned teeth, bulging forehead, depressed nasal bridge and short limbs. Called also *Robinow's dwarfism*
Robinson's disease — cystic neoplasms of the sweat glands occurring on the face in the region of the eyes
Robinson's catheter, circle, stone basket
Robinson-Cohen slide
Robinson-Kepler test
Robinson-Kepler-Power water test
Robison's ester, ester degeneration, ester dehydrogenase
Robles's disease — infestation by worms of the genus *Onchocerca*
Robles's fever
Robson's line, point, position

Roch's lipomatosis
Roche's sign
Rochester's awl, forceps, syringe, tube
Rochester-Carmalt forceps
Rochester-Ewald forceps
Rochester-Ferguson retractor, scissors
Rochester-Harrington forceps
Rochester-Mixter forceps
Rochester-Ochsner forceps
Rochester-Péan forceps
Rochester-Rankin forceps
Rochet's procedure
Rockey's cannula, endoscope, forceps, probe
Rockley's sign
Rocky-Davis incision
Rodman's incision
Rodrigues's aneurysm
Rodriguez-Alvarez catheter
Roe's clamp, solution
Roeder's clamp, forceps, treatment
Roemheld's syndrome — cardiac and gastrointestinal symptoms in excitable persons, most frequently in patients with thyroid disorders
Roffo's test
Roger's disease — ventricular septal defect
Roger's syndrome — continuous excessive secretion of saliva as a result of esophageal carcinoma
Roger's amputation, bruit, dissector, murmur, reaction, reflex, symptom, test
Roger Anderson apparatus
Roger-Josué test
Roger's sphygmomanometer
Rogor-Foot modification of Bielschowsky technique

Röhl's marginal corpuscles
Rohon-Beard cells
Rohr's agranulocytosis, layer, stria
Röhrer's index
Roida's tube
Rokitansky's disease — acute yellow atrophy of the liver
Rokitansky's acute yellow atrophy, diverticulum, hernia, kidney, pelvis
Rokitansky-Aschoff ducts, sinuses
Rokitansky-Cushing ulcers
Rokitansky-Küster-Hauser syndrome — same as *Mayer-Rokitansky-Küster syndrome*
Rolando's angle, area, cells, column, fasciculus, fibers, fissure, funiculus, line, point, substance, tubercle, zone
Rolf's forceps, lance
Roller's nucleus
Rolleston's rule
Rollet's syndrome — sensorimotor ophthalmoplegia and optic atrophy, produced by lesions of the apex of the orbit involving the third, fourth and sixth cranial nerves
Rollet's chancre, incision, irrigator, retractor, stroma
Rollier's formula, radiation, treatment
Romaña's sign
Romano-Ward syndrome — prolonged Q-R interval (atrial activity) in children subject to attacks of unconsciousness resulting from *Adams-Stokes seizures* and ventricular fibrillation
Romanovsky's (Romanowsky's) method, stain

Romberg's disease/syndrome — facial hemiatrophy

Romberg's hemiatrophy, sign, spasm, station, test, trophoneurosis

Romberg-Howship sign, symptom

Römer's reaction, test

Rommel-Hildreth cautery

Rommelaere's sign

Ronchese's test

Rönne's nasal step

Roos's osteotome, retractor

Roper's cannula

Roques's syndrome — parallel sclerosis of the heart and lungs in chronic cor pulmonale in aged patients

Rorschach test

Rosa's law

Rose's operation — removal of the trigeminal ganglion

Rose's position, test, tetanus

Rose-Bradford kidney

Rose-Thompson cleft lip repair

Rose-Waaler test

Rosen's curet, incision, neuralgia, probe, tube

Rosen-Castleman-Liebow syndrome — pulmonary proteinosis

Rosenbach's disease — a skin disease affecting persons coming in contact with meat or dead animals

Rosenbach's syndrome — association of paroxysmal tachycardia with cardiac, gastric and respiratory disturbances

Rosenbach's reaction, sign, test, tuberculin

Rosenbach-Gmelin test

Rosenfield's nomenclature

Rosenheim-Drummond's method, test

Rosenmüller's body, cavity, fossa, gland, node, organ, recess, valve

Rosenow's veal brain broth

Rosenthal's syndrome(s) — hereditary tendency to hemorrhage, resembling hemophilia but caused by plasma thromboplastin deficiency; paralysis on awakening, with inability to move although fully conscious

Rosenthal's canal, degeneration, test, vein

Rosenthal-Kloepfer syndrome — corneal opacities and acromegaloid appearance, with enlargement and thickening of the skin of the scalp so that it lies in folds

Rosenthaler's reagent

Roser's line, mouth gag, sign

Roser-Braun sign

Rosewater's syndrome — a mild form of male familial hypogonadism

Rosi's prosthesis

Rosin's test

Ross's black spores, bodies, catheter, cycle, retractor

Ross-Jones test

Rossbach's disease — hyperchlorhydria

Rossel's test

Rosser's hook

Rössle-Urbach-Wiethe lipoproteinosis

Rossolimo's reflex, sign

Rostan's asthma, shunt

Rot's disease — same as *Rot-Bernhardt disease*

Rot's meralgia

Rot-Bernhardt disease — a condition marked by paresthesia, pain and numbness of the thigh in the region supplied by the lateral femoral cutaneous nerve

Rot-Bielschowsky syndrome — paralysis of the conjugate gaze in one direction

Rotch's sign

Roth's disease — same as *Rot-Bernhardt disease*

Roth's spots

Roth-Bernhardt disease — same as *Rot-Bernhardt disease*

Rothera's test

Rothmann-Makai syndrome — idiopathic circumscribed panniculitis

Rothmund's syndrome — congenital cutaneous dystrophy

Rothmund's dystrophy

Rothmund-Thomson syndrome — a hereditary syndrome marked by poikiloderma and telangiectasia, associated with cataracts, bone defects and hypogonadism

Rothschild's sign

Rotor's syndrome — chronic familial nonhemolytic jaundice

Rotter's nodes, test

Rotter-Erb syndrome — deformities of the bones, joints and tendons, marked by dwarfism, multiple epiphyseal lesions, multiple dislocations, bilateral clubfoot, vertebral deformities and cleft palate

Rouget's bulb, cells, muscle, pericyte

Rougnon-Heberden disease — angina pectoris

Rous-associated virus (RAV)

Rous's sarcoma, test

Roussel's law, sign

Rousselot's caustic

Roussin's test

Roussy-Cornil syndrome — progressive hypertrophic neuritis

Roussy-Déjérine syndrome — same as *Déjérine-Roussy syndrome*

Roussy-Lévy disease — familial ataxia marked by disorders of gait, clubfoot and lack of tendon reflexes

Roussy-Lévy syndrome — same as *Lévy-Roussy syndrome*

Routier's operation — for Dupuytren's contracture

Routte's operation — suturing the saphenous vein so it will open into the peritoneal cavity in order to drain the cavity in cases of ascites with cirrhosis of the liver

Roux's anastomosis, serum

Roux-en-Y anastomosis, incision

Rovighi's sign

Rovsing's syndrome — horseshoe kidney with nausea, abdominal discomfort and pain

Rovsing's sign

Rowland's forceps, keratome, osteotome

Rowley-Rosenberg syndrome — growth retardation, renal aminoaciduria, cor pulmonale and muscular hypoplasia, associated with alveolar hypoventilation, atelectasis and

Rowley-Rosenberg syndrome
(*continued*)
right ventricular hypertrophy
—a familial disorder that has
been observed in the children
of consanguineous parents
Rowntree-Geraghty test
Royce's knife, perforator
Royer's syndrome — association
of diabetes mellitus with
hypogenital dystrophy
Rubin's test
Rubin-Brandborg tube
Rubin-Holth punch
Rubino's reaction, test
Rubins's cannula, needle, test,
tube
Rubinstein's syndrome — a congenital syndrome marked by
mental and motor retardation,
short stature, characteristic
facies, various ocular anomalies, pulmonary stenosis,
keloid formation and abnormalities of the vertebrae and
sternum
Rubinstein-Taybi syndrome —
same as *Rubinstein's syndrome*
Rubner's law, test
Rubovits's clamp
Ruck's watery extract tuberculin
Rud's syndrome — a hereditary
syndrome transmitted as an
autosomal trait, marked by
mental deficiency, epilepsy,
infantilism and congenital
ichthyosis
Ruffini's brushes, corpuscles,
cylinders, organ
Rugby's forceps
Ruge's solution
Ruge-Phillipp test
Ruggeri's reflex, sign

Ruhemann's test, uricometer,
uricometer method
Ruhr's rheumatism
Rulf's convulsions
Rumel's clamp, forceps, splint,
tourniquet
Rumel-Belmont tourniquet
Rummo's disease — downward
displacement of the heart
Rumpel-Leede phenomenon,
sign, test
Rumpf's sign, symptom, traumatic
reaction
Rundles-Falls syndrome — familial
hypochromic microcytic
anemia with erythrocyte
abnormalities, splenomegaly
and sometimes hepatomegaly,
affecting only males
Runeberg's anemia, formula, type
Rusch's catheter, laryngoscope
Rusch-Foley catheter
Ruschelit's bougie, catheter
Rusconi's anus
Rush's clamp, extractor, mallet,
nail, rod
Rushkin's balloon
Ruskin's forceps, rongeur, trocar
Ruskin-Liston forceps
Russe's incision
Russell's syndrome(s) — congenital
dwarfism with short stature,
disproportionately short arms,
cryptorchidism and other
abnormalities; emaciation in
infancy and childhood, caused
by a diencephalic tumor and
associated with initial growth
acceleration, locomotor hyper-
activity, euphoria and pallor
Russell's bodies, double sugar agar,
dwarf, effect, traction, viper,
viper venom

Russell-Buck tractor
Russo's reaction, test
Rust's disease — tuberculous spondylitis of the cervical vertebrae
Rust's syndrome — stiff neck and head with necessity for holding the head with both hands in lying down or rising up—a disorder occurring in tuberculosis, cancer, fracture of the spine, rheumatic or arthritic disease or syphilitic periostitis
Rust's phenomenon, sign
Rustitskii's disease — same as *Kahler's disease*

Rutherford's atom, method
Rutherfurd's syndrome — a familial oculodental disorder of corneal dystrophy, gingival hypertrophy and failure of tooth eruption
Ruttan-Hardisty test
Ruysch's disease — same as *Hirschsprung's disease*
Ruysch's glomeruli, membrane, muscle, tube, tunic, veins
Ryerson's tenotome
Ryle's tube
Rytz's test

S

Saalfield's extractor
Saathoff's test
Sabin's megaloblast, vaccine
Sabin-Feldman syndrome — chorioretinitis and cerebral calcifications—symptoms like those of toxoplasmosis but with negative tests for toxoplasmosis
Sabin-Feldman dye test
Sabouraud's syndrome — a hereditary, congenital disease causing beadlike enlargement and brittleness of hair
Sabouraud's agar, pastille
Sachs's disease — same as *Tay-Sachs disease*
Sachs's antigen, bur, spatula, tube
Sachs-Georgi reaction, test
Sachs-Witebsky reaction, test
Sachsse's test

Saemisch's operation — transfixion of the cornea for cure of accumulation of pus in the eye
Saemisch's section, ulcer
Saenger's macula, reflex, sign, sutures
Saethre-Chotzen syndrome — same as *Chotzen's syndrome*
Safar's bronchoscope
Sage's snare
Sagnac's rays
Sahli's method, reaction, reagent, test
Sahli-Nencki test
St. Agatha's disease — mastitis
St. Anthony's disease — chorea
St. Anthony's dance, fire
St. Appolonia's disease — toothache
St. Avertin's disease — epilepsy

St. Avidus's disease — deafness
St. Blasius's disease — peritonsillar abscess
St. Clair–Thompson curet, forceps
St. Dymphna's disease — insanity
St. Erasmus's disease — colic
St. Fiacre's disease — hemorrhoids
St. Francis's fire
St. Gervasius's disease — rheumatism
St. Gotthard's tunnel disease — hookworm
St. Guy's dance
St. Hubert's disease — rabies
St. Job's disease — syphilis
St. John's dance, evil
St. Luke's retractor, rongeur
St. Main's evil
St. Marks's incision
St. Martin's evil
St. Mathurin's disease — idiocy
St. Modestus's disease — chorea
St. Roch's disease — plague
St. Sement's disease — syphilis
St. Valentine's disease — epilepsy
St. Vitus's dance
St. Zachary's disease — mutism
Saint's triad
Sakaguchi's test
Sakamoto's disease — infantile diarrhea marked by explosive vomiting, milky stools and mild respiratory symptoms, occurring in epidemic form in Japan
Sala's cells
Salah's needle
Salem's sump, tube
Salibi's clamp
Salisbury-Melvin sign
Salk's vaccine
Salkowski's method, test
Salkowski-Arnstein method

Salkowski-Autenrieth-Barth method
Salkowski-Ludwig test
Salkowski-Schipper test
Salmon's catheter
Salomon's test
Salter's incremental lines
Saltzman's method
Salus's arch
Salvatore-Maloney tracheotome
Salvioli's syndrome — a familial syndrome involving the autonomic nervous system, bones, endocrine glands and phosphorus metabolism, causing tremor, chorea, mental disorders, gynecomastia, hypergenitalism and muscular atrophy
Salzmann's nodular corneal dystrophy
Sam Roberts esophagoscope, forceps, laryngoscope
Sampson's cyst, nail, prosthesis
Samuel's position
Sanarelli's serum
Sanarelli-Shwartzman phenomenon
Sanchez Salorio's syndrome — retinal pigmentary dystrophy and cataract, with mental and physical retardation
Sander's disease — a form of paranoia
Sanders's disease — epidemic keratoconjunctivitis
Sanders's bed, forceps, incision, laryngoscope
Sanders-Brown-Shaw needle
Sanderson's polsters
Sandhoff's disease — a form of Tay-Sachs disease marked by a more rapid course

Sandström's bodies, glands
Sandwith's bald tongue
Sanfilippo's syndrome — a form of mucopolysaccharidosis resembling *Hurler's syndrome* but with less severe effects
Sanford's test
Sanger-Brown ataxia
Sansom's sign
Sanson's images
Sansregret modification of Chaussé III method
Santorini's canal, cartilage, caruncle, duct, fissure, ligament, muscle, papilla, parietal vein, plexus, tubercle
Santulli's clamp
Santy's forceps
Sanyal's conjunctivitis
Sappey's fibers, ligament, nucleus, subareolar plexus, veins
Sarbó's sign
Sarmiento's cast
Sarnoff's clamp
Sarns's saw
Sarot's clamp, forceps, thoracoscope
Sarrouy's disease — anemia associated with retarded growth, hepatosplenomegaly, hepatosplenic hematopoiesis, bone marrow hypoplasia and, usually, terminal marasmus
Satinsky's clamp, forceps, scissors
Sato's knife
Satterlee's saw
Satterthwaite's method
Sattler's layer, veil
Satvioni's cryptoscope
Sauer's debrider, forceps, tonsillectome, vaccine
Sauer-Sluder tonsillectome

Sauerbruch's cabinet, prosthesis
Sauerbruch-Coryllos rib shears
Sauerbruch-Lebsche rongeur
Sauerbruch-Zukschwerdt retractor
Saundby's test
Saunders's disease — a dangerous condition of infants with digestive disturbances caused by excessive intake of carbohydrates. It is marked by vomiting, cerebral symptoms and depression of circulation
Saunders's sign
Saunders-Paparella hook, needle, rasp
Saunders-Sutton syndrome — delirium tremens
Saussure's hygrometer
Sauvage's graft, prosthesis
Savill's disease — an acute, infectious disease of unknown cause, marked by vesicular dermatitis followed by desquamation and bodily symptoms of varying severity
Sawtell's applicator, forceps, retractor
Sawtell-Davis forceps, hemostat
Sawyer's retractor
Saxtorph's maneuver
Sayre's operation — application of a plaster-of-Paris jacket for treatment of spondylitis and Pott's disease
Sayre's apparatus, bandage, jacket, splint
Sbarbaro's prosthesis
Scanzoni's operation — forceps rotation of the fetal head in the posterior position of the occiput
Scanzoni's maneuver

Scardino's ureteropelvioplasty

Scarpa's operation — ligation of the femoral artery in Scarpa's triangle

Scarpa's fascia, fluid, foramen, fossa, ganglion, hiatus, ligament, liquor, membrane, nerve, sheath, shoe, staphyloma, triangle

Sceleth's treatment

Schacher's ganglion

Schachowa's spiral tubes

Schaedler's medium

Schaeffer's curet

Schaer's reagent

Schafer's syndrome — a rare, hereditary, congenital disorder marked by gross thickening of the nails, hyperkeratosis of the palms, soles and knees, leukoplakia of the oral mucosa and mental and physical retardation. Called also *Jadassohn-Lewandowsky syndrome*

Schäfer's dumbbell, method

Schäffer's reflex, test

Schalfijew's test

Schall's tube

Schällibaum's solution

Schalm's test

Schamberg's disease — progressive pigmentary dermatosis

Schamberg's dermatosis, extractor

Schanz's disease — traumatic inflammation of Achilles tendon

Schanz's syndrome — weakness of the spinal musculature, marked by fatigue, pain on pressure and a tendency to curvature of the spine

Schanz's brace

Schardinger's enzyme, reaction

Schatz's maneuver

Schatzki's ring

Schaudinn's fluid

Schaumann's disease/syndrome — sarcoidosis

Schaumann's benign lymphogranuloma, bodies, sarcoid, sarcoidosis

Schauta's operation — vaginal hysterectomy for cancer of the cervix uteri

Schauta-Wertheim operation — same as *Wertheim-Schauta operation*

Schede's operation(s) — resection of the thorax for empyema; for varicose veins of leg; excision of the necrosed part of a bone

Schede's clot, method, resection, treatment

Scheibe's deafness

Scheibler's reagent

Scheie's disease — an autosomal recessive condition associated with normal or slightly reduced intellect and stature, with marked hirsutism, broad mouth, retinitis pigmentosa, corneal clouding and joint stiffness

Scheie's operation(s) — scleral cauterization with iridectomy for glaucoma; a technique for needling and aspiration of cataract

Scheie's syndrome — a rare, hereditary mucopolysaccharidosis similar to *Hurler's syndrome* but without mental retardation

Scheiner's experiment

Scheinmann's forceps
Schellong-Strisower phenomenon
Schemm's diet
Schenck's disease — sporotrichosis
Schepelmann's sign
Scherer's method, test
Scheuermann's disease — osteochondrosis of the vertebral epiphyses in youth
Scheuermann's kyphosis
Scheuthauer-Marie-Sainton syndrome — hereditary cleidocranial dysostosis
Schick's reaction, sign, test
Schiefferdecker's disks, symbiosis, theory
Schiemann's selective agar
Schiff's biliary cycle, reaction, reagent, test
Schilder's disease — a subacute or chronic form of leukoencephalopathy of children and adolescents. Its symptoms include blindness, deafness and progressive mental deterioration
Schilder's encephalitis
Schilder-Foix disease — intracerebral symmetrical centrolobar sclerosis
Schiller's iodine, test
Schilling's blood count, leukemia, test
Schimmelbusch's disease — cystic disease of the breast
Schindler's esophagoscope, gastroscope
Schiøtz's tonometer
Schirmer's syndrome — an incomplete form of *Sturge-Kalischer-Weber syndrome,* consisting of angiomas of the face and choroid only, with early appearance of glaucoma

Schirmer's test
Schlange's sign
Schlatter's disease — same as *Osgood-Schlatter disease*
Schlatter's operation — total excision of the stomach for cancer
Schlatter's sprain
Schlatter-Osgood disease — same as *Osgood-Schlatter disease*
Schlein's arthroplasty
Schlemm's canal, ligaments
Schlesinger's phenomenon, sign, test
Schlichting's dystrophy
Schlicter's test
Schloffer's tumor
Schlösser's injection, method, treatment
Schlossmann's method
Schmalz's operation — introducing a thread into the lacrimal duct for cure of stricture
Schmeden's punch, scissors
Schmid-Fraccaro syndrome — congenital clefts of the iris, anal atresia and other malformations. Called also *cat's eye syndrome*
Schmidel's anastomosis
Schmidt's syndrome(s) — unilateral paralysis affecting the vocal cords, the trapezius, and the sternocleidomastoid muscles; an association of thyroid and adrenocortical insufficiency
Schmidt's diet, fibrinoplastin, keratitis, node, test
Schmidt-Lantermann clefts, incisures, segment
Schmidt-Strassburger diet
Schmiedel's ganglion

Schmieden's disease — prolapse of the gastric mucosa into the duodenum

Schmincke's tumor

Schmitt's disease — a lesion of the spinous process of the first thoracic vertebra, with displacement of the apophysis, caused by overstraining

Schmitz's bacillus

Schmorl's disease — herniation of the nucleus pulposus into an adjacent ventral body

Schmorl's bacillus, body, jaundice, method, nodes, nodule, stain

Schmutz's pyorrhea

Schnabel's atrophy, caverns

Schneider's disease — a viral infection that occurs in spring and fall, marked by sudden high fever, chills, nasopharyngitis, arthralgia, malaise, vomiting and headache, often followed by involvement of the central nervous system

Schneider's carmine, indicator, nail, rod

Schnidt's forceps

Schnyder's dystrophy

Schobinger's incision

Schöbl's scleritis

Schoemaker's anastomosis, clamp, gastrectomy, line

Schoenberg's forceps

Scholl's knife, solution

Scholz's disease — a familial leukoencephalopathy marked by demyelination of the cerebral white matter, sensory aphasia, cortical blindness, deafness, spasticity, paralysis and dementia

Schön's theory

Schönbein's operation — staphyloplasty that results in shutting off the nose from the mouth

Schönbein's reaction, test

Schönenberg's syndrome — dwarfism, congenital blepharoptosis, congenital heart defects and mental retardation

Schönlein's disease — same as *Schönlein-Henoch disease*

Schönlein's purpura

Schönlein-Henoch disease — a form of purpura, occurring chiefly in children, due to a vasculitis of unknown cause and marked by urticaria, erythema, arthropathy and renal disturbance

Schönlein-Henoch purpura

Schopfer's test

Schott's bath, treatment

Schottmüller's disease — a general term used for infections caused by *Salmonella* of all groups except *S. typhosa*

Schramm's phenomenon

Schreger's bands, lines, striae

Schreiber's maneuver

Schridde's disease — congenital, generalized dropsy

Schridde's granules

Schroeder's disease — a condition probably caused by deficiency of gonadotropic hormone, marked by hypertrophic endometrium and excessive uterine bleeding

Schroeder's syndrome — high blood pressure, with notable gain in weight, from overactivity of the adrenal glands

Schroeder's curet, forceps, scissors, test
Schroeder-Braun forceps
Schroeder van der Kolk's law
Schroetter's chorea
Schrön's granule
Schrön-Much granules
Schroth's treatment
Schrötter's catheter, chorea
Schubert's forceps, punch
Schubert-Dannmeyer test
Schuchardt's incision
Schüffner's dots, granules, punctuation, stippling
Schuknecht's chisel, excavator, gouge, prosthesis, scissors, speculum
Schüle's sign
Schüller's disease — same as *Hand-Schüller-Christian disease*
Schüller's ducts, glands, method, phenomenon, position
Schüller-Christian disease — same as *Hand-Schüller-Christian disease*
Schulte's test, valve
Schultz's disease — drug-allergic agranulocytosis
Schultz's syndrome — malignant leukopenia
Schultz's angina, method, triad
Schültz-Charlton phenomenon, reaction, test
Schultz-Dale reaction
Schultze's acroparesthesia, bundle, cells, fasciculus, fold, phenomenon, placenta, sign, test, tract, type
Schultze-Chvostek's sign
Schumann's rays
Schumm's test

Schürmann's test
Schütz's bundle, law, micrococcus, rule
Schütz-Borissov law, rule
Schwabach's test
Schwachman's syndrome — primary pancreatic insufficiency with bone-marrow failure
Schwachman-Diamond syndrome — same as *Schwachman's syndrome*
Schwalbe's amygdaloid tubercle, corpuscles, foramen, fissure, line, nucleus, ring, sheath, space
Schwann's cell, cell tumor, membrane, myelin, neurilemma, nucleus, sheath, substance
Schwartz's syndrome — a congenital hereditary disorder marked by myotonic myopathy, dystrophy of epiphyseal cartilage, joint contracture and decrease in the palpebral aperture
Schwartz's leukemia virus, test
Schwartz-Bartter syndrome — inappropriate secretion of antidiuretic hormone
Schwartz-Kerrison rongeur
Schwartz-McNeil test
Schwarz's test
Schweigger's forceps
Schweigger-Seidel sheath
Schweitzer's reagent
Schweizer's forceps
Schweninger's method
Schweninger-Buzzi macular atrophy
Scivoletto's test
Sclavo's serum
Scobee-Allis forceps

Scott's cannula, resectoscope, splint, tube

Scott-Wilson method, reagent

Scoville's curet, forceps, needle, trephine

Scoville-Greenwood forceps

Scoville-Lewis clip

Scribner's shunt

Scriver-Goldbloom-Roy syndrome — a disorder of amino acid metabolism arising from disturbance of renal tubular transport

Scudder's clamp, forceps

Scully's tumor

Scultetus's bandage, binder, dressing, position

Searcy's erysiphake, forceps, tonsillectome, trephine

Sebileau's bands, hollow

Seckel's syndrome — dwarfism marked by small head, narrow birdlike face with a beaklike nose, large eyes and receding lower jaw

Seckel's bird-headed dwarf

Secretan's disease — post-traumatic hard edema of the dorsum of the hand or foot resulting in restriction of digital flexion

Sédillot's operation(s) — correction of a midline cleft in the uvula and soft palate; flap operation for restoring the upper lip

Sédillot's syndrome — changes in the genitalia associated with psychoneurotic disturbances thought to arise from contraception or masturbation

Sédillot's elevator, raspatory

Sedlinger's needle

Seeligmüller's neuralgia, sign

Seessel's pocket, pouch

Séglas's type

Segond's forceps, spatula

Séguin's sign, signal symptom

Sehrt's clamp, compressor

Seibert's tuberculin

Seidel's scotoma, sign, test

Seidelin's bodies

Seidlitz's powder test, powders

Seidlmayer's syndrome — postinfectious purpura of infancy and childhood, marked by elevated lesions

Seifert's reaction

Seiffert's forceps, punch

Seignette's salt

Seiler's knife, scissors

Seitelberger's disease — infantile neuroaxonal dystrophy

Seitz's filter, metamorphosing respiration, sign

Seldinger's technique

Seletz's cannula, catheter, forceps, punch

Seletz-Gelpi retractor

Selivanoff's (Seliwanow's) reaction, test

Selker's reservoir

Sellards's test

Seller's stain

Sellor's clamp, knife, valvulotome

Selman's clamp, forceps

Selter's disease — acrodynia

Selter's tuberculin

Selverstone's clamp, hook, rongeur

Selye's syndrome — the aggregate of all systemic reactions of the body to long-continued exposure to stress. Called also *general adaptation syndrome*

Semb's operation — causing the apex of the lung to collapse for pulmonary tuberculosis

Semb's forceps, retractor, shears
Semb-Sauerbruch rongeur
Semken's forceps
Semon's law, sign
Semon-Hering hypothesis, theory
Semon-Rosenbach law
Semple's treatment, vaccine
Semunya virus
Sen's syndrome — infantile cirrhosis of the liver
Sendai virus
Senear-Usher syndrome — an eruption of scaling erythematous macules, involving the scalp, face and trunk
Sengstaken's balloon, tube
Sengstaken-Blakemore tube
Senn's operation — intestinal anastomosis
Senn's bone plates
Senn-Dingman retractor
Senning's clamp
Senturia's forceps, retractor, speculum
Serature's clip
Sergent's white adrenal line
Serre's operation — correction of skin contractures that distort the angle of the mouth, which involves switching of a skin and subcutaneous tissue flap from one lip to another
Serres's angle, glands
Sertoli-cell-only syndrome — same as *del Castillo's syndrome*
Sertoli's cell tumor, cells, column
Sertoli-Leydig cell tumor
Setchenow's (Sechenoff's) centers, nuclei
Settegast's method
Seutin's bandage
Sever's disease — inflammation of the cartilage of the heel

Sewall's cannula, forceps, trocar
Sexton's knife
Seyderhelm's solution
Sézary's reticulosis syndrome — generalized exfoliative erythroderma caused by cutaneous infiltration by reticular lymphocytes
Sézary's cell, erythroderma, reticulosis
Sforzini's syndrome — a hereditary familial form of exophthalmos not associated with metabolic or endocrine disorders
Shaaf's forceps
Shaeffer's spore stain
Shäfer's syndrome — congenital dyskeratosis
Shaffer's method
Shaffer-Hartmann method
Shaffer-Marriott method
Shaldon's tube
Shallcross's forceps, hemostat
Shambaugh's adenotome, elevator, incision, retractor
Shambaugh-Derlacki chisel, elevator, microscope
Shambaugh-Lempert knife
Shantz's osteotomy
Shapleigh's curet
Sharpey's fibers
Shattock's disease — granuloma caused by foreign-body reaction to implanted silica particles
Shaver's syndrome — bauxite worker's disease, causing interstitial pulmonary fibrosis accompanied by emphysema and pneumothorax
Shay's leukemia, ulcer
Shea's bur, drill, incision, stapedectomy, tube

Shea-Anthony antral balloon

Shear's test

Shearer's forceps, retractor, rongeur

Sheehan's syndrome — postpartum pituitary necrosis

Sheehan's chisel, osteotome, retractor

Sheehy's syndrome — rapidly advancing sensorineural hearing loss in children

Sheehy's forceps, knife, tube

Sheehy-House prosthesis

Shekelton's aneurysm

Sheldon's necrotic purpura

Sheldon-Pudenz dissector, tube

Sheldon-Spatz needle

Sheldon-Swann needle

Shenton's arch, line

Shepard's tube

Shepherd's fracture

Sherman's plate, unit

Sherman-Bourquin unit of vitamin B$_2$

Sherman-Munsell unit of vitamin A

Sherrington's law, phenomenon

Shibley's sign

Shichito disease — scrub typhus

Shier's prosthesis

Shiga's bacillus, toxin

Shiga-Kruse disease — bacillary dysentery

Shiley's shunt, tube

Shiley-Bjork tube

Shiner's tube

Shirodkar's cerclage, needle, procedure

Shirodkar-Page cerclage

Shoemaker's clamp, shears

Shoepinger's incision

Shohl's solution

Shohl-Pedley method

Shone's syndrome — diversion of the tendinous cords of the atrioventricular valves into one papillary muscle instead of two

Shope's fibroma, papilloma

Shorr's stain

Shortbent's scissors

Shrady's saw

Shrapnell's membrane

Shubich-Spatz Bismarck brown stain

Shurly's retractor

Shuster's forceps

Shwartzman's phenomenon, reaction

Shy-Drager syndrome — a progressive encephalomyelopathy involving the autonomic nervous system, marked by atrophy of the iris, incontinence, impotence, tremor and wasting of muscle

Shy-Magee disease — a benign, congenital disease of muscle marked by intramuscular rodlike structures

Sibson's aponeurosis, fascia, furrow, groove, notch, vestibule

Sicar's sign

Sicard's syndrome — same as *Collet-Sicard syndrome*

Sicard-Cantelouble test

Sichel's disease — a type of pseudoptosis, with a fold of skin hanging from the upper lid margin

Sichel's ptosis

Sidler-Huguenin's endothelioma

Siebold's operation — surgical separation of the pubic bone lateral to the median line

Siebold-Bradbury test

Siegert's sign
Siegle's otoscope
Siegrist's spots, streaks
Siegrist-Hutchinson syndrome — post-traumatic chorioretinopathy marked by extreme dilatation of the pupil, macular disorders, choroid rupture, or atrophy of the optic nerve
Siemens's syndrome — a familial type of keratosis involving the face, neck, forearms and backs of the hands
Siemens's dermatosis
Siemens-Bloch pigmented dermatosis
Siemens-Halske cell
Siemerling's nucleus
Sierra-Sheldon tracheotome
Sieur's sign, test
Siffert's method
Sigmund's glands
Signorelli's sign
Sigualt's symphysiotomy
Siker's laryngoscope
Silex's sign
Silver's syndrome — a congenital syndrome marked by low birth weight, short stature, lateral asymmetry, syndactyly, triangular-shaped face and precocious puberty
Silver's bunionectomy, dwarf, osteotome
Silverman's disease — an abnormality of the sternum, marked by pigeon breast
Silverman's needle
Silverskiöld's syndrome — a form of osteochondrodystrophy with slight vertebral changes but curved long bones of the extremities

Silvester's method
Silvestrini-Corda syndrome — failure of the liver to inactivate estrogens, marked by eunuchoid body, atrophy of the testes, defective libido and sterility
Silvestroni-Bianco syndrome — constitutional microcytic anemia
Simmerlin's dystrophy, type
Simmonds's disease — panhypopituitarism
Simmonds's cachexia
Simmons's citrate agar
Simon's dermatome, foci, incision, position, septic factor, sign, speculum, sutures, symptom
Simonart's bands, thread
Simonelli's test
Simons's disease — progressive disappearance of subcutaneous fat above the pelvis, facial emaciation and abnormal deposition of fat about the thighs and buttocks. Also called *lipodystrophy*
Simonsen's phenomenon
Simpson's syndrome — adipose gynandrism affecting either sex
Simpson's forceps, lamp, light, splint
Simpson-Luikart forceps
Sims's position, speculum, suture, test
Singleton's incision
Singley's clamp, forceps
Sinkler's phenomenon
Sipple's syndrome — a hereditary association of pheochromocytoma with medullary thyroid carcinoma

Sippy's diet, method, powder, treatment

Sisto's sign

Sistrunk's operation — removal of thyroglossal cysts and sinuses

Sistrunk's retractor, scissors

Sivash's prosthesis

Sjögren's syndrome — a symptom complex of unknown cause occurring chiefly in older women, marked by keratoconjunctivitis and enlargement of the parotid gland. It is often associated with rheumatoid arthritis and sometimes with systemic lupus erythematosus. Called also *Gougerot-Nulock-Houwer syndrome*

Sjögren-Larsson syndrome — congenital erythroderma in association with mental deficiency and spastic disorders

Sjöqvist's method

Skeele's curet

Skeer's sign, symptom

Skene's catheter, ducts, glands, tubules

Skevas-Zerfus disease — a condition occurring principally among sponge divers who come in contact with the stinging tentacles of sea anemones that are often attached to the base of sponges

Skillern's cannula, forceps, fracture

Skillman's forceps

Skinner's box, line

Skirrow's medium

Sklar-Schiøtz tonometer

Sklowsky's symptom

Skoda's sign, tympany

Slaughter's saw

Slavianski's membrane

Sloan's dissector, incision

Slocum's splint

Slocumb's syndrome — acute disseminated rheumatoid arthritis

Sluder's disease — neuralgia of the sphenopalatine ganglia, causing burning maxillary pain with radiation into the neck and shoulder

Sluder's operation — removal of the tonsil and its capsule

Sluder's guillotine, method, neuralgia, tonsillectome, tonsillectomy

Sluder-Ballenger tonsillectome

Sluder-Demarest tonsillectome

Sluder-Jensen mouth gag

Sluder-Sauer guillotine, tonsillectome

Small-Carrion prosthesis

Smart's forceps, scissors

Smead-Jones closure, sutures

Smedberg's drill

Smee's cell

Smellie's method, scissors

Smeloff-Cutter prosthesis, valve

Smiley-Williams needle

Smillie's meniscotome, retractor

Smith's disease(s) — acute infectious lymphocytosis; mucous colitis

Smith's operation — extraction of an immature cataract with an intact capsule

Smith's dislocation, fracture, pessary, phenomenon, reaction, sign, test

Smith-Dietrich method

Smith-Fisher knife, spatula

Smith-Hodge pessary

Smith-Lemli-Opitz syndrome — a hereditary syndrome marked by multiple congenital anomalies, including microcephaly, mental retardation, defective development of male genitalia, syndactyly and others

Smith-Peterson nail, osteotome, pin, prosthesis

Smith-Strang disease — a defect in methionine absorption, marked by malodorous urine, white hair, mental retardation and convulsions

Smithwick's clamp, dissector, forceps

Smithwick-Hartmann forceps

Sneddon-Wilkinson disease — subcorneal pustular dermatosis

Snell's cell, law

Snellen's chart, reflex, reform eye, sign, test, test type

Snider's match test

Snitman's retractor

Snyder's agar, forceps, hemostat, Hemovac, test

Sobernheim's vaccine

Socin's operation — enucleation of a goitrous or thyroidal tumor from the healthy part of the gland to avoid myxedema

Soemmering's crystalline swelling, foramen, ganglion, gray substance, papilla, process, ring, spot, vein

Sohval-Soffer syndrome — a congenital syndrome marked by male hypogonadism, multiple skeletal abnormalities and mental retardation

Soldaini's reagent, test

Solera's test

Solow's sigmoidoscope

Somers's clamp, forceps

Somerset's bur

Somogyi effect, method, unit

Sondergaard's cleft

Sondermann's canals

Sones's catheter

Sonne's dysentery

Sonne-Duval bacillus

Sonnenschein's test

Sörensen's buffer, method, reagent

Soresi's cannula

Soret's band, effect, phenomenon

Soriano's syndrome — hyperplastic, osteogenic, recurrent osteoperiostitis with pseudotumoral development

Sorondo-Ferre amputation

Sorsby's disease — dystrophy of the fundus beginning in the fifth decade, causing unilateral blurring of central vision and followed by a similar disorder in the other eye

Sorsby's syndrome — a congenital disorder consisting of retinal macular defects, dystrophy of the extremities and abnormal shortness of fingers and toes

Sorsby's macular degeneration

Sorval Porter–Blum ultramicrotome

Soto-Hall sign

Sotos's syndrome — cerebral gigantism

Sottas's disease — progressive hypertrophic interstitial neuropathy

Souligoux-Morestin method

Souques's phenomenon, sign

Souques-Charcot geroderma

Sourdille's keratoplasty

Southey's cannula, trocar, tube

Southey-Leech trocar, tube

Southgate's modification of Mayer's stain

Southwick's clamp, osteotomy

Southworth's symptom complex

Souttar's cautery, tube

Soxhlet's apparatus

Soyka's milk-rice culture medium

Spalding's sign

Spallanzani's law

Spanlang-Tappeiner syndrome — congenital zonular corneal opacity associated with hyperkeratosis of the palms and soles

Spee's curve, embryo

Speed's prosthesis

Spemann's induction

Spence's tail

Spence-Adson forceps

Spencer's disease — a form of epidemic gastroenteritis

Spencer's cannula, forceps, probe, scissors

Spencer-Parker vaccine

Spencer-Wells forceps

Spengler's fragments, immune bodies, tuberculin

Spens's syndrome — same as *Adams's disease*

Speransky-Richen-Siegmund syndrome — necrotizing perforation of the hard palate into the maxillary sinus

Spero's forceps

Spicer's iron diamine method

Spiegelberg's sign

Spieghel's line

Spiegler's reagent, test, tumor

Spiegler-Fendt sarcoid, sarcomatosis

Spielmeyer-Stock disease — retinal atrophy in amaurotic familial idiocy

Spielmeyer-Vogt disease — a late juvenile form of cerebral sphingolipidosis

Spies's punch

Spigelius's line

Spiller's syndrome — epidural ascending spinal paralysis

Spinelli's operation — reversing the prolapsed inverted uterus and restoring it to the correct position

Spira's disease — hypoplasia of the dental enamel caused by drinking water with high fluorine content

Spiro's test

Spitz's nevus

Spitzer's theory

Spitzka's nucleus, tract

Spitzka-Lissauer column, tract

Spivack's operation — cystostomy

Spöndel's foramen

Spondweni virus

Spratt's curet, rasp

Sprengel's deformity

Sprinz-Dubin syndrome — same as *Dubin-Johnson syndrome*

Sprinz-Nelson syndrome — same as *Dubin-Johnson syndrome*

Spritz's bottle

Sprong's sutures

Spurling's forceps, rongeur, sign

Spurling-Kerrison forceps, punch, rongeur

Spurway's syndrome — an inherited condition in which bones are abnormally brittle and subject to fracture

Sputnik-Federov lens

Squire's catheter, sign

Srb's syndrome — aplasia and synostosis of the first two ribs, with a hornlike, bony protrusion of the cranial portion of the sternum

Ssabanejew-Frank operation — same as *Frank's operation*

Stacke's operation — removal of the mastoid and the contents of the tympanum

Stader's splint

Staderini's nucleus

Staehelin's test

Stafne's cyst, mandibular defect

Stahl's ear, No. 1, No. 2

Stähli's line

Stahr's gland

Stallard's sutures

Stamm's gastrostomy, tube

Stammer's method

Stammler's reaction

Stanbury-Hedge defect

Stanford's test

Stanley bacillus

Stanley Kent bundle

Stannius's follicle

Stanton's disease — an infectious disease of rodents transmissible to humans, caused by *Pseudomonas pseudomallei*

Stanton's clamp

Starck's dilator

Stargardt's disease — hereditary degeneration of the retinal macula

Starkey's soap

Starling's hypothesis, law

Starlinger's dilator

Starr-Edwards pacemaker, prosthesis, valve

Stas-Otto method

State's operation — end-to-end anastomosis of the colon for treatment of Hirschsprung's disease

Staub-Traugott effect, phenomenon, test

Staude-Moore forceps, tenaculum

Staunig's method

Staunton's sphymomanometer

Stearns's alcoholic amentia

Stecher's method

Stedman's aspirator, pump, tube

Steele's dilator, elevator

Steele-Richardson-Olszewski syndrome — a progressive neurological disorder occurring in the sixth decade of life, marked by paralysis of the downward gaze, stumbling gait, dystonic rigidity of the trunk and neck and dementia

Steell's murmur

Steenbock's unit of vitamin D

Steer's replicating device

Stehle's method

Stein's operation — reconstruction of the lower lip with flaps taken from the upper lip

Stein's antigen, test

Stein-Abbe lip flap

Stein-Kazanjian flap

Stein-Leventhal syndrome — sclerocystic disease of the ovary marked by hirsutism, obesity, menstrual disturbances, infertility and enlarged ovaries, probably due to excessive androgen secretion. Called also *polycystic ovary syndrome*

Steinach's operation — ligation of the vas deferens with resection of a portion of the vas

Steinach's method

Steinbrocker's syndrome — a disorder of the upper extremity marked by shoulder pain and stiffness and by swelling and pain in the hand, sometimes occurring after myocardial infarction or injury to the neck

Steindler's posterior syndrome — low back pain

Steindler's arthrodesis

Steiner's syndrome — hypertrophy of one side of the entire body. Called also *Curtius's syndrome*

Steiner's tumors

Steiner-Vörner syndrome — multiple, symmetric, red, punctiform angiomas of the skin and mucous membranes with a variety of systemic disorders

Steinert's disease — myotonic dystrophy

Steinle-Kahlenberg test

Steinmann's extension, pin

Stellwag's brawny edema, sign, symptom

Stender's dish

Stenger's test

Stensen's canal, duct, experiment, foramen, plexus, veins

Stent's graft, mass

Stenvers's method, position, view

Stenzel's prosthesis, rod

Stephen's spots

Stepita's clamp

Sterles's sign

Sterling-Okuniewski sign

Stern's position, test

Stern-McCarthy electrotome, panendoscope, resectoscope

Sternberg's disease — same as *Hodgkin's disease*

Sternberg's giant cells, sign

Sternberg-Reed cells

Sternheimer-Malbin stain

Stevens's forceps, hook, scissors

Stevens-Johnson syndrome — same as *Johnson-Stevens disease*

Stevenson's clamp, forceps, scissors

Stewart's purple, test

Stewart-Holmes sign

Stewart-Morel syndrome — same as *Morgagni's syndrome*

Stewart-Treves syndrome — lymphangiosarcoma occurring in upper extremities affected by postmastectomy lymphedema

Sticker's disease — a mildly contagious disease of children marked by a rose-colored, lacelike macular rash

Sticker's sarcoma

Stickler's syndrome — a hereditary syndrome marked by progressive myopia and by abnormal epiphyseal development in the vertebrae and long bones

Stieda's disease — same as *Pellegrini's disease*

Stieda's fracture, process

Stieda-Pellegrini syndrome — traumatic calcification of the collateral tibial ligament

Stierlin's sign, symptom

Stifel's figure

Still's disease — a form of chronic arthritis affecting children, marked by enlargement of lymph nodes and intermittent fever

Still's syndrome — juvenile rheumatoid arthritis

Still's murmur
Still-Chauffard syndrome — same as *Chauffard's syndrome*
Stille's clamp, forceps, gouge, osteotome, shears, trephine
Stille-Adson forceps
Stille-Bjork forceps
Stille-Horsley forceps
Stille-Leksell rongeur
Stille-Liston forceps
Still-Luer forceps, rongeur
Stiller's asthenia, rib, sign
Stilling's syndrome — same as *Duane's syndrome*
Stilling's canal, column, fibers, fleece, nucleus
Stilling-Turk-Duane syndrome — same as *Duane's syndrome*
Stimson's sign
Stintzing's tables
Stitt's catheter
Stock's test
Stock-Spielmeyer-Vogt syndrome — juvenile amaurotic familial idiocy
Stocker's line, sign
Stockholm-Koch method
Stockman's clamp
Stoerck's loop
Stoerk's blennorrhea
Stoker's treatment
Stokes's disease — same as *Graves's disease*
Stokes's operation — Gritti-Stokes amputation
Stokes's amputation, collar, expectorant, law, reagent, sign, test
Stokes-Adams disease — same as *Adams-Stokes disease*
Stokvis's disease — a syndrome caused by absorption of

Stokvis's disease (*continued*) nitrites and sulfides from the intestine, marked by excessive methemoglobin in the circulating blood associated with cyanosis and by severe enteritis, dyspnea, syncope, anemia and occasionally by digital clubbing
Stokvis's test
Stokvis-Talma syndrome — same as *Stokvis's disease*
Stoll's test
Stoltz's pubiotomy
Stone's eye implant
Stone-Holcombe clamp
Stoneman's forceps
Stookey's reflex
Storck's test
Storey's forceps
Storm Van Leeuwen chamber
Stormer's viscosimeter
Storz's bronchoscope, telescope
Storz-Beck snare
Storz-Iglesias resectoscope
Stout's wiring
Strachan-Scott syndrome — nutritional deficiencies, particularly of vitamin B_2, with pain, numbness and paresthesia of the palms, soles, joints and shoulders, dimmed vision, deafness and emaciation
Strange's test
Stransky-Regala syndrome — chronic familial hemolytic anemia, marked by erythroblastosis of the bone marrow with a profusion of immature erythroblasts
Strasburger's cell plate
Strassburg's test

Stratte's clamp, forceps
Straus's biological test, phenomenon, reaction
Strauss's cannula, needle, sign, test
Strayer's knife
Street's pin
Streeter's horizons
Stroganoff's (Stroganov's) treatment
Strombeck's breast reduction, incision
Stromeyer's cephalhematocele, splint
Strong's bacillus
Struempel's forceps, rongeur
Strully's curet, hook, scissors
Strully-Kerrison rongeur
Strümpell's disease(s) — a hereditary form of lateral sclerosis in which spasticity is limited to the legs; polioencephalomyelitis
Strümpell's phenomenon, reflex, sign, type
Strümpell-Leichtenstern disease — hemorrhagic encephalitis
Strümpell-Lorrain disease — spinocerebellar degeneration
Strümpell-Marie disease — rheumatoid spondylitis
Strümpell-Westphal disease — the cerebral changes of hepatolenticular degeneration
Strümpell-Westphal pseudosclerosis
Strunsky's sign
Struve's test
Struyken's forceps, punch
Stryker's dermabrader, dermatome, frame, saw
Stryker-Halbeisen syndrome — a scaling, macular eruption on

Stryker-Halbeisen syndrome (*continued*)
the face and upper trunk from vitamin B complex deficiency, associated with macrocytic anemia
Stuart's broth, factor, transport medium
Stuart-Bras disease — veno-occlusive disease of the liver
Stuart-Prower factor
Stubbs's curet
Stühmer's disease — atrophy of the glans penis, resulting in stricture of the urethral meatus
Sturge's disease — same as *Sturge-Weber syndrome*
Sturge's syndrome — same as *Sturge-Kalischer-Weber syndrome*
Sturge-Kalischer-Weber syndrome — a congenital syndrome consisting of angiomas of the face, leptomeninges, and choroid and glaucoma—often associated with intracranial calcification, mental retardation, hemiplegia and epilepsy. Called also *Dimitri's disease*
Sturge-Weber syndrome — same as *Sturge-Kalischer-Weber syndrome*
Sturge-Weber-Dimitri disease — same as *Sturge-Weber syndrome*
Sturm's conoid, interval
Sturmdorf's operation — excision of diseased endocervix
Stutsman's snare
Sucquet-Hoyer anastomosis, canal
Sudeck's disease — post-traumatic osteoporosis

Sudeck's atrophy, critical point, porosis

Sudeck-Leriche syndrome — posttraumatic osteoporosis with vasospasm

Sugg's catheter

Suker's sign

Sulkowitch's test

Sullivan's test

Sulzberger-Chase phenomenon

Sulzberger-Garbe syndrome — an exudative lichenoid dermatitis associated with other cutaneous and systemic manifestations

Sumner's method, reagent, sign

Sundt's clip

Suranyi's test

Surgaloy's sutures

Sutter's blood groups

Sutton's disease — a severe form of disease of the oral mucosa, marked by ulcerative lesions surrounded by a red border, caused by local injury, allergic reaction, endocrine imbalance and emotional stress

Sutton's nevus

Sutton-Gull disease — arteriocapillary fibrosis

Suzanne's gland

Švec's leukemia

Svedberg's unit

Swan's syndrome — blind spot syndrome

Swan-Ganz catheter

Swank-Davenport method

Swanson's implant, prosthesis

Swediaur's (Schwediauer's) disease — inflammation of the calcaneal bursa

Sweeney's retractor, speculum

Sweet's disease — a rare disease predominant in women, marked by sudden onset of plaque-like lesions of the face, neck and upper extremities accompanied by conjunctivitis, fever, malaise and arthralgia

Sweet's forceps, punch, scissors

Swenson's operation — removal of the rectum and the aganglionic segment of the bowel for Hirschsprung's disease

Swenson's procedure

Swift's disease — same as *Swift-Feer disease*

Swift-Feer disease — acrodynia

Swyer-James syndrome — chronic obstructive pseudoemphysema

Sydenham's disease — an acute, toxic, infective disorder of the nervous system, usually associated with acute rheumatic fever in young persons, marked by involuntary, jerky movements of the face, neck and limbs

Sydenham's chorea, cough

Sydney crease, line

Sylva's irrigator

Sylvest's disease — epidemic pleurodynia

Sylvest's syndrome — an acute, infectious disease caused by the Coxsackie B virus, marked by sudden onset of fever and severe pain in the muscles of the lower chest or abdomen

Sylvius's angle, aqueduct, cistern, fissure, fossa, iter, valve, ventricle

Syme's operation(s) — amputation of the foot at the ankle joint,

Syme's operation (*continued*)
  with removal of both malleoli;
  external urethrotomy
Syme's amputation
Symington's body
Symmers's disease — giant follicular lymphoma

Syms's tractor
Syrian ulcer
Szabo's test
Szent-Györgyi reaction
Sztehlo's clamp

T

Tabb's curet, knife
Taenzer's disease — a skin disorder marked by redness and roughness of the eyebrows and spreading to the face and scalp
Tahyna virus
Taillefer's valve
Takahara's disease — a rare disease occurring principally in Japan, caused by congenital absence of the enzyme catalase. It is marked by recurrent infections of the gingiva, but more often than not no symptoms are present
Takahara's syndrome — a congenital deficiency of blood catalase, with malignant alveolar pyorrhea and gangrene, seen in Japan and Switzerland
Takahashi's forceps
Takata's reagent
Takata-Ara test
Takayasu's disease/syndrome — pulseless disease, same as *Martorell's syndrome*
Takayasu's arteritis
Talbot's law
Tallerman's apparatus, treatment
Tallqvist's scale
Talma's disease — delayed relaxation of muscle following con-

Talma's disease (*continued*)
  traction, from either injury or disease
Talma's operation — surgical production of artificial adhesions between the liver and spleen and the omentum and abdominal wall for ascites from cirrhosis of the liver
Tamura-Takahashi disease — hereditary black blood disease
Tanner's operation — procedure in which the left and short gastric veins are divided and the stomach is bisected and resutured, for bleeding esophageal varices
Tanner's method
Tanret's reaction, reagent, test
Tansini's operation(s) — amputation of the breast; removing a cyst of the liver; gastric resection
Tapia's syndrome — unilateral paralysis of the larynx and tongue, with atrophy of the tongue
Tar's symptom
Tardieu's spots, test
Targowla's reaction, test
Tarin's fascia, foramen, fossa, space

Tarini's recess
Tarinus's band, valve, velum
Tarlov's cyst
Tarnier's forceps
Tarrant's method
Tashkent ulcer
Tatum's clamp
Tauber's catheter, speculum
Taussig-Bing syndrome — complete transposition of the aorta, with ventricular septal defect, right ventricular hypertrophy, anterior situation of the aorta and posterior situation of the pulmonary artery
Taussig-Bing complex, heart
Taussig-Snellen-Albers syndrome — drainage of the pulmonary vein into the inferior vena cava, associated with septal defects
Tawara's node
Tay's disease — degeneration of the choroid seen in advanced life, thought to be from an atheromatous condition of arteries
Tay's choroiditis, sign, spot
Tay-Sachs disease — the infantile form of cerebral sphingolipidosis, marked by degeneration of brain cells leading eventually to dementia, blindness, paralysis and death
Taybi's syndrome — bone dysplasia, dwarfism, cleft palate, peculiar facies, deafness and mental retardation
Taylor's syndrome — hyperemia of the ovary
Taylor's apparatus, curet, diet, method, speculum, splint, sutures, test

Taylor-Hulton method
Teale's operation — amputation that preserves a long, rectangular flap of muscle and integument on one side of the limb and a short, rectangular flap on the other
Teale's amputation, forceps
Teevan's law
Teichmann's crystals, test
Tellais's sign
Tellyesniczky's fluid, mixture
Temple-Fay retractor
Tenckhoff's catheter
Tenner's cannula
Tenon's capsule, fascia, membrane, space
Terry's syndrome — retrolental fibroplasia
Terson's disease — cerebral aneurysms, subarachnoid hemorrhage, ocular venous stenosis and venous saccular dilatation of the eye
Terson's forceps, speculum
Teschen's virus
Tesla's current
Testivin's sign
Teufel's method
Teutleben's ligaments
Teutschländer's syndrome — dystrophic metalipoid calcinosis
Textor's operation — removal of thin, split-thickness skin grafts by razor, knife or dermatome
Thamm's tuberculin
Thane's method
Thatcher's nail
Thayer-Doisy unit
Thayer-Martin medium
Thaysen's disease — nontropical sprue, or celiac disease

Thaysen's syndrome — attacks of severe pain in the region of the anorectal ring and the internal anal sphincter

Thebesius's veins

Theden's bandage

Theile's canal, glands

Theiler's mouse encephalomyelitis, virus

Theimich's lip sign

Theis's retractor

Theobald's probe

Theobald Smith's phenomenon

Thévenard's disease — same as *Hick's syndrome*

Thézac-Porsmeur method

Thibierge-Weissenbach syndrome — calcinosis

Thiele's syndrome — pain and tenderness in the lower portion of the sacrum and coccyx and in contiguous tissues

Thiemann's disease — familial necrosis of the phalangeal epiphysis, resulting in deformity of the interphalangeal joints

Thiersch's operation — removal of skin grafts with a razor

Thiersch's canaliculus, graft, sutures, wire

Thiersch-Duplay urethroplasty

Thiry's fistula

Thiry-Vella fistula

Thoma's ampulla, fluid

Thoma-Zeiss counting cell, counting chamber

Thomas's syndrome(s) — a combination of disorders of equilibrium, adiadochokinesia, halting speech, ataxia, reflex and sensitivity disorders and often cerebral catalepsy; hypo-

Thomas's syndrome (*continued*) thyroidism, with secondary hypertrophic osteoarthropathy and exophthalmos following partial thyroidectomy

Thomas's cryoextractor, heel, keratome, pessary, sign, splint, test

Thomas-Binetti test

Thomas-Warren incision

Thomayer's sign

Thompson's syndrome — congenital optic atrophy

Thompson's catheter, line, lithotrite, prosthesis, resectoscope, test

Thompson, F. R., hip prosthesis, rasp

Thoms's forceps, pelvimeter, tenaculum

Thoms-Allis forceps

Thoms-Gaylor forceps, punch

Thomsen's disease — a congenital, hereditary disease marked by tonic spasm and rigidity of muscles upon movement after rest

Thomsen's phenomenon

Thomson's disease — a hereditary developmental disease marked by hyperkeratotic lesions and xerodermatous changes

Thomson's clamp, sign

Thoraeus's filter

Thorek's aspirator, scissors

Thorek-Feldman scissors

Thorek-Mixter forceps

Thorel's bundle

Thormählen's test

Thorn's syndrome — a rare disorder caused by renal tubular damage of unknown origin,

Thorn's syndrome (*continued*)
resulting in loss of sodium
chloride, acidosis, dehydration
and vascular collapse

Thornton's nail, screw, sign

Thornwald's irrigator, perforator

Thornwaldt's (Tornwaldt's)
disease — chronic inflammation of the pharyngeal bursa,
accompanied by formation of
pustular cyst and nasopharyngeal stenosis

Thornwaldt's (Tornwaldt's) abscess, bursa, bursitis, cyst

Thorpe's curet, forceps, scissors

Thorpe-Castroviejo scissors

Thorpe-Westcott scissors

Throckmorton's reflex

Thudichum's test

Thunberg's tube

Thygeson's disease — epithelial
punctate keratitis associated
with viral conjunctivitis

Tidy's test

Tiedemann's nerve

Tiemann's catheter

Tietze's syndrome — idiopathic,
painful, nonsuppurative swellings of the costal cartilages

Tillaux's disease — mastitis with
multiple tumors of the breast

Tillaux-Phocas disease — same as
Cheatle's disease

Timberlake's evacuator, obturator,
resectoscope

Timbrall-Fisher incision

Timme's syndrome — ovarian and
adrenal insufficiency

Timofeew's apparatus, corpuscles

Tindale's medium

Tinel's sign

Tischler's forceps, punch

Tisdall's method

Tiselius's apparatus

Titterington's method, position

Tizzoni's test

Tobey's rongeur

Tobey-Ayer maneuver, test

Tobold's apparatus, forceps

Tobold-Fauvel forceps

Todd's bodies, button, cautery,
cirrhosis, needle, palsy, paralysis, process

Todd-Hewitt broth

Toison's fluid, solution

Tollens's test

Tollens, Neuberg and Schwket test

Tolosa-Hunt syndrome — unilateral paralysis of the eye muscles

Tom Jones sutures

Toma's sign

Tomes's fibers, fibrils, granular
layer, process

Tommaselli's disease — pyrexia
and hematuria associated with
excessive intake of quinine

Tommasi's sign

Tooke's knife, spatula

Toomey's evacuator, syringe, tube

Tooth's disease — progressive
neuropathic muscular atrophy

Tooth's atrophy, type

Töpfer's test

Topinard's angle, line

Torek's operation(s) — for unde-
scended testicle; for excision
of the thoracic part of the esophagus

Torkildsen's operation — ventric-
ulocisternostomy

Tornwaldt's (Thornwaldt's)
disease — chronic inflammation of the pharyngeal bursa,
accompanied by formation of
pustular cyst and nasopharyngeal stenosis

Torquay's test

Torre's syndrome — multiple tumors of the sebaceous glands associated with visceral malignancy

Torres-Teixeira bodies

Torsten-Sjögren's syndrome — same as *Marinesco-Garland syndrome*

Toti's operation — dacryocystorhinostomy

Touraine's syndrome — angioid streaks in cardiovascular disorders

Touraine-Solente-Golé syndrome — thickening of the skin of the face and scalp, thickening of the bones of the limbs and clubbing of the fingers

Tourette's disease — same as *Gilles de la Tourette's syndrome*

Tournay's sign

Tourtual's canal

Touton's giant cells

Tower's forceps, retractor

Towne's projection roentgenogram

Townley's forceps, prosthesis

Townsend's ionization

Toyama's disease — pityriasis

Toynbee's corpuscles, experiment, law, ligament, maneuver, otoscope

Tracy-Welker method

Trambusti's reaction, test

Trantas's dots

Trapp's coefficient, factor, formula

Traquair's scotom

Trattner's catheter

Traube's corpuscles, curves, double tone, dyspnea, heart, membrane, murmur, plugs, resonance theory, semilunar space, sign

Traube-Hering curves, waves

Trautmann's triangle

Treacher Collins syndrome — defective mandibulofacial bone formation

Treitz's angle, arch, fossa, hernia, ligament, muscle

Trélat's speculum

Trendelenburg's operation(s) — excision of varicose veins; ligation of the great saphenous vein for varicose veins; synchondroseotomy; pulmonary embolectomy for the treatment of postoperative embolism

Trendelenburg's cannula, gait, position, sign, symptom, tampon, test

Trendelenburg-Crafoord clamp

Tresilian's sign

Tretop's test

Treves's operation — opening of abscess through the loin, irrigating and curetting the sac and scraping away dead bone for Pott's disease

Treves's fold

Trevor's disease — a rare condition characterized by swellings of the extremities constituted by epiphyseal cartilage, resulting in limitation of joint movement

Triboulet's reagent, test

Trillat's method

Trimadeau's sign

Tripier's amputation

Troell-Junet syndrome — a combination of acromegaly, toxic goiter, diabetes mellitus and hyperostosis of the cranial vault

Troeltsch's speculum

Troisier's syndrome — severe debility associated with diabetes

Troisier's ganglion, node, sign

Troisier-Hanot-Chauffard syndrome — diabetes mellitus, with hypertrophic cirrhosis of the liver and dark-brown skin pigmentation

Trolard's net, plexus, vein

Tröltsch's corpuscles, pouch, recesses, spaces

Trommer's test

Trömner's sign

Trotter's syndrome — unilateral neuralgia in the region of the mandible, tongue and ear

Trousseau's syndrome — slowly advancing thrombophlebitis associated with visceral malignancy

Trousseau's apophysiary points, dilator, forceps, phenomenon, sign, spot, test, twitching

Trousseau-Jackson dilator

Trousseau-Lallemand bodies

Troutman's eye implant, forceps, gouge, scissors

Trudeau's medium

Trueta's method, technique, treatment

Trümmerfeld line

Trusler's clamp

Tschernogowbou's test

Tschmarke's treatment

Tsuchiya's test

Tswett's method

Tubbs's dilator

Tucker's bronchoscope, esophagoscope, laryngoscope, telescope, tube

Tucker-McClean forceps

Tudor-Edwards costotome

Tuffier's ligament, method, test

Tuffier-Raney retractor

Tuffnell's bandage, treatment

Tulpius's valve

Tuohy's catheter, needle

Türck's bundle, cell, column, degeneration, fasciculus, trachoma

Turck's zone

Turcot's syndrome — a hereditary syndrome marked by development of polyps of the brain and colon

Turek's spreader

Turell's forceps, proctoscope, sigmoidoscope

Türk's cell, irritation leukocyte, lymphomatosis

Turkel's trephine, tube

Turkestan ulcer

Turlington's balsam

Turnbull's blue reaction

Turner's syndrome — a hereditary chromosomal anomaly marked by gonadal dysgenesis, short stature, neck webbing, elbow deformity and cardiac defects

Turner's cerate, dilator, hypoplasia, marginal gyrus, prosthesis, sign, sulcus, tooth

Turner-Warwick urethroplasty

Turpin's syndrome — congenital bronchiectasis, megaesophagus, tracheoesophageal fistula, vertebral deformities, rib malformations and heterotopic ductus thoracicus

Turyn's sign

Tuttle's forceps, proctoscope, sigmoidoscope, test

Twining's method

Twort-d'Herelle phenomenon

Tycos's sphygmomanometer

Tyding's forceps, knife, tonsillec-
tome
Tydings-Lakeside forceps
Tyndall's cone, effect, light, phe-
nomenon
Tyrode's solution
Tyrrell's fascia, hook

Tyson's crypts, glands, test
Tyzzer's disease — necrosis of the
liver and intestine caused by
Bacillus piliformis, occurring
in many mammals and occa-
sionally in humans
Tzanck's cell, test

U

Uchida's incision, technique
Uden's syndrome — coronary dis-
orders resulting from high
position of the diaphragm
Udránszky's test
Uebe's applicator
Uehlinger's syndrome — thickening
of the skin of the face, scalp
and extremities, clubbing of
the fingers and deformity of
the long bones
Uffelmann's reagent, test
Uganda S virus
Uhl's anomaly
Uhlenhuth's test
Uhthoff's sign
Ullmann's line
Ullrich's syndrome — congenital,
atonic, sclerotic muscular
dystrophy
Ullrich's retractor
Ullrich-Feichtiger syndrome —
micrognathia, occurrence of
an extra finger or toe, genital
abnormalities and other de-
fects
Ullrich and Fremerey-Dohna syn-
drome — same as *Hallermann-
Streiff syndrome*
Ullrich-Turner syndrome — same
as *Noonan's syndrome*

Ulrich's test
Ultzmann's test
Umber's test
Underwood's disease — a disorder
of lipid metabolism usually
present at birth or shortly
after, characterized by harden-
ing of subcutaneous fat and
development of multiple, firm
nodules on the buttocks,
trunk, thighs, cheeks, arms
and feet
Undritz anomaly
Unna's disease — a chronic inflammatory disease of the skin
marked by yellowish patches,
greasy, moist or dry scales and
itching
Unna's syndrome — an inherited,
familial form of hypotrichosis,
with eyelashes and eyebrows
often missing at birth
Unna's alkaline methylene blue
stain, boot, cell, dermatosis,
layer, nevus, paste, vesicle,
wrap
Unna-Pappenheim stain
Unna-Taenzer disease — same as
Taenzer's disease
Unna-Taenzer stain

Unna-Thost syndrome — a congenital disease marked by symmetrical thickening of the epidermal horny layers of the palms and soles, often extending to the dorsal surfaces of the knuckles

Unschuld's sign

Unverricht's disease — progressive familial myoclonic epilepsy

Unverricht-Lafora disease — same as *Unverricht's disease*

Updegraff's needle

Uppsala virus

Urbach's lipoproteinosis

Urbach-Oppenheim disease — a dermatosis occurring in diabetes, marked by necrosis of the elastic and connective tissue of the skin with degeneration of collagen

Urbach-Wiethe syndrome — a rare familial and congenital lipid storage disease characterized by multiple lipoid infiltrations

Urbach-Wiethe syndrome (*continued*)
that produce waxiness and thickening of the skin and mucous membranes of the mouth, pharynx, larynx and hypopharynx, resulting in hoarseness

Urbantschitsch's bougie

Uriolla's sign, test

Urov's disease — same as *Kashin-Beck disease*

Uruma virus

Uschinsky's culture medium

Usher's syndrome — congenital nerve deafness and progressive degeneration of the neuro-epithelium

Uskow's pillars

Ussing's equation

Uyemura's syndrome — a combination of night blindness, epithelial xerosis, multiple white spots on the retina and faulty dark adaptation

V

Vahlquist-Gasser syndrome — a chronic, benign form of granulocytopenia of children without systemic manifestations

Vail's syndrome — neuralgic pain in the nose, face, eye, ear, head, neck and shoulder, usually unilateral, often nocturnal, associated with symptoms of nasal sinusitis

Valdini's method

Valenta's test

Valentin's corpuscles, ganglion, pseudoganglion

Valentine's position, splint, tube

Valleix's points

Vallery-Radot and Blamoutier lipomatosis

Vallet's mass

Valli-Ritter law

Valsalva's experiment, ligaments, maneuver, sinus, test, zone

Valsuani's disease — progressive pernicious anemia in puerperal women

Van Alyea's cannula, tube

van Bogaert's encephalitis, sclerosing leukoencephalitis

van Bogaert–Bertrand syndrome — same as *Canavan's disease*

van Bogaert–Divry syndrome — hereditary, diffuse, cortico-meningeal venous angiomatosis, characterized by mental deficiency, epilepsy, pyramidal and extrapyramidal disorders, hemianopsia, pigmentation disorders and telangiectasia

van Bogaert–Hozay syndrome — sudden arrest of growth of the extremities, followed by decalcification and osteolysis of various bones of the hands and feet

van Bogaert–Scherer-Epstein syndrome — familial hypercholesterolemia

van Buchem's syndrome — a hereditary disorder marked by osteosclerosis of the skull, mandible, clavicles, ribs and long bones, associated with elevated blood alkaline phosphatase and sometimes leading to optic atrophy and deafness

van Buren's disease — same as *Peyronie's disease*

van Buren's forceps

van Deen's test

Van de Graaff's generator

van den Bergh's test

van den Velden's test

van der Hoeve's syndrome — a hereditary syndrome consisting of blue scleras, osteogenesis imperfecta, and otosclerotic deafness, usually transmitted as an autosomal dominant trait Also called *Adair-Dighton syndrome* and *Dighton-Adair syndrome*

van der Kolk's law

Van der Waals bond, forces, radius

van der Woude's syndrome — a hereditary syndrome marked by cleft lip or cleft palate occurring in association with cysts of the lower lip

Van Doren's forceps

van Gehuchten's cells, method

van Gieson's stain

van Helmont's mirror

van Hook's operation — uretero-ureterostomy

Van Hoorn's maneuver

van Hoorne's canal

Van Lint's akinesia, block

Van Lint and Atkinson akinesia, block

Van Neck's disease — nonspecific ischiopubic osteochondritis in children of both sexes

Van Neck–Odelberg syndrome — same as *Van Neck's disease*

van Ness's rotation

Van Osdel's guillotine

Van Slyke's formula, method, test

Van Slyke–Cullen method, test

Van Slyke–Fitz method

Van Slyke–Meyer method

Van Slyke–Palmer method

Van Struycken forceps, punch

Vanderbilt's clamp, forceps

Vanghetti's prosthesis

Vannas's knife, scissors

van't Hoff's law, rule

Vanzetti's sign

Vaquez's disease — same as *Vaquez-Osler disease*

Vaquez-Osler disease — polycythemia vera

Varolius's bridge, valve

Vasconcelos-Baretto clamp

Vasiliev's disease — same as *Weil's disease*

Vater's ampulla, corpuscles, duct, papilla

Vater-Pacini corpuscles

Vaudremer's tuberculin

Vaughan's disease — anemia characterized by immature leukocytes and nucleated red cells, usually observed in metastatic carcinoma of the bone marrow

Vaughan's split products

Vaughan-Novy test

Veau's elevator, palatoplasty

Vedder's agar, culture medium, sign

Veeneklaas's syndrome — chronic bronchitis associated with dental caries

Veenema's retractor

Veenema-Gusberg needle, punch

Veillon's tube

Vella's fistula

Velpeau's bandage, deformity, hernia

Venable's plate

Venable-Stuck nail

Venning Browne test

Venus's girdle

Veraguth's fold

Verbiest's syndrome — narrowing of the lumbar vertebral canal, characterized by symptoms of compression of the caudal nerve roots

Verbrugge's clamp

Verbrycke's syndrome — cholecystohepatic flexure adhesions

Verdan's syndrome — limited action of flexor activity of the uninvolved fingers in adhesive tenosynovitis

Verga's lacrimal groove, ventricle

Verheyen's stars

Verhoeff's operation — posterior sclerotomy followed by electrolytic punctures

Verhoeff's elastic method, forceps, scissors, stain, sutures

Vermale's operation — amputation by double-flap transfixion

Verner-Morrison syndrome — diarrhea, hypokalemia and achlorhydria, associated with secretion of a toxin by a pancreatic islet-cell tumor

Vernes's test

Vernet's syndrome — paralysis of the motor components of glossopharyngeal, vagal and accessory cranial nerves, occurring most frequently as a result of head injury

Verneuil's disease — syphilitic disease of the bursa

Verneuil's canals, neuroma

Vernon's tube

Vernon-David proctoscope, sigmoidoscope

Verocay's bodies

Verres's needle, trocar

Verse's disease — deposit of calcium in one or more intervertebral disks

Verstraeten's bruit

Vesalius's foramen, ligament

Vesely-Street nail

Vezien's scissors

Viamonte-Hobbs electrosurgical unit

Viamonte-Jutzy electrosurgical unit

Vickers's hyperbaric bed

Vicq d'Azyr's band, body, bundle, fasciculus, foramen, stripe, tract

Vidal's disease — a skin disease of psychogenic origin, marked by a confluent lichen and papular eruption

Vidal's operation — subcutaneous ligation of the veins for varicocele

Vierordt-Mesh formula

Viers's erysiphake

Vieth-Müller horopter

Vieussens's annulus, ansa, foramen, isthmus, limbus, loop, ring, valve, veins, ventricle

Vignal's cells

Vigouroux's sign

Vilanova-Cañadell syndrome — a combination of a papular, dry, skin eruption, hypothyroidism and vitamin A deficiency

Vilanova-Piñol Aguadé syndrome — a dermatological disorder characterized by pea-sized, subcutaneous nodules of the legs

Villard's button

Villaret's syndrome — unilateral paralysis of the ninth, tenth, eleventh and twelfth cranial nerves, producing paralysis or anesthesia of the pharynx, soft palate, larynx and vocal cords

Villemin's theory

Vim's needle

Vim-Silverman needle

Vincent's disease — necrotizing ulcerative gingivostomatitis

Vincent's angina, gingivitis, infection, spirillium, stomatitis, tonsillitis

Vineberg's operation — to establish a collateral blood supply to the heart in which an in-

Vineberg's operation (*continued*) ternal mammary artery is implanted into the myocardium

Vinke's tongs, tractor

Vinson's syndrome — same as *Plummer-Vinson syndrome*

Vinson-Plummer syndrome — same as *Plummer-Vinson syndrome*

Virchow's disease — acute congenital encephalitis

Virchow's angle, cells, corpuscle, crystals, degeneration, gland, granulations, hydatid, law, line, node

Virchow-Robin spaces

Virchow-Seckel dwarfism

Virden's catheter

Vischer's lumboiliac incision

Visscher-Bowman test

Vitali's test

Vladimiroff-Mikulicz amputation

Vleminckx's solution

Voegtlin's unit

Voelcker-Joseph test

Vogel's curet

Vogel-Lee test

Voges-Proskauer reaction, test

Vogt's disease — a form of corneal dystrophy characterized by glints of a golden hue under indirect light

Vogt's syndrome — a condition associated with birth trauma, marked by involuntary hand movements, difficulty in walking, outbursts of laughter or tears, speech disorders and sometimes mental deficiency

Vogt's angle, bone-free projection, cataract, cephalodactyly, cornea, degeneration, point, white limbal girdle

Vogt-Hueter point

Vogt-Koyanagi syndrome — uveo-meningitis marked by exudative inflammation of the iris and choroid, associated with patchy depigmentation of the skin and hair and sometimes with retinal detachment and deafness

Vogt-Spielmeyer disease — the juvenile form of cerebral sphingolipidosis

Vohwinkel's syndrome — a mutilating disease characterized by hyperkeratosis and keratotic lesions on the dorsal surfaces of the hands and feet, knees and elbows, and by constricted digits

Voigt's boundary lines

Voillemier's point

Voit's nucleus

Volavsek's syndrome — keratosis of the palms, with involvement of the periarticular areas of the fingers

Volhard's nephritis, test

Volhard-Arnold method

Volhard-Harvey method

Volkmann's disease — congenital deformity of the foot, caused by tibiotarsal dislocation

Volkmann's operation — incision of the tunica vaginalis for hydrocele

Volkmann's syndrome — post-traumatic muscular hypertonia and degenerative neuritis. Also known as *Volkmann's contracture*

Volkmann's canals, cheilitis, contracture, deformity, ischemic paralysis, membrane, retractor, splint, spoon, subluxation

Volkovitsch's sign

Vollmer's test

Voltolini's disease — acute, purulent inflammation of the inner ear with severe pain, followed by involvement of the meninges with fever, delirium and unconsciousness

Voltolini's sign, tube

von Aldor's test

Von Apathy's gum syrup medium

von Bardeleben's prefrontal bone

von Behring's fluid

Von Bergmann's hernia

von Bezold's abscess

von Economo's disease — lethargic encephalitis

von Economo's encephalitis

von Eichen's cannula

von Fürth–Charnass method

von Gierke's disease — glycogen storage disease, accompanied by enlargement of the liver and heart with progressive muscular degeneration

von Gies joint

von Graefe's cautery, forceps, sign, speculum

von Haberer's gastrectomy

von Haberer–Aguirre gastrectomy

von Haberer–Finney gastrectomy, gastroenterostomy

von Hippel's disease — angiomatosis confined to the retina. With cerebral involvement it is known as *Hippel-Lindau disease* or *von Hippel-Lindau disease*

von Hippel–Lindau disease — hereditary phakomatosis, characterized by congenital angiomatosis of the retina and cerebellum

von Jaksch's disease — an anemia of young children, accompanied by poikilocytosis, peripheral red blood cell immaturity, leukocytosis and hepatosplenomegaly

von Jaksch's anemia, test

von Kossa's stain

von Kupffer's cells

von Langenbeck's bipedicle mucoperiosteal flap

von Leber's atrophy

von Maschke's test

von Mering's reflex

von Meyenburg's disease — a degenerative disease of cartilage producing many and bizarre forms of arthritis

von Monakow's fibers

von Mondak's forceps

von Petz's clamp

von Pirquet's cutireaction, reaction, test

von Recklinghausen's disease — same as *Recklinghausen's disease*

von Recklinghausen's test

von Saal's pin

von Weber's triangle

von Willebrand's disease/syndrome — a congenital hereditary tendency to hemorrhage, marked by prolonged bleeding time and deficiency of Hageman coagulation factor

von Zeynek and Mencki test

von Zumbusch's psoriasis

Voorhees's bag, needle

Voorhoeve's disease — linear striation in the metaphyses of long and flat bones

Voorhoeve's dyschondroplasia

Vörner's heloderma

Voronoff's operation — transplantation into a man of the testes of an anthropoid ape in an effort to rejuvenate the recipient

Vossius's keratitis, lenticular ring

Vrolik's disease/syndrome — an inherited condition in which the bones are brittle and subject to fracture, sometimes accompanied by otosclerotic deafness

Vulpian's atrophy, law, test

W. Dean McDonald clamp

Waaler-Rose test

Waardenburg's syndrome(s) — a hereditary disorder marked by abnormal width of the nasal bridge, pigmentary disturbances, leukoderma and sometimes cochlear deafness; a hereditary disorder marked by

Waardenburg's syndrome(s) (*continued*) acrocephaly, orbital and facial deformities, syndactyly, cleft palate, muscular contraction and cardiac malformation

Waardenburg-Jonkers disease — progressive corneal dystrophy of young infants, character-

Waardenburg-Jonkers disease
(*continued*)
   ized by the appearance of
   minute dots on the paren-
   chyma occupying the entire
   surface of the cornea
Wachendorf's membrane
Wachenheim-Reder sign
Wachsberger's bur
Wachtenfeldt's clip, forceps
Wada's prosthesis, test
Wade's balsam, staining method
Wade-Fite staining method
Wade-Fite-Faraco staining method
Wadsworth-Todd cautery
Waelsch's urethritis
Wagener's retinitis
Wagner's disease — a familial form
   of retinal dystrophy characterized by progressive myopia
   associated with sclerosis and
   atrophy of the vessels of the
   choroid, macular degeneration
   and patches of retinal detach-
   ment
Wagner's operation — osteoplastic
   resection of the skull
Wagner's corpuscles, hammer, line,
   osteogenic sarcoma, polymyositis, punch, resection, spot,
   test, theory
Wagner-Jauregg treatment
Wagner-Unverricht syndrome — an
   association of myositis with
   dermatitis, characterized by
   erythema of the face and eyelids and muscular pain and
   weakness
Wagstaffe's fracture
Wahl's sign
Walcher's position
Walcheren fever

Waldeau's forceps
Waldenberg's apparatus
Waldenström's disease(s) — an
   acute form of thyrotoxicosis
   with muscular and cerebral
   complications; osteochondrosis of the capital femoral
   epiphysis
Waldenström's syndrome — same
   as *Calvé-Legg-Perthes syndrome*
Waldenström's hepatitis, macroglobulinemia, uveoparotitis
Waldeyer's colon, fluid, fossa,
   gland, layer, ligament, ring,
   sulcus
Wales's bougie, dilator
Walker's forceps, method, retractor, scissors, trephine
Walker-Apple scissors
Walker-Atkinson scissors
Wallace-Diamond method
Walldius's prosthesis
Wallenberg's syndrome — a condition due to occlusion of the
   posterior inferior cerebellar
   artery, marked by loss of pain
   sensation in the face and extremities and muscular incoordination
Waller's law
Wallgren's disease — obstruction
   of the splenic vein, with
   venous stasis of the spleen,
   resultant splenomegaly and
   development of collateral
   circulation
Wallhauser-Whitehead method
Walpole's sodium acetate buffer
Walsh's curet
Walsh-Ogura orbital decompression

Walsham's forceps
Walter's bromide test, forceps, spud
Walter-Bohmann syndrome — tachycardia, hypothermia, polypnea, pallor and cold sweat following cholecystectomy or cholecystoduodenostomy
Walter-Deaver retractor
Walthard's cell rests, inclusions, islets
Walther's clamp, dilator, ducts, forceps, ganglion, oblique ligament, sound
Walther-Crenshaw clamp
Walton's forceps, knife, law, rongeur, scissors
Walton-Schubert forceps, punch
Wang's test
Wangensteen's apparatus, clamp, colostomy, drainage, forceps, suction, tube
Wanner's symptom
Wanscher's mask
Wappler's cystoscope, electrode
Warburg's apparatus, coenzyme, ferment
Ward's syndrome — multiple, nevoid, basal cell carcinomata associated with dyskeratosis palmaris et plantaris
Ward's triangle
Ward-French needle
Wardill four-flap method, palatoplasty
Wardrop's disease — acute inflammation of the matrix of the nails, occurring spontaneously in debilitated states or as the result of an injury
Waring's method, system

Warren's fat columns, incision, test
Wartenberg's disease — neuritis of the superficial ramus of the radial nerve
Wartenberg's sign, symptom
Warthen's clamp
Warthin's tumor
Warthin-Finkeldey cells
Warthin-Starry-Faulkner method
Wasko's probe
Wassermann's reaction, test
Wassermann-positive pneumonia, pulmonary infiltrations
Wassilieff's disease — leptospiral jaundice
Water's operation — a form of extraperitoneal cesarean section
Waterhouse's urethroplasty
Waterhouse-Friderichsen syndrome — a rapidly fulminating meningococcal septicemia marked by massive purpura, bilateral adrenal hemorrhage and shock
Waterman's bronchoscope
Waters's position, view roentgenogram
Waters-Waldron position
Watkins's operation — for prolapse and procidentia uteri, in which the bladder is separated from the anterior wall of the uterus
Watson's forceps, method, speculum
Watson-Cheyne dissector
Watson-Crick helix
Watson-Jones gouge, incision
Watson-Schwartz test
Watson-Williams forceps, needle, rasp, rongeur
Watts's clamp, tenaculum

Weary's hook, spatula
Weaver's clamp
Webb's bolt, retractor, stripper
Weber's disease — same as *Sturge-Kalischer-Weber syndrome*
Weber's syndrome — paralysis of the oculomotor nerve, producing ptosis, strabismus and loss of light reflex. Also called *Weber's paralysis*
Weber's catheter, circle, corpuscle, douche, glands, implant, insufflator, law, method, organ, paradox, paralysis, retractor, scissors, sign, symptom, test, tubercle, zone
Weber-Christian disease — relapsing, febrile, nodular, nonsuppurative panniculitis
Weber-Christian syndrome — subcutaneous nodules and plaques resulting in atrophy of the subcutaneous fatty layer of the skin
Weber-Christian panniculitis
Weber-Cockayne syndrome — a form of epidermolysis in which large vescicles and erosions appear on the hands and feet in response to very slight injury
Weber-Dimitri disease — same as *Sturge-Kalischer-Weber syndrome*
Weber-Dimitri syndrome — same as *Sturge-Weber syndrome*
Weber-Dubler syndrome — same as *Weber's syndrome*
Weber-Fechner law
Weber-Fergusson incision
Weber-Fergusson-Longmire incision
Weber-Leyden syndrome — same as *Leyden's paralysis*

Webril's bandage
Webster's operation — for retrodisplacement of the uterus
Webster's knife, retractor, test, tube
Wechsler Adult Intelligence Scale, Intelligence Scale for Children
Weck's clamp, shears, tube
Wecker's spatula
Wedensky's facilitation, inhibition, phenomenon
Weder's retractor
Weder-Solenberger retractor
Wedl's cells
Weech's syndrome — same as *Christ-Siemens-Touraine syndrome*
Weeks's bacillus, needle, speculum
Wegener's syndrome — a progressive disease marked by granulomatous lesions of the respiratory tract and, finally, by widespread inflammation of all organs of the body
Wegener's granulomatosis
Wegierko's coma
Wegner's disease — osteochondrotic separation of epiphyses in hereditary syphilis
Wegner's osteochondritis, sign
Weichardt's antikenotoxin, reagent
Weichbrodt's reaction, test
Weichselbaum's diplococcus
Weidel's test
Weigert's fibrin stain, iron hematoxylin stain, law, method, myelin sheath staining method, neuroglia fiber stain, resorcinfuchsin stain
Weigert-Pal technique
Weigl's vaccine
Weil's disease — leptospiral jaundice

Weil's syndrome — same as *Larrey-Weil disease*

Weil's basal layer, forceps, icterus, rongeur, splint, stain, test, zone

Weil-Felix reaction, test

Weill's syndrome — same as *Adie's syndrome*

Weill's sign

Weill-Marchesani syndrome — a congenital disorder of connective tissues, transmitted as an autosomal dominant or recessive trait and marked by short fingers and toes, short stature and brachydactyly

Weill-Reys syndrome — same as *Adie's syndrome*

Weill-Reys-Adie syndrome — same as *Adie's syndrome*

Weinberg's reaction, retractor, rule, spreader, test

Weinberg-Himelfarb syndrome — fetal endocardial fibroelastosis

Weiner's method

Weingarten's syndrome — tropical pulmonary eosinophilia

Weingartner's forceps, rongeur

Weir's operation — appendicostomy

Weir Mitchell's disease — bilateral vasodilatation of the extremities, with burning pain and increased skin temperature

Weir Mitchell's treatment

Weis's forceps

Weisbach's angle

Weisenbach's forceps

Weisman's forceps, tenaculum

Weisman-Graves speculum

Weismann's theory

Weismann-Netter's syndrome — congenital, familial anteropos-

Weismann-Netter's syndrome (*continued*) terior curvature and thickening of the tibia and fibula of both legs

Weismann-Netter's dysostosis

Weismann-Netter and Stuhl syndrome — same as *Weismann-Netter's syndrome*

Weiss's reflex, sign, test

Weiss-Baker syndrome — same as *Charcot-Weiss-Baker syndrome*

Weissmann's bundle, fibers

Weitbrecht's cartilage, cord, foramen, ligament, retinaculum

Weitlaner's retractor

Welch's bacillus

Welch Allyn forceps, laryngoscope, otoscope, proctoscope, retinoscope, sigmoidoscope, transilluminatory tube

Welcher's angle

Welcker's method

Welin's technique

Welker's method

Welker-Marsh method

Wellaminski's perforator

Welland's test

Wells's clamp, forceps, tractor

Welsh's abscess

Wenckebach's disease — downward displacement of the heart

Wenckebach's block, heart block, period, phenomenon

Wender's test

Wenzell's test

Weppen's test

Werdnig's disease — same as *Werdnig-Hoffmann syndrome*

Werdnig-Hoffmann disease/syndrome — a heritary, progressive, infantile form of muscular

Werdnig-Hoffmann disease/syndrome (*continued*)
atrophy resulting from degeneration of the anterior horn cells of the spinal cord

Werdnig-Hoffmann atrophy, paralysis, type

Werlhof's disease — idiopathic thrombocytopenic purpura

Werlhof-Wichmann syndrome — same as *Werlhof's disease*

Wermer's syndrome — polyendocrine adenomatosis

Werner's disease — a rare hereditary condition marked by premature aging

Werner's syndrome — premature senility of adults, marked by cataracts, hyperkeratinization and sclerodermatous changes in the skin

Werner-His disease — an infection caused by *Rickettsia quintana* transmitted by lice and marked by attacks of headache, hyperesthesia and intermittent fever; called also *trench fever*

Werner-Schultz disease — agranulocytosis

Wernicke's disease — an inflammatory, hemorrhagic encephalopathy with lesions of the hypothalamus and periventricular region

Wernicke's syndrome — a mental condition, usually of old age, marked by defective memory, loss of sense of location, confusion and bewilderment

Wernicke's aphasia, area, center, cramp, dementia, encephalopathy, field, fissure, reaction, sign, symptom, test, triangle, zone

Wernicke-Korsakoff syndrome — the coexistence of *Wernicke's syndrome* with *Korsakoff's disease*

Wernicke-Mann hemiplegia, type

Wertheim's operation — for cancer of the cervix

Wertheim's clamp, forceps, hysterectomy, ointment, splint

Wertheim-Cullen clamp, forceps

Wertheim-Navratil needle

Wertheim-Reverdin clamp

Wertheim-Schauta operation — for cystocele, with interposition of the uterus between the base of the bladder and the anterior vaginal wall

Wesolowski's prosthesis

Wesselsbron's disease — a mosquito-borne, fatal disease of lambs, transmissible to humans, in whom it causes a mild, febrile illness

Wesselsbron's virus

Wesson's mouth gag, retractor

West's syndrome — an encephalopathy of infants causing spasms and arrest of psychomotor development

West's chisel, gouge

Westberg's space

Westcott's scissors

Wester's clamp, scissors

Westergren's method

Westermark's sign

Westphal's disease — same as *Strümpell-Westphal disease*

Westphal's syndrome — familial paroxysmal paralysis

Westphal's ataxia, neurosis, nucleus, phenomenon, pupillary reflex, sign, symptom, zone

Westphal-Leyden syndrome — an acute form of ataxia of unknown origin

Westphal-Piltz phenomenon, reflex

Westphal-Strümpell disease — hepatolenticular degeneration

Westphal-Strümpell syndrome — same as *Wilson's disease*

Westphal-Strümpell pseudosclerosis

Wetzel's grid, test

Wever-Bray phenomenon

Weyers's syndrome(s) — congenital gastrointestinal atresia of parts of the gastrointestinal system, with obstruction of the adjoining vessels; iridodental dysplasia

Weyers's oligodactyly syndrome — a congenital syndrome consisting of deficiency of the ulna and ulnar rays, abnormal membrane in the interpalpebral fissure, malformations of the kidney and spleen and cleft palate

Weyers-Fulling syndrome — multiple oculodentofacial abnormalities, including hypoplasia of the dental root and early loss of teeth, cataract, microphthalmia, glaucoma and peculiar facies

Weyers-Thier syndrome — a congenital syndrome consisting of abnormal smallness of eyes, twisted face due to maxillary dysplasia, malocclusion of teeth and vertebral malformations

Weyl's test

Wharton's duct, gelatin, jelly

Whatman's filter paper

Wheatstone's bridge

Wheeler's eye implant, knife, spatula

Wheeler-Johnson test

Wheelhouse's operation — perineal section for impermeable stricture of the urethra

Whipple's disease/syndrome — a malabsorption syndrome marked by diarrhea, steatorrhea, arthritis, lymphadenopathy and central nervous system lesions

Whipple's operation — radical pancreatoduodenectomy

Whipple's incision, intestinal lipodystrophy, method, pancreatoduodenectomy, test, triad

Whitcomb-Kerrison punch

White's disease — a familial eruption, beginning in childhood, in which keratotic papules of the trunk, face, scalp and axillae become crusted with wartlike elevations

White's operation — castration for hypertrophy of the prostate

White's chisel, forceps, mallet, scissors

White-Lillie forceps

White-Oslay forceps

White-Proud retractor

White-Smith forceps

Whitehead's operation(s) — excision of hemorrhoids; removal of the tongue with scissors

Whitehorn's method

Whiteside's test

Whitfield's ointment

Whiting's rongeur, tonsillectome

Whitman's operation(s) — arthroplasty of the hip; a method of astragalectomy

Whitman's frame

Whitmore's disease — an infectious disease of rodents transmissible to humans, in whom it causes either a chronic granulomatous pneumonia or a fulminant septicemia with high mortality

Whitmore's bacillus, bag, fever

Whitnall's tubercle

Whitten's effect

Whitver's clamp

Whytt's disease — tuberculous meningitis causing acute hydrocephalus

Wichmann's asthma

Wickersheimer's fluid, medium

Wickham's striae

Widal's disease/syndrome — same as *Hayem-Widal syndrome*

Widal's reaction, test

Widal-Abrami disease — acquired hemolytic anemia

Widal-Abrami syndrome — same as *Hayem-Widal syndrome*

Wideroe's test

Widmark's conjunctivitis, test

Widowitz's sign

Wiechowski-Handorsky method

Wiedemann's syndrome — thalidomide embryopathy

Wiener's breast reduction, genetic theory, keratome, speculum

Wiener-Pierce rasp, trocar

Wigand's maneuver, version

Wigby-Taylor method

Wigmore's saw

Wijs's test

Wilbrand's prism test

Wilbur-Addis test

Wildbolz reaction, test

Wilde's cords, forceps, incision, punch

Wilde-Blakesley forceps

Wilde-Bruening snare

Wilder's cystotome, diet, dilator, law, sign, trephine

Wildermuth's ear

Wildervanck's syndrome — a hereditary familial syndrome marked by deaf-mutism, short neck and paralysis of the external ocular muscles

Wildervanck-Waardenburg-Franceschetti-Klein syndrome — same as *Wildervanck's syndrome*

Wildgen-Reck locator, magnet

Wilke's brace

Wilkerson's bur

Wilkie's disease — partial or complete block of the third segment of the duodenum

Wilkins's disease — congenital adrenal hyperplasia

Wilkinson's anemia

Wilkinson-Peter test

Wilks's disease — a form of cutaneous tuberculosis marked by verrucous lesions of the fingers

Willan's lepra

Willan-Plumbe syndrome — same as *Willan's lepra*

Willauer's raspatory, scissors

Willebrand's syndrome — same as *Willebrand-Jurgens syndrome*

Willebrand-Jurgens syndrome — hemorrhagic diathesis inherited as a simple dominant trait, characterized by prolonged bleeding time and associated with epistaxis and

Willebrand-Jurgens syndrome (*continued*)
  bleeding from the gastrointestinal tract, gums, uterus and at the sites of surgical operations
Willett's clamp, forceps
Williams's syndrome — a congenital disorder characterized by physical and mental deficiency, elfin facies, aortic stenosis and occasionally, elevated blood calcium. It may be associated with hypersensitivity to vitamin D
Williams's colpopoiesis, craniotome, method, phenomenon, position, probe, sign, speculum, tracheal tone
Williams-Campbell syndrome — congenital deficiency in the cartilaginous wall of the trachea or of a bronchus, leading either to obstructive emphysema or bronchiectasis
Williamson's blood test, sign
Willis's disease — diabetes mellitus
Willis's antrum, circle, cords, nerve, pancreas, paracusis, pouch, valve
Willner's spots
Willock's respiratory jacket
Wills's anemia, factor
Willy Meyer incision, radical mastectomy
Wilman's clamp
Wilmer's chisel, retractor, scissors
Wilms's nephroblastoma, tumor
Wilson's disease(s) — dermatitis exfoliativa; hepatolenticular degeneration
Wilson's syndrome — hepatolenticular degeneration

Wilson's awl, clamp, degeneration, leads, modification of Bowie's stain, muscle, spreader, trocar, wrench
Wilson-Blair culture medium
Wilson-Mikity syndrome — a rare and often fatal form of pulmonary insufficiency in low-birth-weight infants, marked by abnormal respiratory action and cyanosis
Wiltberger's spreader
Wimberger's sign
Wimshurst's machine
Winckel's disease — a fatal disease of newborn infants, marked by jaundice, hemoglobinuria, hemorrhage, cyanosis, convulsions and collapse
Winckler's test
Wincor's scissors
Windscheid's disease — neurologic symptoms of arteriosclerosis
Winer's catheter
Winiwarter's operation — cholecystoenterostomy
Winiwarter-Buerger disease/syndrome — thromboangiitis obliterans (same as *Buerger's disease*)
Winkelstein's alkalinized milk drip
Winkler's disease — a painful disorder of the ear, marked by hard nodules involving the skin and cartilage
Winkler's body
Winkler-Waldeyer closing ring
Winogradsky's culture medium
Winslow's collateral fibers, foramen, hiatus, ligament, pancreas, star, test
Winter's syndrome — a congenital syndrome consisting of renal

Winter's syndrome (*continued*)
hypoplasia, anomalies of the
genitalia, especially vaginal
atresia, and abnormalities of
the middle-ear ossicles

Winterbottom's sign, symptom

Winternitz's sound

Wintersteiner's compound

Wintrich's sign

Wintrobe's method, tube

Wintrobe-Landsberg method

Wirsung's canal, duct

Wis-Foregger laryngoscope

Wis-Hipple laryngoscope

Wise's disease — same as *Mucha-Habermann syndrome*

Wise-Rein disease — same as *Kaposi's disease*

Wiseman-Doan syndrome — primary splenic neutropenia

Wishard's catheter

Wishart's disease — tumors of the spinal nerve roots and auditory nerves

Wishart's test

Wiskott-Aldrich syndrome — a rare and usually fatal hereditary syndrome, transmitted as an X-linked recessive trait and characterized by chronic eczema, chronic suppurative otitis media, anemia and thrombocytopenic purpura

Wiskott-Aldrich-Huntley syndrome — same as *Wiskott-Aldrich syndrome*

Wissler-Fanconi syndrome — high intermittent fever, exanthemata, arthralgia, carditis, pleurisy, neutrophil leukocytosis and increased sedimentation rate

Wistar's pyramid

Witkop's disease — hereditary benign premature keratinization in individual cells

Witkop-Von Sallmann disease — same as *Witkop's disease*

Witkop-Von Sallmann syndrome — a hereditary congenital disease of the oral mucosa and bulbar conjunctiva, characterized by gelatinous plaques of the conjunctiva and thickening of the oral mucosa

Wittmaack-Ekbom syndrome — same as *Ekbom's syndrome*

Wittner's forceps

Witts's anemia

Witz's test

Witzel's operation — gastrostomy

Wladimiroff's operation — same as *Mikulicz's operation*

Wladimiroff's tarsectomy

Woakes's saw

Wohlfart-Kugelberg-Welander disease — progressive muscular dystrophy with fibrillary twitching

Wohlgemuth's test

Wohlwill-Corino Andrade syndrome — same as *Andrade's syndrome*

Woillez's disease — acute idiopathic pulmonary congestion

Woldman's test

Wolf's syndrome — an association of multiple anomalies caused by partial deletion of the short arm of a chromosome of the B group

Wolf's catheter, method

Wolf-Hirschhorn syndrome — chromosomal abnormality,

Wolf-Hirschhorn syndrome (*continued*)
marked by microcephaly, a vertical skin fold on either side of the nose, cleft palate, micrognathia, cryptorchidism and hypospadias

Wolf-Schindler gastroscope

Wolfe's forceps, graft

Wolfe-Krause graft

Wolfenden's position

Wolff's duct, law, reagent

Wolff-Calmette reaction

Wolff-Chaikoff effect

Wolff-Eisner reaction, test

Wolff-Junghans test

Wolff-Parkinson-White syndrome — paroxysmal tachycardia, shown in an electrocardiographic pattern of short P-R interval (atrial activity) and prolonged QRS complex (ventricular activity)

Wölfler's operation — anterior gastrojejunostomy for pyloric obstruction

Wölfler's sign, sutures

Wolfram's syndrome — a hereditary association of diabetes mellitus, diabetes insipidus, optic atrophy and neural deafness

Wolfring's glands

Wolfson's clamp, retractor

Wolkowitsch's sign

Wollaston's doublet

Wolman's disease — primary familial xanthomatosis in infants, usually leading to early death

Wolman's xanthomatosis

Wolters's method, nevus

Wong's method

Wood's filter, glass, lamp, light, metal, sign, test

Woodbridge's sutures, treatment

Woodbury's test

Woodruff's catheter

Woods-Fildes hypothesis, theory

Woodson's elevator, spoon

Woodward's forceps, sound

Woolner's tip

Woringer's disease — a manifestation of faulty fat assimilation occurring in children fed fat-rich food, characterized by hepatomegaly with colicky pain, headache, vomiting, nausea, fatigability and pallor

Woringer-Kolopp disease — a form of reticulosis, with multiple cutaneous tumors

Worm-Müller's test

Wormley's test

Worth's chisel, forceps

Woulfe's bottle

Wreden's sign

Wright's syndrome — a neurovascular syndrome caused by occlusion of the subclavian artery, resulting from malposition of the arm

Wright's method, plate, stain, version

Wrisberg's cartilage, ganglion, ligament, line, nerve, staff, tubercle

Wuhrmann's disease — myocardial fibrosis

Wullen's stone dislodger

Wullstein's forceps, knife, retractor, scissors, tympanoplasty

Wullstein-House forceps

Wunderlich's syndrome — hemorrhage surrounding the kidney

Wunderlich's curve
Wundt's tetanus
Wundt-Lamansky law
Wurd's catheter
Wurster's test
Wurth's vein stripper
Wützer's operation — for the radical cure of inguinal hernia
Wutzler's scissors
Wyatt's disease — a systemic disorder of the neonatal period, from infection with a cyto-

Wyatt's disease (*continued*) megalovirus acquired before birth
Wyburn-Mason's syndrome — arteriovenous aneurysm of the midbrain, with retinal, facial and mental changes
Wyeth's operation — amputation at the hip joint
Wylie's drain, forceps, pessary
Wynn's method
Wysler's sutures

Yankauer's operation — curettement of the bony end of the eustachian tube
Yankauer's bronchoscope, esophagoscope, forceps, nasopharyngoscope, tube
Yankauer-Little forceps
Yasargil's forceps, raspatory, scissors, technique
Yazujian's bur
Yellen's clamp
Yemen ulcer
Yeo's treatment
Yeomans's forceps, proctoscope, sigmoidoscope
Yerkes discrimination box
Yerkes-Bridges test
Yersin's serum
Yoshida's dissector, sarcoma, tumor

Young's operation(s) — partial prostatectomy; total excision of seminal vesicles and partial excision of ejaculatory ducts
Young's syndrome — amyotrophic bulbar lateral sclerosis
Young's clamp, dilator, forceps, retractor, rule, test
Young-Helmholtz theory
Young-Millin needle holder
Youssef's syndrome — a rare syndrome combining urinary incontinence and menstrual hematuria, caused by a vesicouterine fistula appearing after lower segment cesarean section
Yvon's coefficient, test

Z

Zachary–Cope DeMartel clamp

Zahn's infarct, lines, pockets, ribs

Zahorsky's disease — an acute mild viral disease of young children, marked by fever and followed by rash

Zahorsky's syndrome — an acute infectious disease of childhood caused by Coxsackie A viruses, characterized by sudden high fever and vesicular ulcerative lesions of the soft palate and faucial areas

Zak's reaction

Zaleski's test

Zambesi ulcer

Zander's apparatus, cells

Zanelli's method

Zang's space

Zange-Kindler syndrome — block of the cerebrospinal fluid in the cisterna magna, from space-occupying lesions of the posterior cranial fossa

Zangemeister's test

Zanoli-Vecchi syndrome — convulsions with apnea and loss of consciousness, appearing suddenly two to three hours after surgery

Zappacosta's test

Zappert's syndrome — a cerebellar disorder characterized by ataxia of station and gait, intention tremor, nystagmus and slurred speech. The onset is sudden in normal children or in children recovering from infectious diseases

Zappert's chamber

Zaufal's sign

Zeeman's effect

Zeis's glands

Zeisel's test

Zeissel's layer

Zeller's test

Zellweger's syndrome — a rare syndrome marked by muscular hypotonia, incomplete myelinization of nerve tissues, craniofacial malformations and glomerular cysts of the kidney

Zenker's crystals, degeneration, diverticulum, fixative, fluid, necrosis, pouch, solution

Zero family

Zeune's law

Ziegler's operation — V-shaped iridectomy

Ziegler's cautery, forceps, speculum

Ziegler-Furniss clamp

Ziehen's test

Ziehen-Oppenheim disease — a progressive disorder of children marked by muscular contractions producing bizarre distortions of the spine and hips

Ziehl's carbolfuchsin stain, solution

Ziehl-Neelsen method, stain

Ziemssen's motor points

Zieve's syndrome — hypercholesterolemia, hepatosplenomegaly, fatty infiltration of the liver, hemolytic anemia and hypertriglyceridemia following the intake of large amounts of alcohol

Ziffern's test
Zika virus
Zimaloy's prosthesis
Zimany's bilobed flap
Zimmer's clamp, prosthesis, splint
Zimmerlin's atrophy, type
Zimmermann's arch, corpuscle, decoction, elementary particles, virus
Zinn's aponeurosis, artery, cap, circle, corona, ligament, membrane, ring, tendon, zone, zonule
Zinsser's inconsistency
Zinsser-Engman-Cole syndrome — a congenital syndrome characterized by dyskeratosis, pigmentation of the skin, nail dystrophy, aplastic anemia, hypersplenism, acrocyanosis, hyperhidrosis of the palms and soles and leukoplakia of the tongue and hard palate
Zipser's clamp
Zittmann's decoction
Zoellner's needle, raspatory, scissors
Zoepffel's edema
Zoll's pacemaker
Zollinger-Ellison syndrome — a complex of symptoms consisting of intractable, fulminating peptic ulcer, severe gastric hyperacidity and islet-cell tumors of the pancreas that may be benign or malignant
Zöllner's figures, lines
Zondek-Aschheim test
Zondek-Bromberg-Rozin syndrome — galactorrhea and hyperthyroidism
Zoon's erythroplasia

Zouchlos's test
Zsigmondy's gold number method, test
Zuckerkandl's bodies, convolution, dehiscences, gland, organs
Zuelzer's syndrome — eosinophilia, leukocytosis and hypergammaglobulinemia in infants and young children, with manifestations that include hepatomegaly, pulmonary infiltrations, asthma, joint lesions, urticaria and convulsions
Zuelzer's awl, plate
Zuelzer-Kaplan syndrome(s) — a congenital familial form of chronic hemolytic anemia, characterized by jaundice, hepatosplenomegaly, osseous changes and a tendency toward development of mongoloid facies; a severe, chronic hypochromic microcytic anemia attributed to the interaction of the hemoglobin C gene with the thalassemia gene
Zuelzer-Ogden syndrome — a combination of hematopoietic disorders, characterized by progressive macrocytic anemia, leukopenia and thrombocytopenia
Zuntz's theory
Zutt's clamp
Zwahlen's syndrome — same as *Franceschetti's syndrome*
Zwanck's pessary
Zweifel-DeLee cranioclast
Zwenger's test

Appendices

Appendix 1
TABLE OF ELEMENTS

NAME	SYMBOL	AT. NO.	AT. WT.*
Actinium	Ac	89	(227)
Aluminum	Al	13	26.982
Americium	Am	95	(243)
Antimony	Sb	51	121.75
Argon	Ar	18	39.948
Arsenic	As	33	74.922
Astatine	At	85	(210)
Barium	Ba	56	137.34
Berkelium	Bk	97	(247)
Beryllium	Be	4	9.012
Bismuth	Bi	83	208.980
Boron	B	5	10.811
Bromine	Br	35	79.909
Cadmium	Cd	48	112.40
Calcium	Ca	20	40.08
Californium	Cf	98	(249)
Carbon	C	6	12.011
Cerium	Ce	58	140.12
Cesium	Cs	55	132.905
Chlorine	Cl	17	35.453
Chromium	Cr	24	51.996
Cobalt	Co	27	58.933
Copper	Cu	29	63.54
Curium	Cm	96	(247)
Dysprosium	Dy	66	162.50
Einsteinium	Es	99	(254)
Erbium	Er	68	167.26
Europium	Eu	63	151.96
Fermium	Fm	100	(253)
Fluorine	F	9	18.998
Francium	Fr	87	(223)
Gadolinium	Gd	64	157.25
Gallium	Ga	31	69.72
Germanium	Ge	32	72.59
Gold	Au	79	196.967
Hafnium	Hf	72	178.49
Hahnium	Ha	105	(260)
Helium	He	2	4.003
Holmium	Ho	67	164.930
Hydrogen	H	1	1.008
Indium	In	49	114.82
Iodine	I	53	126.904
Iridium	Ir	77	192.2
Iron	Fe	26	55.847
Krypton	Kr	36	83.80
Lanthanum	La	57	138.91
Lawrencium	Lw	103	(257)
Lead	Pb	82	207.19
Lithium	Li	3	6.939
Lutetium	Lu	71	174.97
Magnesium	Mg	12	24.312
Manganese	Mn	25	54.938
Mendelevium	Md	101	(256)

*Atomic weights are corrected to conform with the 1961 values of the Commission on Atomic Weights, expressed to the fourth decimal point, rounded off to the nearest thousandth. The numbers in parentheses are the mass numbers of the most stable or most common isotope.

NAME	SYMBOL	AT. NO.	AT. WT.*
Mercury	Hg	80	200.59
Molybdenum	Mo	42	95.94
Neodymium	Nd	60	144.24
Neon	Ne	10	20.183
Neptunium	Np	93	(237)
Nickel	Ni	28	58.71
Niobium	Nb	41	92.906
Nitrogen	N	7	14.007
Nobelium	No	102	(253)
Osmium	Os	76	190.2
Oxygen	O	8	15.999
Palladium	Pd	46	106.4
Phosphorus	P	15	30.974
Platinum	Pt	78	195.09
Plutonium	Pu	94	(242)
Polonium	Po	84	(210)
Potassium	K	19	39.102
Praseodymium	Pr	59	140.907
Promethium	Pm	61	(147)
Protactinium	Pa	91	(231)
Radium	Ra	88	(226)
Radon	Rn	86	(222)
Rhenium	Re	75	186.2
Rhodium	Rh	45	102.905
Rubidium	Rb	37	85.47
Ruthenium	Ru	44	101.07
Rutherfordium	Rf	104	(261)
Samarium	Sm	62	150.35
Scandium	Sc	21	44.956
Selenium	Se	34	78.96
Silicon	Si	14	28.086
Silver	Ag	47	107.870
Sodium	Na	11	22.990
Strontium	Sr	38	87.62
Sulfur	S	16	32.064
Tantalum	Ta	73	180.948
Technetium	Tc	43	(99)
Tellurium	Te	52	127.60
Terbium	Tb	65	158.924
Thallium	Tl	81	204.37
Thorium	Th	90	232.038
Thulium	Tm	69	168.934
Tin	Sn	50	118.69
Titanium	Ti	22	47.90
Tungsten	W	74	183.85
Uranium	U	92	238.03
Vanadium	V	23	50.942
Xenon	Xe	54	131.30
Ytterbium	Yb	70	173.04
Yttrium	Y	39	88.905
Zinc	Zn	30	65.37
Zirconium	Zr	40	91.22

*Atomic weights are corrected to conform with the 1961 values of the Commission on Atomic Weights, expressed to the fourth decimal point, rounded off to the nearest thousandth. The numbers in parentheses are the mass numbers of the most stable or most common isotope.

Appendix 2
SYMBOLS

Symbols consisting of letters of the alphabet appear in Abbreviations.

Ⓛ	left
®	right, trademark
Ⓜ	murmur
⊙	start of operation
⊗	end of operation
□	male
○	female
♂	male
♀	female
*	birth
†	death
α	alpha particle, is proportional to
Δ	prism diopter
Δt	time interval
ΔA	change in absorbance
ΔpH	change in pH
Ω	ohm
π	3.1416−ratio of circumference of a circle to its diameter
σ	1/100 of a second, standard deviation
χ^2	chi square (test)
τ	life (time)
$\tau\frac{1}{2}$	half-life (time)
?	question of, questionable, possible
$>$	greater than
$\not>$	not greater than
$\geq$	greater than or equal to
$<$	less than
$\not<$	not less than
$\leq$	less than or equal to
$\sim$	approximate
$\simeq$	approximately equal to
$\pm$	not definite, plus/minus
(+)	significant
(−)	insignificant
(±)	possibly significant
↓	decreased, depression
↑	elevation, increased

⇧	up	2×	twice
↑V	increase due to *in vivo* effect	×2	twice
↓V	decrease due to *in vivo* effect	′	foot, minute, primary accent, univalent
↑C	increase due to chemical interference during the assay	″	inch, second, secondary accent, bivalent
		.. ‖	two
↓C	decrease due to chemical interference during the assay	/	of, per
→	causes, no change, transfer to	:	ratio (is to)
		::	equality between ratios, "as"
←	is due to	∴	therefore
⇌	reversible reaction	+	plus, positive, present
⊖	normal	−	minus, negative, absent
√c̄	check with	÷	divided by
φ	none	=	equals
V	systolic blood pressure	≠	does not equal, not equal to
∧	diastolic blood pressure	≅	approximately equals
#	gauge, number, weight, pound(s)	%	per cent
℞	recipe, take	℥	ounce
°	degree	f℥	fluid ounce
24°	24 hours	Ə	scruple
1°	primary	m	minim
2°	secondary	ʒ	drachm, dram
2d	second	fʒ	fluidrachm, fluidram
2ndry	secondary	√	root, square root, radical
1×	once	²√	square root

$\sqrt[3]{}$	cube root	606	arsphenamine
∞	infinity	914	neoarsphenamine
⌣	combined with		

Appendix 3
PREFIXES

Prefixes for Metric System Multiples and Submultiples

Symbol	Name	Value
T	tera	10^{12}
G	giga	10^{9}
M	mega	10^{6}
my	myria	10^{4}
k	kilo	10^{3}
h	hecto	10^{2}
dk	deka	10
d	deci	10^{-1}
c	centi	10^{-2}
m	milli	10^{-3}
μ	micro	10^{-6}
n	nano	10^{-9}
p	pico	10^{-12}
f	femto	10^{-15}
a	atto	10^{-18}

Appendix 4
GREEK ALPHABET

The Greek alphabet has 24 letters:			
Printed			
Capital	*Small*	**Names of Letters**	
Α	α	"Αλφα	alpha
Β	β	Βῆτα	beta
Γ	γ	Γάμμα	gamma
Δ	δ	Δέλτα	delta
Ε	ε	"Εψιλον	epsilon
Ζ	ζ	Ζῆτα	zeta
Η	η	ᵀΗτα	eta
Θ	θ	Θῆτα	theta
Ι	ι	'Ιῶτα	iota
Κ	κ	Κάππα	kappa
Λ	λ	Λάμϐδα	lambda
Μ	μ	Μῦ	mu
Ν	ν	Νῦ	nu
Ξ	ξ	Ξῦ	xi
Ο	ο	"Ομικρον	omicron
Π	π	Πῖ	pi
Ρ	ρ	Ρῶ	rho
Σ	σ, ς	Σῖγμα	sigma
Τ	τ	Ταῦ	tau
Υ	υ	"Υψιλον	upsilon
Φ	φ	Φῖ	phi
Χ	χ	Χῖ	khi
Ψ	ψ	Ψῖ	psi
Ω	ω	'Ωμέγα	omega

Appendix 5
POSITIONS OF FETUS

Cephalic Presentation

1. Vertex—occiput, the point of direction

Left occipitoanterior	L.O.A.
Left occipitotransverse	L.O.T.
Right occipitoposterior	R.O.P.
Right occipitotransverse	R.O.T.
Right occipitoanterior	R.O.A.
Left occipitoposterior	L.O.P.

2. Face—chin, the point of direction

Right mentoposterior	R.M.P.
Left mentoanterior	L.M.A.
Right mentotransverse	R.M.T.
Right mentoanterior	R.M.A.
Left mentotransverse	L.M.T.
Left mentoposterior	L.M.P.

3. Brow—the point of direction

Right frontoposterior	R.F.P.
Left frontoanterior	L.F.A.
Right frontotransverse	R.F.T.
Right frontoanterior	R.F.A.
Left frontotransverse	L.F.T.
Left frontoposterior	L.F.P.

Breech or Pelvic Presentation

1. Complete breech—sacrum, the point of direction
(feet crossed and thighs flexed on abdomen)

Left sacroanterior	L.S.A.
Left sacrotransverse	L.S.T.
Right sacroposterior	R.S.P.
Right sacroanterior	R.S.A.
Right sacrotransverse	R.S.T.
Left sacroposterior	L.S.P.

2. Incomplete breech—sacrum, the point of direction. Same designations as above, adding the qualifications footling, knee, etc.

Transverse Lie or Shoulder Presentation

Shoulder—scapula, the point of direction

Left scapuloanterior	L.Sc.A.	} Back anterior positions
Right scapuloanterior	R.Sc.A.	
Right scapuloposterior	R.Sc.P.	} Back posterior positions
Left scapuloposterior	L.Sc.P.